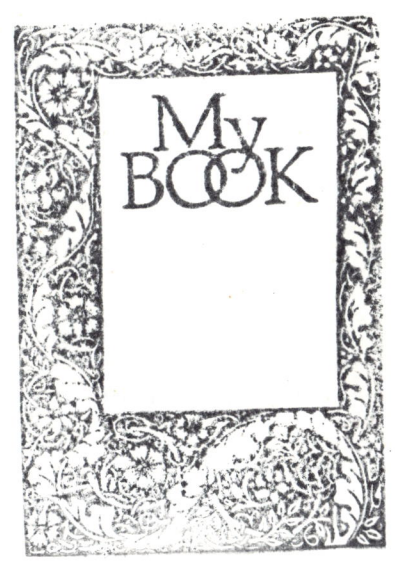

My
BOOK

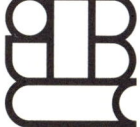

"This book offers a wealth of knowledge from a broad spectrum of contributors—both renowned researchers and clinicians—who share wisdom gained from years of work in the field and countless hours spent serving clients affected by the AIDS crisis. Michael O'Connor's *Treating the Psychological Consequences of HIV* is an essential resource and should be in the library of every practitioner who works with HIV-infected and -effected clients."
—SETH C. KALICHMAN, PH.D., *assistant professor, Georgia State University, Atlanta, and author of* Understanding AIDS

"*Treating the Psychological Consequences of HIV* provides health and mental health practitioners with a sophisticated and comprehensive presentation of treatment for the psychological and psychosocial consequences of HIV/AIDS. It represents a major step forward in the field."
—JOHN R. ANDERSON, PH.D., *director, American Psychological Association Office on AIDS*

"This book will be an extremely useful resource for all counselors, psychologists, and psychiatrists who are confronted with the diverse challenges of HIV disease among their clients. It is comprehensive, up-to-date, thoughtful, and makes a unique contribution to the field."
—ANKE A. EHRHARDT, PH.D., *director, HIV Center for Clinical and Behavioral Studies, and professor of clinical psychology, Department of Psychiatry, Columbia University*

TREATING
THE PSYCHOLOGICAL
CONSEQUENCES OF HIV

THE JOSSEY-BASS LIBRARY OF CURRENT CLINICAL TECHNIQUE

IRVIN D. YALOM, GENERAL EDITOR

NOW AVAILABLE

Treating Alcoholism
Stephanie Brown, Editor

Treating Schizophrenia
Sophia Vinogradov, Editor

Treating Women Molested in Childhood
Catherine Classen, Editor

Treating Depression
Ira D. Glick, Editor

Treating Eating Disorders
Joellen Werne, Editor

Treating Dissociative Identity Disorder
James L. Spira, Editor

Treating Couples
Hilda Kessler, Editor

Treating Adolescents
Hans Steiner, Editor

Treating the Elderly
Javaid I. Sheikh, Editor

Treating Sexual Disorders
Randolph S. Charlton, Editor

Treating Difficult Personality Disorders
Michael Rosenbluth, Editor

Treating Anxiety Disorders
Walton T. Roth, Editor

Treating the Psychological Consequences of HIV
Michael F. O'Connor, Editor

FORTHCOMING

Treating Children
Hans Steiner, Editor

TREATING THE PSYCHOLOGICAL CONSEQUENCES OF HIV

A VOLUME IN THE JOSSEY-BASS LIBRARY OF CURRENT CLINICAL TECHNIQUE

Michael F. O'Connor, EDITOR
Irvin D. Yalom, GENERAL EDITOR

Jossey-Bass Publishers • San Francisco

Substantial discounts on bulk quantities of Jossey-Bass books are available to corporations, professional associations, and other organizations. For details and discount information, contact the special sales department at Jossey-Bass Inc., Publishers (415) 433–1740; Fax (800) 605–2665.

For sales outside the United States, please contact your local Simon & Schuster International Office.

 Manufactured in the United States of America on Lyons Falls Turin Book. This paper is acid-free and 100 percent totally chlorine-free.

Library of Congress Cataloging-in-Publication Data

Treating the psychological consequences of HIV/Michael F. O'Connor, editor; Irvin D. Yalom, general editor.
   p.   cm.—(The Jossey-Bass library of current clinical technique)
   Includes bibliographical references and index.
   ISBN 0-7879-0314-0 (alk. paper)
   1. HIV infections—Psychological aspects. I. O'Connor, Michael Francis.
   II. Yalom, Irvin D., date. III. Series.
RC607.A26T73 1996
616.97'92'0019—dc20   96-31519
                                                              CIP

FIRST EDITION
PB Printing   10 9 8 7 6 5 4 3 2 1

CONTENTS

CHAPTER 8

TREATING HIV IN DUAL DIAGNOSIS PATIENTS 269
Philip A. Bialer, Steven Bluestine, and Jeffrey J. Richards

CHAPTER 9

LEGAL AND ETHICAL ISSUES IN THE TREATMENT OF HIV 309
Jeff Stryker

APPENDIX

SELECTED LIST OF MEDICATIONS USED IN HIV AND THEIR MENTAL HEALTH CONSEQUENCES 329

ABOUT THE AUTHORS 337

INDEX 341

FOREWORD

At a recent meeting of clinical practitioners, a senior practitioner declared that more change had occurred in his practice of psychotherapy in the past year than in the twenty preceding years. Nodding assent, the others all agreed.

And was that a good thing for their practice? A resounding "No!" Again, unanimous concurrence—too much interference from managed care; too much bureaucracy; too much paper work; too many limits set on fees, length, and format of therapy; too much competition from new psychotherapy professions.

Were these changes a good or a bad thing for the general public? Less unanimity on this question. Some pointed to recent positive developments. Psychotherapy was becoming more mainstream, more available, and more acceptable to larger segments of the American public. It was being subjected to closer scrutiny and accountability—uncomfortable for the practitioner but, if done properly, of potential benefit to the quality and efficiency of behavioral health care delivery.

But without dissent this discussion group agreed—and every aggregate of therapists would concur—that astounding changes are looming for our profession: changes in the reasons that clients request therapy; changes in the perception and practice of mental health care; changes in therapeutic theory and technique; and changes in the training, certification, and supervision of professional therapists.

From the perspective of the clientele, several important currents are apparent. A major development is the de-stigmatization of psychotherapy. No longer is psychotherapy invariably a hush-hush affair, laced with shame and conducted in offices with separate entrance and exit doors to prevent the uncomfortable possibility of clients meeting one another.

Today such shame and secrecy have been exploded. Television talk shows—Oprah, Geraldo, Donahue—have normalized

ix

psychopathology and psychotherapy by presenting a continuous public parade of dysfunctional human situations: hardly a day passes without television fare of confessions and audience interactions with deadbeat fathers, sex addicts, adult children of alcoholics, battering husbands and abused wives, drug dealers and substance abusers, food bingers and purgers, thieving children, abusing parents, victimized children suing parents.

The implications of such de-stigmatization have not been lost on professionals who no longer concentrate their efforts on the increasingly elusive analytically suitable neurotic patient. Clinics everywhere are dealing with a far broader spectrum of problem areas and must be prepared to offer help to substance abusers and their families, to patients with a wide variety of eating disorders, adult survivors of incest, victims and perpetrators of domestic abuse. No longer do trauma victims or substance abusers furtively seek counseling. Public awareness of the noxious long-term effects of trauma has been so sensitized that there is an increasing call for public counseling facilities and a growing demand, as well, for adequate counseling provisions in health care plans.

The mental health profession is changing as well. No longer is there such automatic adoration of lengthy "depth" psychotherapy where "deep" or "profound" is equated with a focus on the earliest years of the patient's life. The contemporary field is more pluralistic: many diverse approaches have proven therapeutically effective and the therapist of today is more apt to tailor the therapy to fit the particular clinical needs of each patient.

In past years there was an unproductive emphasis on territoriality and on the maintaining of hierarchy and status—with the more prestigious professions like psychiatry and doctoral-level psychology expending considerable energy toward excluding master's level therapists. But those battles belong more to the psychotherapists of yesterday; today there is a significant shift toward a more collaborative interdisciplinary climate.

Managed care and cost containment is driving some of these changes. The role of the psychiatrist has been particularly affected as cost efficiency has decreed that psychiatrists will less frequently deliver psychotherapy personally but, instead, limit their activities to supervision and to psychopharmacological treatment.

In its efforts to contain costs, managed care has asked therapists to deliver a briefer, focused therapy. But gradually managed care is realizing that the bulk of mental health treatment cost is consumed by inpatient care and that outpatient treatment, even long-term therapy, is not only salubrious for the patient but far less costly. Another looming change is that the field is turning more frequently toward the group therapies. How much longer can we ignore the many comparative research studies demonstrating that the group therapy format is equally or more effective than higher cost individual therapies?

Some of these cost-driven edicts may prove to be good for the patients; but many of the changes that issue from medical model mimicry—for example, efforts at extreme brevity and overly precise treatment plans and goals that are inappropriate to the therapy endeavor and provide only the illusion of efficiency—can hamper the therapeutic work. Consequently, it is of paramount importance that therapists gain control of their field and that managed care administrators not be permitted to dictate how psychotherapy or, for that matter, any other form of health care be conducted. That is one of the goals of this series of texts: to provide mental health professionals with such a deep grounding in theory and such a clear vision of effective therapeutic technique that they will be empowered to fight confidently for the highest standards of patient care.

The Jossey-Bass Library of Current Clinical Technique is directed and dedicated to the front-line therapist—to master's and doctoral-level clinicians who personally provide the great bulk of mental health care. The purpose of this entire series is to offer state-of-the-art instruction in treatment techniques for the most commonly encountered clinical conditions. Each volume offers a focused theoretical background as a foundation for practice and then dedicates itself to the practical task of what to do for the patient—how to assess, diagnose, and treat.

I have selected volume editors who are either nationally recognized experts or are rising young stars. In either case, they possess a comprehensive view of their specialty field and have selected leading therapists of a variety of persuasions to describe their therapeutic approaches.

Although all the contributors have incorporated the most recent and relevant clinical research in their chapters, the emphasis in these volumes is the practical technique of therapy. We shall offer specific therapeutic guidelines, and augment concrete suggestions with the liberal use of clinical vignettes and detailed case histories. Our intention is not to impress or to awe the reader, and not to add footnotes to arcane academic debates. Instead, each chapter is designed to communicate guidelines of immediate pragmatic value to the practicing clinician. In fact, the general editor, the volume editors, and the chapter contributors have all accepted our assignments for that very reason: a rare opportunity to make a significant, immediate, and concrete contribution to the lives of our patients.

Irvin D. Yalom, M.D.
Professor Emeritus of Psychiatry
Stanford University

INTRODUCTION

Michael F. O'Connor

The worst medical disaster of the twentieth century is now well into its second decade. Daily headlines remind us that infection rates and deaths from the disease continue to rise around the world. AIDS is now the leading cause of death among U.S. twenty-five- to forty-four-year-olds. As of 1993, one in every ninety-two American men between the ages of twenty-seven and thirty-nine, and one in every thirty-three young African-American men, were thought to be infected. AIDS is spreading among teens and among heterosexuals. And women are the fastest-growing segment of the population afflicted. The numbers climb. And as they do, more and more of us are affected, one way or another, by the dreaded plague.

This volume addresses the psychological consequences of HIV for all of us. For that reason, the uninfected, the families and friends, the caregivers, and the worried well, as well as those infected, are the focus here. AIDS is no longer "only a gay disease," or one that affects only individuals on the "fringe" of society. The Reagan administration's desire to stop the advance of the disease "before it reaches the heterosexual population and the general population" has become an absurd and rather transparent fantasy, if it was ever anything else. We are all in it now.

The enormity of HIV—the incredible changes in our reality, the amazing medical and research developments related to virology and the immune system, the tragic losses—all affect us daily. There now exists a generation that has not lived in a world without AIDS. We now think differently about health, sex, relationships, love, mortality, and the limitations of science. We think differently about infection and contagion. We better understand the difference between a virus and bacteria. We have been forced to grapple with moral, ethical, and legal issues in a way few could have comprehended twenty years ago. Who would have thought in 1978 that there would one day be "safe sex" messages on the backs of buses in every major urban center? Who would have guessed then that a debate would soon rage over educating our seventh graders about condoms? Who would have worried about our blood supply, or asked their loved ones to donate untainted blood for their surgery? Was there anyone who could have predicted that a modern plague would get the better of modern humanity? Perhaps, but there was once a time when few of us were concerned about such issues. Now, these and other concerns related to HIV are a fact of life.

Some general information will be useful to you in preparation for the chapters that follow. I will briefly discuss disease demographics and the nature of the disease, recent changes in how the disease is approached medically, some considerations in treating ethnic minority group individuals, the likely impact on providers, and the orientation of our approach to this book, before reviewing the chapter contributions.

DEMOGRAPHICS

HIV and AIDS refer to two different conditions, as defined by medical markers. AIDS is all but conclusively thought to be caused by the human immunodeficiency virus or HIV. One may be infected with HIV for many years without symptoms. Once symptoms occur, progression to full-blown AIDS is likely. Actual cases of AIDS therefore reflect the development of physiological changes resulting from a compromised immune system that are potentially serious enough to debilitate the individual significantly. Consequently, estimates of current HIV infections do not reflect the number of individuals who have succumbed to AIDS, and estimates of AIDS cases likewise do not reflect the even larger number of those infected with HIV.

Relevant statistics can be difficult to interpret for other reasons. There is a difference between AIDS estimates for those who remain alive, as opposed to "cumulative" cases, which include those who have died from the disease. The mortality rate is also different than the cumulative case rate. Rates for minority groups may include both men and women or refer only to men or only to women ("Latino/a" versus "Latino or Latina"). Likewise, distinct categories may overlap, such as homosexual men who also use IV drugs. Finally, age estimates may be confusing, in that one may become infected well before being found to be seropositive or diagnosed with AIDS. I encourage you to review carefully the numbers that follow to avoid confusion.

World Estimates

The World Health Organization (WHO) reported a cumulative estimate of HIV infection prevalence totaling 20 million cases worldwide as of April 1996, with an expectation of thirty to forty million cases worldwide by the year 2000.

As of December 1995, WHO reported a provisional world estimate for cumulative AIDS cases of approximately 6 million. Approximately 1.3 million AIDS cases were reported in 1995, up 26 percent from the number reported in 1994. Although infection rates are stabilizing and even decreasing among some groups in the United States, the world is likely yet to see the worst ravages of the disease.

How bad will it get? Approximately ten thousand new infections are thought to occur worldwide every day. About 60 percent of these infections occur in the developing world, where preventive education and medical treatments are least available, and where populations are often large and already beset by many health problems. In Asia, where heterosexual transmission is the most common mode, some 3.5 million are thought to be infected.

The pandemic is particularly troublesome when one looks at the estimated 333 million new cases of curable (non-HIV) sexually transmitted diseases that are thought to have occurred in 1995 alone. This staggering number is very important to epidemiologists, who note that such prevalence, in addition to reflecting instances wherein HIV could have been transmitted, also reflects individuals who, because of the possibility of genital lesions and inflammation, are at greater risk for HIV infection of self and others.

National Estimates

An estimated one million Americans (or 1 in every 250 Americans) are currently alive and infected with HIV. In the United States, the Centers for Disease Control and Prevention (CDC) report a cumulative total of 513,486 cases of AIDS as of December 1995. Over 320,000 people have now died in the United States from AIDS as of that date.

The majority of cases of AIDS, 42 percent by these estimates, have occurred among men who have sex with men. The majority are no longer white, however, with approximately 175,000 African Americans and 90,000 Hispanic individuals so diagnosed. Those who inject drugs currently account for about 130,000, or 26 percent, of AIDS cases in the United States. Other groups affected include Asians, Native Americans, Pacific Islanders, and individuals who are infected via blood transfusion or tissue (including hemophiliacs). Although these latter groups certainly compose an important segment of those affected by the disease, they represent relatively smaller percentages of individuals infected in the United States.

The vast majority of AIDS cases are male, but women represent almost 76,000 cases of AIDS in the United States. As mentioned previously, women represent the fastest-growing group of new infections, and for the first time, in 1992, the number of women infected through heterosexual contact exceeded those infected through IV drug use. The current CDC estimate of heterosexually acquired AIDS cases is 35,683. Two-thirds of these cases are women. This means that the virus is increasingly spreading to the "general" population in the United States.

Children are also increasingly affected by the disease, and in this country more than 3,600 children had died from the disease as of June 1995. Children under the age of thirteen currently account for approximately 7,000 AIDS cases. But perhaps most alarming is the estimate, found in the first presidential report on young people and AIDS, that 25 percent of new HIV infections now occur among individuals between the ages of thirteen and twenty. Obviously, our young people are at significant risk.

Overall then, HIV poses a growing threat to the developing world community, to women, to children and adolescents, to minority group members, and to heterosexuals. In other words, enormous numbers of individuals are now, or will be, touched by the disease—perhaps through a relative's infection, or that of a loved one or a friend at work—but inevitably touched.

As the epidemic broadens, more and more clients presenting for counseling and psychotherapy will have concerns related to HIV. Clinicians, even those who formerly have had little or no contact with such issues, will be increasingly called on to help with the crisis.

NATURE OF THE DISEASE

As you might expect, HIV infection and AIDS share some characteristics with other infections and diseases; in other ways, they are unique. Like most serious illnesses, the disease is likely to worsen symptomatically over time. Many symptoms, such as fatigue and weight loss, are similar to those of other diseases. Other symptoms, such as Kaposi's Sarcoma lesions, result in physically deforming and unfortunately emblematic evidence of the plague. HIV often involves a very long waiting game. Symptoms may not appear for several years, if they appear at all. The patient is left to wonder and wait for the onset of symptoms, a torturous experience for anyone. Perhaps worse yet, the individual may have little reason to think he or she is infected, consequently infecting others unknowingly. Imagine the realization that one has infected one's life partner, or even a casual friend!

At present the disease has no cure. The disease strikes certain disenfranchised groups disproportionately. Like many others, this disease is highly stigmatized. As the following chapters will show, there are many idiosyncratic factors common to HIV infection and AIDS that have a significant impact on the physical and psychological health of those affected.

Notions of how to approach the virus change almost daily. Whereas we formerly talked about AIDS-Related Complex (ARC) for example, referring to people who were in the early symptomatic stage but not yet suffering from "full-blown" AIDS, we have now begun to refer to infections in terms of the degree of viral activity and other markers. The diagnosis of ARC no longer exists. Similarly, measurements of "helper T-cells" are no longer the only consideration for gauging the progression of infection. Meanwhile, medications are now more often used in combination rather than alone. Many opportunistic illnesses can be prophylactically treated. For example, *Pneumocystis carinii* pneumonia, a formidable and highly deadly infection in the early years, is now fairly easily prevented through medical procedures.

Although the nature of the disease itself changes little, despite mutations in the virus, our approach to the disease is constantly in flux. This reality makes coping with the disease not unlike an on-going experiment, and on the receiving end is the patient who wishes only to be well, or perhaps just to survive.

Individuals with HIV are often searching for the newest information on treatment. They may be enrolled in several studies over the course of the infection. They may also be rejected for involvement. The mental health clinician needs to understand that at heart, HIV is an infection of uncertainty—obviously for the patient, but also for friends and loved ones.

Disease Progression

Disease progression and symptoms vary widely among those infected. There are at least several different strains of the virus, which is capable of mutating rapidly with time. Disease progression is thought to be affected by a wide variety of factors, including among others the strain of the virus, the condition of the immune system, genetics, viral load, and psychosocial factors.

It is increasingly the case that we speak of HIV and AIDS in relation to the estimated stage of infection. The following is a typical model, although there is some variation depending on the source of information:

Stage 0	The worried well
Stage I	Acute stage—recently infected, possibly with flu-like symptoms; term also used to refer to the period of first diagnosis
Stage II	Asymptomatic ("latent") stage
Stage III	Early symptomatic stage
Stage IV	AIDS

Until recently, the blood count of CD4 helper/inducer T-lymphocytes, or T-cells, was the most frequently used estimate of disease progression. These cells work on behalf of the immune system to fight off infection. The virus attacks these cells and others progressively, thereby compromising the system's protective response. A compromised immune system eventually leaves the individual susceptible to numerous opportunistic infections, which may ultimately lead to death. An individual is diagnosed with AIDS once these T-cells have dropped below 200 per cubic milliliter of blood. As the average individual carries about 800 to 1,200 T-cells per cubic milliliter of blood normally, and the disease may progress relatively slowly, many people have lived with the HIV infection for many years without a diagnosis of AIDS.

Antiretrovirals, Protease Inhibitors, and Combinant Drug Therapies

Without treatment, the HIV virus typically will invade and destroy cells in the body as it replicates and increases its presence. Drug treatments designed to interrupt the action and production of the virus have been developed over the years and continue to emerge on a regular basis. (For information on specific medications, including their functions and side effects, the reader is referred to the Appendix and to David Ostrow's review of medical treatments in Chapter Two.) Some drugs, such as Zidovudine (AZT), didanosine (ddI), and dideoxycitidine (ddC), can forestall the action of the virus or halt its progress, at least for a time. Combinant therapies using these and other drugs have become popular in recent years and will be further elaborated on here. The newest type of drugs designed to alter or prevent the virus's replication is the protease inhibitor. These drugs act on an entirely different site in viral production than do the earlier antiretrovirals, which worked to inhibit the action of reverse transcriptase, thereby interrupting the ability of the virus to replace the host cell's genetic code (DNA) with its own. Protease inhibitors interrupt the dispersal of viable virus from the infected cell by blocking the action of an enzyme called protease. To the extent protease inhibitors are effective at their task—and they are not 100 percent effective—the actual amount of virus in the body can be reduced, perhaps even to zero. This does not mean that the virus cannot reemerge when medications are stopped, and the immune system may or may not recover from any damage already done. The advantage of using several drugs in different combinations over time comes from the imperfect action of any one medication in eliminating the virus. As well, because HIV replicates at a very high rate, mutations in the virus are relatively common. This allows the virus to become resistant to existing medications in relatively short periods of time. Consequently, patients may often change their drug regimens after a year or two in response to poor performance or the development of side effects. The patient is rarely without some worry about what's ahead, even when current medications appear to be helping.

Paralleling these new drug developments, measurements of *viral load* have become important indicators of the patient's health. Whereas the number of T-cells tells us something about the damage to the patient's immune system, viral load tells us the rate at which the virus is actively replicating and, therefore, actively destructive to the host. We once thought of HIV as lying dormant during the asymptomatic or "latent" phase, but we now know that the virus may actively replicate for years before symptoms are apparent. As a result, medical opinion now advocates treating the virus more aggressively and sooner. This is one very good reason for encouraging those who have not yet been tested for HIV to prepare to find out their serostatus. Again, it is not clear how much help drug treatments can provide if the immune system is severely damaged because treatment was not obtained in a timely manner.

Naturally, the development of combinant and protease inhibitor therapies is viewed as a godsend by patients and doctors alike. People who have been diagnosed with HIV or AIDS, sometimes years ago, may now be able to lead a relatively normal life with regular medication. There are cautions, however. Not everyone will tolerate or benefit from these therapies. Currently, the therapies are quite demanding, in some cases requiring the patient to take one of a variety of medications almost hourly. A major danger is the risk involved in failing to maintain such a rigorous drug regimen; the virus could develop a strain resistant to the prescribed medications. This might occur if the patient's viral load increases even briefly—say for two or three days. Finally, the financial cost of these medications is very high. Whereas affluent patients and patients with good insurance coverage might be able to afford ongoing treatment, patients of lesser means might not. In regard to the global problem of HIV in particular, such medications will likely remain utterly out of reach for millions.

Those who do benefit from these therapies might be faced with new, albeit preferable, dillemas. Many have left careers and used retirement funds for their treatment. They must find a way to reenter the world in some cases. They must continue to pay for their treatments. At the very least, they must make the transition from an expectation of dying soon to one of surviving indefinitely. Perhaps these survivors will suffer from guilt as they come to grips with having been rescued from the disease that took their less-fortunate loved ones and friends. Counselors must be sensitive to these dynamics, even while celebrating the good news.

Psychological Influence on Illness

Some studies have shown that disease and psychological processes may be deeply linked. Psychosomatic illness has been described for many years. Recent exploration in this area relative to HIV has proven quite interesting, and has shown that such social considerations and psychological conditions as drug abuse, depression, stress, and anxiety may affect disease progression and symptomatology. A positive outlook, social support, stress reduction, and a cognitive adaptation to the disease have all been shown to positively affect health in HIV infection. Although this area of research is relatively new, several possible physiological pathways of influence are being considered, including the neuroendocrine and autonomic nervous systems.

Naturally, the illness also affects one's psychological state. Additional effects—for example, an increase in symptoms, more contact with doctors as the disease progresses, the effects of medical treatments, and bereavement—also have been and are currently being studied. It has been shown that having a way to make sense of the disease is crucial to positive adjustment. This refers to an existential resolution of the infection—a way to understand the question "Why me?" It has also been shown that the level of positive adjustment is related to the number of physical symptoms, as we might expect. These and other considerations will be explored in the chapters that follow.

A NOTE ON ETHNIC MINORITY CONCERNS

It was with some difficulty that Chapter Five on treating ethnic minority group members was obtained. Despite my best efforts and consultation with numerous individuals and organizations,

I was unable to identify a final contributor for this chapter until well after first drafts of all the other chapters had been submitted. This was the unfortunate result of a combination of problems and circumstances. From the start, individuals I contacted for this effort were generally overwhelmed with other work. Many expressed an interest in tackling such a project but were unable to find the time to do so. As well, the first contributor who committed to write this chapter did not follow through. One conclusion to be drawn from these events is that minority researchers and practitioners in this area are in short supply and work under a heavy burden of demands to speak to multiple problems. In addition, as Dr. Gutierrez notes in his chapter, one minority group member is often asked to speak for all. I have now asked myself if I would be willing to represent this nation's Caucasians with my voice. My answer is a resounding "no." So I may have made the mistake of asking too much of these contributors.

In any case, I believe we must address a number of issues if we are to adequately provide for the treatment of ethnic minority populations. With the limited perspective I can offer after reviewing at least some of the literature, I will try here to highlight some important considerations for this population that are not fully addressed elsewhere in the volume.

To begin with, we are reminded that people of African-American and Latino descent in this country are currently becoming infected with HIV at a greater rate than are most other groups. What's more, because socioeconomic factors may preclude treatment for a number of reasons, these individuals are likely to receive fewer of the benefits of the newer emerging therapies. Requests and complaints concerning more funding for and more attunement to minority concerns and needs relative to HIV have been heard for years. The response has clearly not been adequate.

Our approach to research and treatment of HIV in minority groups is also flawed. For example, investigators have noted the importance of distinguishing cultural identity or ethnicity from race. Racial status does not necessarily tell us much about the

culture from which an individual is derived, yet this consideration is not normally imbedded in research protocols. Such information about enculturation can be extremely important, as Dr.
Gutierrez notes in Chapter Five. A single, middle-class, Hispanic
woman, for example, will likely have different health and financial priorities, capacities for seeking assistance, and financial
means than a poor mother of five who lives in the barrio with
her family of origin. Likewise, individuals who are of mixed race
are often not well-differentiated by research methodology, leaving us with unanswered questions and possibly spurious conclusions about how race relates to HIV infection.

Despite the fact that many findings must be approached cautiously, we do have some useful information to bring to bear. For
example, African-American women have been shown to yield
greater benefit from prevention efforts delivered by other
African-American women than by the efforts of non-matched
presenters. On follow-up, these women were found to be significantly more sensitized to AIDS, more likely to have talked to
friends about AIDS, and more likely to have been tested for HIV
than women informed by non-matched presenters. High-risk,
non-minority women have been found to be more concerned
about AIDS than are high-risk, minority women. The latter
group does not differ from low-risk minority women in this
regard. While the reasons for this may not be entirely clear, the
facts remain and are important in formulating interventions for
this group. Ethnic minority group members have also been
shown to be more reticent to discuss common spiritual beliefs
about the cause of illness with white majority individuals. Naturally, if one believes illness is related to divine intervention,
one's attitudes toward the infected individual and his or her
treatment, among other things, may be affected.

More important, perhaps, is the increased distance and potential distrust the insensitive investigator or service provider creates with minority group members by trampling on or ignoring
such important values. Values and other differences may be quite
localized as well, as one study comparing New England and
Florida IV-drug users has shown. Some groups, such as African

Americans, have reason to be distrustful of research and treatment efforts, given the historical withholding of treatment—for example, for syphilis among African-American participants in the Tuskegee study earlier this century.

Research findings in this arena can also be complex and not easily categorized on the basis of race. As previously noted, ethnic culture apparently is not considered in studies of patterns of infection and risk behavior. Relative risk for AIDS, for example, was shown to be higher among IV-drug–using ethnic minority group members than among white individuals who engaged in similar behavior. This may be due to higher rates of needle-sharing, greater difficulty in obtaining sterile equipment, and/or poorer health status among members of ethnic minority populations as compared to whites. Hence, the same behavior—in this case IV-drug use—may have different risks associated with it in different contexts. In another example, a study comparing races in relation to extra-marital behavior found that African-American men without a partner were the group most likely to have sex with multiple partners, while ethnic minority women with primary partners were the least likely to do so. According to one study, African-American men may be more likely to engage in unprotected anal intercourse in spite of a correct perception of their risk for infection. This research also showed, however, that unprotected anal intercourse was more likely for individuals who had low incomes, had been paid for sex, and/or had injected drugs. These findings point to some of the subtleties to which the researcher and clinician must be sensitive in reviewing global findings that are often relayed in the form of racial group statistics.

Bisexual behavior has been linked to risk behavior. As Dr. Gutierrez notes, Latino men are more likely to engage in bisexual behavior than other males, in part for cultural reasons, and, therefore, to be at greater risk for infection and for spreading of the virus.

Social stigma, fear of discrimination, and fear of potential adverse effects have been shown to be obstacles to testing and counseling for HIV/AIDS among African Americans and

Latinos/as, as has general denial of risk. But other more obvious factors may also be involved. For example, a posteriori analyses of data from a 1988 study found that African Americans and Latinos/as were more likely to report having been tested or planning to be tested compared to individuals from other racial or ethnic groups. However over one-third of Latinos/as and African Americans in this study had not heard of a test to detect the HIV virus. Although the latter finding has likely improved with time—more people are likely aware of the HIV antibody test now than in 1988—these results show that intended compliance can be influenced by factors that are relatively simple. Another example of this point is the finding that issuing coupons for redemption may compel otherwise resistant, drug-using, high–HIV-risk individuals to come to outpatient detoxification treatment. This study also found that individuals at higher risk for HIV on the basis of recent IV-drug use and an absence of previous treatment will be more likely to utilize such inducements, and that these individuals are more likely to be members of ethnic minorities and men. Again, a relatively simple, pragmatic response to the realities of an individual's circumstances and priorities can make an enormous difference in the outcome of our efforts. Within ethnic minority communities, we must be especially sensitive to financial, temporal, and transportation concerns, personal values, and social constraints as well as other barriers to services. In many cases, these must be addressed first if our therapeutic interventions are to be effective.

A final note on Asian and Pacific Islanders is in order. Although according to current statistics this group appears to be at comparatively low risk for HIV, there is some evidence that their risk is increasing. One recent study reported that 27 percent of individuals in this group reported engaging in unprotected sex in the last three months. Substance abuse was found to be the greatest influence on unsafe sexual practices. This study also found that 11 percent of subjects had engaged in sex for money. Additionally, the Asian-American gay population has been assimilated, to a greater or lesser extent, into the larger gay community. Therefore, grief and loss may be significant problems in this community even though Asian-American infections and deaths remain relatively low. Naturally, such losses may be assumed to affect other gay minority group members in a similar manner.

Programs have been created to help educate providers in developing greater cultural sensitivity and the ability to consider such issues in designing and implementing treatment services. Providers are encouraged to get further consultation and training in this area as necessary and available.

CLINICAL APPROACH

This volume is eclectic in its theoretical approach, reflecting the various orientations of the contributors. However, there are at least a few assumptions that all of the contributors share.

First, it is important when working with people with HIV infection to maintain a developmentally and culturally sensitive point of view. Few would argue that infection for a pregnant woman would have the same meaning as for a gay man, or that the infected Hispanic man will have the same experience as a six-year-old Caucasian. Individual development, sexual orientation, cultural background, ethnicity, sex, age, introversion or extroversion, degree of isolation, emotional support, and numerous other factors influence and diversify the likely experience of the HIV-infected individual.

Second, it is crucial that the clinician be aware of the rapidly changing medical circumstances surrounding HIV infection. New treatments are constantly emerging, the most recent suggesting very positive changes in how we will manage the disease. It is important to remain up-to-date on available treatments and resources for the individual infected with HIV, both to better understand the client and to allow the clinician to focus on issues that may be significant for the individual. A client who tells the therapist that his T-cells have dropped to under 200 has also just told her he has AIDS. Although he may know he has done so, the clinician may not, and an important crisis in the client's health and therapy could go undetected.

Third, events such as a diagnosis of HIV infection are likely to raise strong emotional reactions in the client. As such, they are also likely to raise previously unresolved concerns, and even historical traumas. This process of cueing is particularly devastating for certain individuals, depending on their background. As the chapter on treating gay men notes, it is a relatively common problem among individuals in this group. It is known that the likelihood of psychiatric symptoms among those infected with HIV typically correlates with the experience of symptoms before diagnosis. Hence those who have suffered from depression prior to infection, for example, are more likely to experience such symptoms after infection.

Finally, virtually every contributor has noted the enormous opportunities presented to the individual who is tackling an HIV-related diagnosis: perhaps to resolve past conflicts with him- or herself, with family, or with others or to finally do something about a long-standing substance abuse problem, for example. This fact becomes all the more true as the potential arises that HIV disorders might be chronic, treatable, medical conditions rather than death sentences.

IMPACT ON THE PROVIDER

We begin this book with a chapter on transference and countertransference. We do so for a variety of reasons, not the least of which is the need to understand the enormous impact HIV work typically has on the mental health professional. For the average clinician, the effects of working with HIV-positive clients will be difficult enough. For clinicians who treat a large number of such cases, who are at risk or infected themselves, or who have lost loved ones to the disease, the impact can be overwhelming. In these cases, case load management, down-time, consultation, and support are essential. There may even come a time, now some fifteen years into the pandemic, when some clinicians will need to change roles completely. In any case, professional distress and burnout are very real problems for the mental health professional who works with HIV.

Overview of the Contents

The best and the brightest HIV researchers and clinicians have lent their extensive expertise to build this volume. The quality of their contributions will be obvious to the reader. They have been asked here to offer something different from the typical publication. In addition to relaying important facts about the disease, they have been asked to speak in plain English and from personal experience about the treatment needs of those afflicted. They have had to adopt a new posture, to set aside a purely academic orientation in some instances, and to relate their own human experience with the disease, in hopes of better and more fully communicating the wealth of information they have to share. The results have surpassed my own greatest hopes.

We begin this volume with a chapter by Steven Cadwell on transference and countertransference, as noted previously. This chapter provides an excellent sampling of the experiences of the client and therapist working with HIV and the likely issues that arise, as well as direction for the practitioner concerning treatment, consultation, and managing burnout.

Chapter Two is David Ostrow's excellent and extensive review of HIV disease, prognosis, and medical treatments. This chapter includes an up-to-date review of current literature on psychiatric symptoms and treatments.

In Chapter Three, Roberta Ann Olson, Heather Huszti, and Jeffrey Parsons present a very thorough review of pediatric and adolescent HIV. This chapter is extremely important, given the increasing impact of HIV on our children and youth.

My own chapter on treating gay men with HIV follows. This chapter focuses on the psychological impact of HIV on the individual; in it, I have attempted to integrate issues relevant to gay men generally with those specific to living with HIV.

In Chapter Five, Fernando Gutierrez has provided us with a review of the culturally sensitive treatment of HIV, discussing such issues as cultural influences on behavior and identity, individual identity versus group identity, and cultural aspects of sexuality, among others. This chapter is most important, given the demographic trends we have already noted.

Kathleen Goggin and Judith Rabkin in Chapter Six discuss women and HIV, extensively reviewing the literature for the most recent information on this, the fastest-growing group of those infected.

Douglas Rait, Joan Ross, and Stephen Rao have contributed an excellent chapter on family and couples treatment, including considerations for HIV-affected families, heterosexual and gay couples, and serodiscordant couples.

In Chapter Eight, Philip Bialer, Steven Bluestine, and Jeffrey Richards have prepared a concise and thorough review of treatment for dual diagnosis patients, including the treatment of HIV for substance abusers, the mentally ill, and homeless populations.

We end the volume with Jeff Stryker's discussion of ethical and legal issues in the treatment of HIV. This is an important area of concern for the clinician, given the many issues raised by HIV infection, including confidentiality, reporting requirements, and assessment of competence.

The world is different, thanks to HIV. This volume is designed to reflect that difference. We also hope to provide herein the best and most current assistance we can to those who work on the front lines of psychological treatment for HIV. This volume is for the psychotherapists, the social workers, the lay counselors, and the many other dedicated mental health professionals who deal with the impact HIV has on all of us. We have done our best to make this the most current and accessible guide possible to the psychological treatment of HIV. In this different world, we hope it will help you make a difference.

ACKNOWLEDGMENTS

Many individuals have assisted me in making this book possible. First, I must acknowledge the extraordinary efforts of the contributors, who were willing to extend themselves and their worldviews to create what I hope is a truly accessible and useful volume. Special thanks to Alan Rinzler for his vision, his clear and constructive editorial suggestions, and his general support in the process. Thanks also to editorial assistant Katie Levine, who helped so much with the numerous details involved in getting this volume to press. Ann Rutherford and the American Psychological Association's Office on AIDS must also be acknowledged for their assistance in helping to identify appropriate contributors for certain chapters, and for supplying additional topical references. My thanks go to Vicki Mays for her assistance in the area of treatment for people of color. My appreciation also goes to the Stanford Lane and Green library staff, whose assistance was consistently helpful and timely, and to the Department of Psychiatry and Behavioral Sciences of the Stanford School of Medicine.

None of this would have been possible were it not for Dr. Yalom. My great thanks go to him for trusting me with this compelling and challenging task. Also thanks to Carlos Greaves for his encouragement to take on this project. Finally, special thanks to my partner, Spencer Stratton, for believing in and supporting me in this process, and for so much more.

NOTES

P. xiii, *As of 1993, one in every ninety-two American men . . . were thought to be infected:* Study says one in ninety-two young men may have HIV. (1995, November 24). *San Francisco Chronicle*, p. 1.

P. xiii, *women are the fastest-growing segment of the population afflicted:* See Chapter Six of this volume.

P. xv, *The World Health Organization (WHO) reported . . . worldwide by the year 2000:* Centers for Disease Control and Prevention (CDC). (1996, April). *AIDS information: International protections/statistics.* Washington, DC: Author.

P. xv, *In Asia, . . . some 3.5 million are thought to be infected:* Quinn, T. (1996, November). Paper presented at the meeting of the American Association for the Advancement of Science, Baltimore, MD.

P. xv, *estimated 333 million new cases of curable (non-HIV) sexually transmitted diseases:* World Health Oragnization. (1995). *The current global situation of the HIV/AIDS pandemic as of 15 December, 1995.* Geneva, Swit.: Global Programme on AIDS.

P. xvi, *In the United States, the Centers for Disease Control and Prevention (CDC) report . . . in the United States from AIDS as of that date:* Centers for Disease Control and Prevention (CDC). (1995). *HIV/AIDS Surveillance Report,* 7 (2), 19.

P. xvii, *found in the first presidential report on young people and AIDS:* Centers for Disease Control and Prevention (CDC). (1995), *ibid;* Fleming, P. S. (1996). *Youth and HIV/AIDS: An American agenda* (A Report to the President). Washington, D. C.: Office of National AIDS Policy.

P. xviii, *researchers have noted the importance of distinguishing cultural identity or ethnicity from race:* Jue, S., and Kain, C. (1989). Culturally sensitive AIDS counseling. In C. Kain (Ed.) *No longer immune: A counselor's guide to AIDS* (pp. 131–148). Alexandria, VA: American Counseling Association Press; Wyatt, G. (1991). Examining ethnicity versus race in AIDS related sex research. *Social Science and Medicine, 33*(1), 37–45.

P. xviii, *individuals who are of mixed race are often not well-differentiated by research methodology:* Wyatt, G. (1991). Examining ethnicity versus race in AIDS related sex research. *Social Science and Medicine, 33*(1), 37–45.

P. xix, *African-American women have been shown . . . delivered by other African-American women:* Kalichman, S. C., Kelley, J., Hunter, T. L., Murphy, D. A., & Tyler, R. (1993). Culturally tailored HIV-AIDS risk-reduction messages to African American urban women: Impact on risk sensitization and risk reduction. *Journal of Consulting and Clinical Psychology, 61*(2), 291–295.

P. xix, *High-risk, non-minority women have been found to be more concerned about AIDS than are high-risk, minority women:* Kalichman, S. C., Hunter, T. L., & Kelley, J. (1992). Perceptions of AIDS susceptibility among minority and non-minority women at risk for HIV infection. *Journal of Consulting and Clinical Psychology, 60*(5), 725–732.

P. xix, *Ethnic minority group members have also been shown . . . with white majority individuals:* Klonoff, E. A. (1994). Culture and gender diversity in common sense beliefs about the causes of six illnesses. *Journal of Behavioral Medicine, 17* (4), 407–418.

P. xix *Values and other differences may be quite localized as well:* Merrill, S. (1991). Confronting the AIDS epidemic among IV-drug users: Does ethnic culture matter? *AIDS Education and Prevention, 3*(3), 258–283.

P. xix, *African Americans, have reason to be distrustful of research and treatment efforts:* Thomas, S. B. (1991). The Tuskegee Syphilis Study, 1932 to 1972: Implications for HIV education and AIDS risk programs in the Black community. *American Journal of Public Health, 81*(11), 1498–1505.

P. xix, *ethnic culture apparently is not considered in studies of patterns of infection and risk behavior:* Merrill, S. (1991). Confronting the AIDS epidemic among IV-drug users: Does ethnic culture matter? *AIDS Education and Prevention, 3*(3), 258–283.

P. xx, *due to higher rates of needlesharing, . . . as compared to whites:* Peterson, J. L., & Bakeman, R. (1989). AIDS and IV-drug use among ethnic minorities: Intravenous-drug use and AIDS. [Special issue]. *Journal of Drug Issues, 19*(1) 27–37.

P. xx, *African-American men without a partner were the group most likely to have sex with multiple partners:* Dolcini, M. M., Coates, T. J., Catania, J. A., Kegeles, S. M., & Hauck, W. W. (1995). Multiple sexual partners and their psychosocial correlates: The population-based AIDS in Multiethnic Neighborhoods (AMEN) study. *Health Psychology, 14*(1), 22–31.

P. xx, *African-American men may be more likely to engage in unprotected anal intercourse:* Peterson, J. L., Coates, T. J., Catania, J. A., Middleton, L., Hilliard, B., & Hearst, N. (1992). High-risk sexual behavior and condom use among gay and bisexual African-American men. *American Journal of Public Health, 82*(11), 1490–1494.

P. xx, *Bisexual behavior has been linked to risk behavior:* Diaz, T., Chu, S. Y., Frederick, M., Hermann, P., Levy, A., Mokotoff, E., Whyte, B., Conte, L., Herr, M., Checko, P. J., Rietmeijer, F., Sorvillo, F., & Mukhtar, Q. (1993). Sociodemographics and HIV risk behaviors of bisexual men with AIDS: Results from a multistate interview project. *AIDS, 7* (9), 1227–1232.

P. xx, *Social stigma, fear of discrimination, . . . as has general denial of risk:* Phillips, K. A., & Coates, T. J. (1995). HIV counseling and testing: Research and policy issues. Special section: HIV testing ten years on. *AIDS Care, 7*(2), 115–124.

P. xx, *over one-third of Latinos/as and African Americans in this study had not heard of a test to detect the HIV virus:* Phillips, K. A. (1993). Factors associated with voluntary HIV testing for African-Americans and Hispanics. *AIDS Education and Prevention, 5*(2), 95–103.

P. xxi, *issuing coupons for redemption may compel . . . to come to outpatient detoxification treatment:* Sorenson, J. L., Costantini, M. F., Wall, T. L., & Gibson, D. R. (1993). Coupons attract high-risk heroin users into detoxification. *Drug and Alcohol Dependence, 31*(3), 247–252.

P. xxi, *A final note on Asian and Pacific Islanders . . . there is some evidence that their risk is increasing:* Diaz, T., Chu, S. Y., Frederick, M., Hermann, P., Levy, A., Mokotoff, E., Whyte, B., Conte, L., Herr, M., Checko, P. J., Rietmeijer, F., Sorvillo, F., & Mukhtar, Q. (1993). Sociodemographics and HIV risk behaviors of bisexual men with AIDS: Results from a multistate interview project. *AIDS, 7* (9), 1227–1232.

P. xxi, *Programs have been created . . . in designing and implementing treatment services:* Day, N. A. (1990). Training providers to serve culturally different AIDS patients: AIDS: A clinical perspective. [Special issue]. *Family and Community Health, 13*(2), 46–53.

P. xxii, *Whereas we formerly talked about AIDS-Related Complex (ARC):* See Chapter Two of this volume.

P. xxvi, *Some studies have shown . . . are deeply linked:* Kameny, M. E. (1994). Psychoneuroimmunology of HIV infection. In Zegans, L. S., & Coates, T. J. (Eds.), *Psychiatric manifestations of HIV disease. The Psychiatric Clinics of North America, 17*(1), 55–68.

P. xxvi, *Although this area of research is relatively new:* Kameny, M. E. (1994). Psychoneuroimmunology of HIV infection. In L. S. Zegans & T. J. Coates (Eds.), *Psychiatric Manifestations of HIV disease. The Psychiatric Clinics of North America, 17*(1), 55–68.

P. xxvii, *In has been shown that having a way:* See Chapter Four of this volume.

P. xxvii, *It has also been shown that the level of positive adjustment:* See Chapter Four of this volume.

TREATING
THE PSYCHOLOGICAL
CONSEQUENCES OF HIV

This volume is dedicated to
the profound strength and optimism of the human spirit,
which, like all in nature, desires only to grow.

I

TRANSFERENCE AND COUNTERTRANSFERENCE

Steven A. Cadwell

A client with HIV and a therapist are in an office together. Unexpressed and intense feelings flood the room. Imagine being inside both of their heads:

Inside the client with HIV, the following feelings race—some conscious, others unconscious: "I'm terrified of what's happening to me. I'm afraid of this pain . . . of dying. I feel repulsive. How can I trust that you aren't repulsed? Who could care about me? I feel so much shame. Sometimes I feel I deserve this and you think so too. Why should I risk depending on you?"

Inside the therapist's head, there is bound to be an equally entangling mix of conscious and unconscious feelings: "How can I help? He's so scared. His sores are hard to look at. He needs so much. Will he die? I wish I had the power to cure him. I've seen too much of this. There but for the grace of God go I. . . . I'm afraid."

Given this flood of feeling on both sides, how do any of us do this work?

Work with HIV can pull at all of our client's deepest vulnerabilities and our own: fear of death, body shame, confusion about sexuality, the repulsiveness of disease, dread of loss of control, fear of dependency, and moral conflicts, to name a few. As we enter this work with our clients, we are choosing to work with their deepest vulnerabilities and must be prepared to deal with our own. Vital to remaining effective in the work is our tracking and management of the client's transference and our own countertransference.

TRANSFERENCE AND COUNTERTRANSFERENCE DEFINED

Although there are many ways *transference* has been understood, I will take an object relations perspective and use transference to mean the misperception of reality in relationship to others. In the therapy relationship, transference is about the patient's need for you the therapist "to be other than who you are." In positive transference, the patient hopes you are the "good" parent he never had. This dynamic is risky—the honeymoon is bound to end—but it also allows for the possibility of a strong alliance in the treatment.

Negative transference is the dread that the therapist is the "bad" negligent or abusive parent the patient did have. This negative transference threatens the possibility of making a healthy relationship with the therapist. Equally unfounded in current reality, both positive and negative transference can be used as tools for understanding the patient's experience and to help him accept what is real. By working transference through with the patient, we can develop a "good enough" relationship, helping the patient trust his capacity to discern what is real and who can be trusted to help him bear it. Notice that transference is another way of understanding the patient's resistance to engaging in the relationship with you.

A particularly pernicious kind of transference is projective identification; the client projects (or transfers) what she dreads about herself onto you the therapist and invites you to bear that unbearable part of herself. We will ultimately want to help the client develop a less toxic means of binding her shifting sense of self.

By *countertransference* I mean the therapist's (yours or my) mis-perception of reality, specifically the conscious and unconscious responses of the therapist to his client's "presentation, person, and material. Both the therapist's responses (affective, cognitive, somatic) and his defenses against these influence his interper-sonal responses. His responses will be stirred by his response to the reality of HIV, disease and death, the impact of hearing the details of his client's experience with HIV, the severity of the symptoms and adaptations to HIV, and his own personality, his-tory, and current circumstances and their overlap with his client."

Countertransference can work in two directions, which par-allel the valences of transference. In my positive countertrans-ference, I could idealize the client as only good, and I could hope to be the Good Parent for my patient. Although seemingly benign, this illusion is based on my grandiosity. The patient is bound to be more complex than only "good"; he's bound to be a mixture of good and bad. Furthermore, I can't be that fanta-sized Good Parent. My desire to be his Good Parent can pro-mote unrealistic, damaging boundary problems for the patient and myself.

My negative countertransference includes my irrational dread about the patient. In the case of working with a patient with HIV, my dread will be affected my own history—my experience or lack of experience with death and disease—and my conflicts about the issues raised by HIV. Rather than staying with the client's need, I may dread her vulnerability, identify too closely due to my own dreaded vulnerability, and want to act too quickly to ease her symptoms and thus avoid a deeper look at her pain and conflict. In my haste, I'd be acting more to avoid my own anxiety than in her best interest. This may be true even though I might appear to be very involved in solving her problems. This phenomenon is referred to as *countertransference resistance:* the therapist's resistance to what the client is delivering to the rela-tionship, both real and transferred.

My behavior may be triggered by my idiosyncratic response to a particular client; in which case, I'd better know myself well enough to keep my feelings from getting in the way of the treatment. At the same time, analyzing my response can be illuminating. It can offer a window into the patient's earlier experience with abuse or neglect by parents or others. My job is to make use of this data to position myself in an empathic alliance with him.

This alliance will be affected both by the transference *and* by the real relationship between us. In work related to HIV, life and death are at stake. Both members of the therapeutic relationship may experience a profound encounter with the other person. The therapist must not overlook the real relationship and her authentic feelings in it—including deep caring and love. Again, part of our task is to determine where to focus the work while sustaining the relationship. Particularly when working with HIV, we must pay attention to the irrational, unconscious, transferential feelings that threaten to distort the relationship from both sides of the room. We also need to support the relationship and its safety. How do we sustain this balance?

Although negative transference and countertransference reactions are painful for both sides, we should not avoid them. Uncovering them or being hit over the head by them can be a critical piece of the therapeutic process. Analyzing such reactions may reveal the block that has interfered with many other relationships in the client's life, or in our own.

The ongoing process of untangling the primitive hope and dread from the real aspect of a relationship is the therapeutic work. It is also what makes therapy effective. The dynamics of positive and negative transference and countertransference are inevitable in any treatment. These dynamics are exacerbated in HIV work in part because of the stigma associated with the disease. Consequently, intense hope and dread may be engendered in the client and ourselves. In this chapter, I will be examining those issues and reactions particular to work with clients with HIV.

CORE ISSUES

In psychotherapy with people with HIV, the transference and countertransference themes develop from the core issues—death and dying, disease, sexuality, and IV drug use—the epidemic forces on us. These are issues that we'd rather deny or avoid, which makes the work all the more charged.

Death and Dying

For both members of the relationship, a prominent and charged issue will be death itself. Ernest Becker, in his Pulitzer prize–winning book, *The Denial of Death*, powerfully exposes our terror of death and the elaborate cultural and psychological defenses we use to deny it. He views one's core striving for identity as the creation and sustenance of one's being; that is, this striving is the basis of a "healthy" narcissistic investment in Being. Death is seen as the major threat and the most compelling human problem. HIV rips through our denial and exposes this core problem for all involved.

In the HIV epidemic, death comes at an unpredictable time, out of synch with the "expected" life span of the "normal" adult. With the elderly, rationalizing comments often cushion our horror: "At least she lived a good, long life." Most often, HIV does not affect people in old age. HIV kills children, young adults, anyone in its way. Furthermore, in the case of HIV we are confronted with our mortality by an often prolonged and debilitating dying process.

Disease

Disease can be dreaded as the vehicle of death and a threat to our autonomy and sense of control. Disease can feel disgusting for the diseased and those who witness it.

HIV is often painful in excruciating ways. The symptoms are often undeniable: emaciation, fungal infections, lesions, incontinence. Our patient may dread being seen in such a compromised state. We ourselves may have difficulty sitting with the patient's disfigurement.

The disease also threatens the integrity of the patient's mind. We all invest our very sense of selfhood in the smooth working of our mind. The threat of losing our mind is the stuff of horror movies. Patient and therapist are both vulnerable to this terror.

Sexuality

Our sexual urges have the power to pull us beyond our vision of ourselves as transcendent and rational. Reckoning with this power can be disturbing. At certain times, sexuality can feel dangerous. At other times, sex can feel liberating.

To work with clients with HIV, we must be able to look frankly at sexuality even if it takes forms that make us squirm. We must also be able to respect and embrace the power of sex. Our culture and most of us in it have intensely mixed feelings about sex: puritanical repulsion combined with commercially exploited preoccupation. Shame will encumber our patients as they bring the disease and their sexuality to us. We may be challenged to stretch our sexual comfort zone to include bisexuality; multiple sex partners ("promiscuity"); nonmonogamy; the sex industry; and varieties of sexual behavior, including anal sex, oral sex, rimming, fisting, or sadomasochism.

IV Drug Use

We may be repelled by the notion of injecting drugs. Drug use itself is criminal. Drug users often feed their habit through illegal behavior that violates others. We may be prejudiced in belief that all drug users are psychopathic criminals or are stupid and unattractive. Our own issues about dependency, lack of control, deviance, self-destruction, pleasure, and pain can cloud our ability to work with IV drug users. Our own wish to be able to solve others' problems may be sorely tried if we expect to bring quick sobriety to clients with addictions.

In each of these highly charged areas, we and our clients are bound to encounter many misconceptions and prejudices reflective of the homophobic, sexist, racist, death phobic culture in which most of us were raised. To better understand the range of complex transferential issues that may crop up, it will be useful to look at the context and history of this epidemic—a core issue in its own right.

THE IMPACT OF STIGMA

Some argue that HIV is "just a virus." But it has particular meaning in our culture. The meaning we give HIV is derived from how it was originally perceived, who was first affected, and the way the larger culture sought to distance itself from the disease.

In the United States, HIV was first identified among gays, already a stigmatized minority. It was next seen to endanger other marginalized minorities: IV drug users (through shared needles), women (through sex and IV drugs), ethnic minorities (who are more often drug users), youth (through their high risk for unsafe sex and drug use), and people with hemophilia (who are already "different" because of their medical condition). Each of these groups carries a dimension of being an outsider. Each came into the epidemic already marginalized. As the epidemic spread, the majority used the disease to further marginalize minorities and distance itself from the perils of disease.

HIV, Morality, and Homophobia

The link between HIV and morality is crucial to the social meaning we have attributed to HIV, and that link creeps into our clients' transference to us and our countertransference to them. As in the case of syphilis, HIV has become a label that stigmatizes those with HIV as promiscuous, immoral, and dangerous. Because the cause of HIV disease is misperceived to be sexual behavior rather than a virus, an anxious public has been forced to struggle with its sexual taboos. Just as the individual psyche requires certain defenses to remain "sane," society develops mores and norms to create and maintain order. When an individual or subgroup is perceived as transgressing the norms or breaking taboos, the social order is threatened, and society reacts to restore order.

In popular consciousness, gay people with HIV are judged to have broken an important taboo and transgressed a significant norm: they prefer sexual relations with the same sex and are assumed to be promiscuous in their sexual expression. Homophobia, the irrational fear of homosexual thoughts and behaviors, further intensifies this rigid rejection. IV drug users are also seen as worthless and expendable. By denying their humanity, they are written off. The IV drug users' risk for HIV is another characteristic that distances them and reinforces their marginalization.

Impact of Stigma on Transference

The experience of being marginalized can lead to the real experience of being neglected and abused by the larger culture. The patient is apt to feel shame and a sense of being bad. In this way, this traumatic disease is retraumatizing an already traumatized minority. Shame and trauma may become hurdles to seeking help at all, breeding negative transference that prevents the client from entering our office.

In a newly diagnosed client, this shame may be expressed in rage, and this rage may be projected onto the therapist. The client can't believe that you can be trusted. His dread is that you will not care for him as a person. Instead he believes that you, just like everyone else, will marginalize him further.

Rejection. Prejudice. Rejection. A woman, a person of color, a gay man, even a child with HIV can experience this.

The work of the therapist is to shore up real resources (both internal and external) that the client can enlist. The therapist must also attend to the unconscious meanings of the disease and of death that may interfere with the client's capacity to call upon these resources. The therapist must uncover the transferred meaning the client gives to the disease. What is the client reexperiencing as a result of this disease? What helplessness? What dreaded earlier relationship of abuse or neglect is being resurrected?

In this epidemic, gay men often experience new versions of old injuries. The gay man may return to an old familiar closet of isolation or inauthenticity as a result.

RICK

Rick, a forty-eight-year-old African-American bodybuilder who is a nurse, interviews with me to join a gay men's psychotherapy group I run. All of his friends have died of HIV. He is completely isolated and not dating. He feels that their deaths are *his* fault, just as *he* was to blame for his father's death of brain cancer (another secret the family never talked about). He has always been the caretaker. He is overwhelmed with hopelessness and dread because he has been helpless to CURE his friends. (Just so, he was unable to cure himself of his homosexuality and still feels bad about it.) He isolates himself in another closet. He asks me for help to come out of it by joining the group.

Reenacting Prior Abuse:
The Impact of Intrapersonal Stigma

One meaning of persistent high-risk sex is the compulsive reenacting of the internalized rejecting other. The hate is now directed against the self. Risky sex can be a suicide attempt; the individual is following the twisted orders from a core sense of badness.

AMBROSIO

Ambrosio, a thirty-eight-year-old Latino HIV educator I've seen in treatment for over three years, is HIV-negative. His ex-lover is HIV-positive. He comes in panicked about canker sores in his mouth. He'd tasted blood when sucking a trick's penis and woke up to see sores on the man's penis the next morning. As he talks through his panic, we both come to understand that he's telling me another version of his feeling that if he does get HIV, it's further confirmation that he's bad, thereby matching the intense rejection he'd felt from his abusive father and brother. We review what he believes to be his acceptable sexual risk practice. We resume our pursuit of understanding what he gets and doesn't get from his conquest of handsome men.

All too often for gay men what may lurk is the ghost of a traumatizing abusive father. Studies are tracking the prevalence of childhood physical and sexual abuse in gay men who become HIV-positive.

MIKE

Mike is a thirty-three-year-old gay man who has HIV. He looks like the boy next door. I've seen him for five years, during which time he discovered he was infected with the virus, then was diagnosed with AIDS; he retired on disability at thirty-two.

Mike's parents divorced when he was three. His mother died when he was seven. He was left with his father. Until that time, he only knew his father as a gift giver at Christmas. Santa Claus turned out to be alcoholic, sadistic, and emotionally and physically abusive, as did a series of stepmothers.

Mike survived through dissociation, and has a deep sense of being bad, as though he deserved the abuse. We have spent painful times searching through the terror that haunts him. Although a very compliant "best boy" on the outside, inside he has always felt bad. He could describe a part of him that was dressed in black leather who rebelled against everyone; a rebel with what cause? He described his pattern of being attracted to older, bigger men. He was often overwhelmed by them, feeling that he couldn't say no. In one such encounter, which included unprotected anal sex, he was infected.

Our work has been slow and steady in building his positive sense of self. He has worked through his shame about his past and uncovered many contemporary versions of this earlier shame; at one point he was fired from a job for stealing money. He has worked hard to trust me through all this. He yearns that I will be good, nurturing, caring, and loving. He dreads that I will retaliate and judge him. He dreads that my pursuit of him will be invasive and abusive: that I will become his bad dad all over again. He has grown to trust that I am with him, not against him. He doesn't have to hide, dissociate, subvert, rebel, or be alone.

He also is able to talk about HIV as the perpetrator. He dreads that the virus is abusing him. By facing his dread directly, he's been able to hope again. He started dating a man six months ago, finally pushing through his dread that to love someone would mean to infect them. On Mike's proposal, the man he's dated has moved in with him from out of town one month ago. We are still at work with his fear of the new intimacy. We are also celebrating his delight in love he had only hoped for before.

Your client may misconstrue infection as the return of dreaded abuse. The client then has a negative transference to HIV as the perpetrator. HIV is tragic, but it need not become the childhood trauma revisited alone. This time, you can be with the client, examining the unconscious meaning, the meaning that is transferred to the disease, to death, and to the experience of becoming dependent on you, the care provider.

Normalizing the Transference

It is critical that you anticipate and normalize these transferred feelings. Your initial work is to invite the client to create a safe relationship. You need to recognize the positive transference—the client's hope to be cured. Some of that wish will be the lifeblood of the therapeutic alliance. You need to hold that transference carefully, as you anticipate that the client is inevitably going to be disappointed with your inability to cure or rescue her.

At the same time, you need to be alert to negative transference—the client's dread of being neglected by you or abused by you. The client could fear you will neglect her by not really caring. Or she could be terrified that you will violate her integrity or some other boundary and further shame or stigmatize her.

The valence and intensity of these transference reactions may vary over the mercurial course of the disease. Issues of autonomy, dependence, shame, and trust may flair when the client is hospitalized and then subside when he returns home. Distrust of the therapist may seem to occur out of the blue but in fact may be directly tied to times when the client has to give up some sense of autonomy elsewhere in his life. The therapist needs to be attentive to how changes in the client's life will change the meaning of the therapeutic relationship.

The rigidity of the transference distortion may depend on how long the therapist and client have worked together, whether or not there was a period of work before the onset of debilitating illness, and the preexistent personality of the client.

PSYCHOLOGICAL IMPLICATIONS FOR THE THERAPIST

Other authors have delineated the different, difficult countertransference reactions to psychosis, to suicidality, to terminal illness, to cancer patients, and to dying patients. Work with clients with HIV is difficult because the likely inevitability of death is brutally apparent, as is the specter of deterioration, waste, and excruciating pain. Furthermore, working with patients with HIV may mean working with all these difficult clinical challenges at once: primitive issues (if the client has characterological problems or regresses under stress), the issues of psychosis (stemming from organic complications), issues of suicidality, and the issues of terminal illness.

Clinicians are not immune to the impact of the stigma against HIV. Fear of contagion, death, and homosexuality all have been documented in the countertransference responses of clinicians. Fear of the contagion of stigmatization is also important to track. A therapist may worry, "Will my practice collapse if I'm seen as an AIDS therapist? Will I get any other referrals?" Awareness of these anxieties and our capacity to manage them are critical in clinical work with persons with AIDS. Our own shame and our impulse to distance from the one stigmatized may be overwhelming at times.

On the other hand, we may overidentify with the marginalized client. We may have a wish to cure, to control, or to work on a more health-focused outcome. In our own grandiosity, we may wish to be the savior. In this manner, we take on the client's positive transference wish by trying to gratify it. This is both delusional and exhausting.

Monitoring Our Boundaries

An important gauge for determining the interference of our countertransference will be our appropriate use of boundaries in the relationship. The term *boundaries* refers to the flexible and secure capacity to distinguish between the self and the outside world. For the therapist, loss of boundaries leads to overidentification and fusion with the client. On the other hand, the therapist's overly rigid boundaries lead to an ineffective empathic relationship with the client.

The therapist working with clients with HIV needs to constantly gauge her own feelings. Her feelings may be consciously and effectively expressed in her *crossing* the boundary of the conventional frame of therapy in the service of the client (by making a home visit when the client is sick, for example). Or the therapist's feelings may be unconsciously and ineffectively acted out by *breaking* the boundary (for example, by offering free service in a wish to be nice to the client) or by erecting insurmountably *rigid* boundaries (for example, by refusing to see anyone out of the office or for a reduced fee). Our own comfort level with the range of issues involved will affect how we deal with them. Negotiating the boundary in the service of the client and tracking our own impulses to keep the boundary too rigid or too permeable take constant self-analysis, which can be enhanced through consultation.

Just as HIV threatens our clients' core sense of self, so too will it threaten ours. We too will be faced with our own feelings about death, disease, and security. We'll be torn by our own instinct to preserve ourselves and flee our client whose life is so horrifying and endangered. We then may become flooded with guilt for having wished to flee, and we may overcompensate by doing too much for the patient.

Our work is to continue to manage the boundaries with a realistic sense of the limits and resources of the therapeutic relationship. We thereby do not replicate the bad others in our client's past. Nor are we reenacting any of our own.

Complication of Shared Characteristics

Although the therapist's capacity to identify with the client is a critical component of empathy, identification can also be hazardous. In this work, the risk of overidentification is very high because of the high probability that therapists working with people with HIV will themselves be affected by the disease: by being a member of a risk group, or by being infected ourselves, or by having partners, family members, or friends who have been infected or are at high risk.

One gay therapist describes his vulnerability as provoked by sitting with his clients' experiences of loss: "I often sit with clients who've lost forty or fifty friends. Their whole friendship network is wiped out, and I feel like I have something in common with them. I've lost colleagues, friends, family. It's very hard to be with them in their anxiety because it really hits close to home."

Another gay therapist struggles with the impact of his lover's HIV illness: "Sometimes I feel like I can manage a certain kind of attachment in my clinical work and also a certain objectivity. But having a partner who has HIV makes me feel the pain too much at times—both in my work and in my personal life. I get overwhelmed by the sense of so much loss. I can't imagine life without my lover. My dread of losing him is bound to slip into my clinical work."

Other matches between the therapist's characteristics and those of the client also can be powerful. Shared gender, age, race, religion, or life circumstance may all pull for a stronger identification that can equally facilitate and complicate the empathic bond:

A twenty-five-year-old Polish-American woman was seen in therapy by a forty-eight-year-old Polish-American female therapist. The client was infected by her husband, who she didn't know had been an IV drug user. She was overcome with shame and depression. She'd kept her infection a secret from her family, who sustained their denial about her status, never asking her about it even after her husband died of HIV.

The therapist found her to be lovely, bright and engaging. "She could have been my daughter or my friend." The therapist found herself clearly more affected by this client than by her gay male clients.

Just as shared characteristics may activate a capacity to identify with the client, they may also complicate the impact of the work unconsciously. The therapist's rescue fantasies may erupt in a way they never have with other, less similar clients. Or survivor guilt may be more intense: "We are just alike. Why aren't I the one who is infected?" The intensity of these concerns may vary for the clinician at different points in the course of the disease.

The "Real" Relationship

Even as I emphasize the importance of recognizing the unconscious, irrational countertransferential meaning of what is enacted by the therapist in the treatment relationship, again I want to acknowledge the impact of what can be a devastatingly real encounter with disease, death, trauma, and multiple loss.

Just as it is important to acknowledge and validate the real relationship with the client for the client's sake, so it is important that we acknowledge and validate the real relationship for the therapist's sake.

Research suggests that the "real" features of the therapist—the personal qualities and interpersonal skills of the clinician—account for at least as much treatment outcome as specific techniques and theories employed. The meaningful encounter between the therapist and patient is facilitated primarily by the core personhood of the psychotherapist. A therapist uses herself to connect to the client. Her self is bound to be affected in the interchange.

Fortunately, the contemporary theory of therapeutic interaction is burgeoning on this front and can be a great resource of affirmation for the therapist who works with people with HIV. Contemporary psychoanalytic theories and relational theorists (such as Stephen Mitchell and Jean Baker Miller), intersubjectivists (such as Robert Stolorow and George Atwood), interpersonalists (such as Edgar Levenson), and interactive theorists (such as Christopher Bollas) have all moved to add to the two former modes of therapeutic action (that is, insight into drive conflicts and corrective experience of deficits) a third mode: the relationship, which includes empathic attunement *and* authentic engagement. An essential aspect of this third mode of therapeutic action is its emphasis on the presence of two persons in the clinical relationship and on the importance of attending to both, not just the client. Often we are enriched; we grow with our clients. But sometimes we can be overwhelmed and become impaired by the intensity of what the real relationship takes out of us.

TRAUMATIC STRESS SYNDROME

Depending on the therapist's previous experience with death and disease, work with HIV may be a first intimate encounter with mortality. The level of personal anxiety, the intensity of the stress this work may deliver, the horror, dread, and repulsion may all be highly individual. At different points in a career of doing this work, the therapist may experience the work at varying intensity. The first HIV case, the twentieth, or the ninety-eighth will each have an impact, but the particular impact will vary.

Chronic Traumatic Stress Syndrome

In doing this work, the therapist needs to be keenly aware of the effect on himself of both his exposure to distinct traumatic clinical episodes and the cumulative impact of repeated exposure to trauma over time. The epidemic delivers trauma over and over again, rather than discretely delivering it in one incident. This creates a chronic traumatic stress syndrome. A therapist talks about this: "It feels so endless. I mean, you don't get a chance to recover from one death before the next one hits. So I don't know where the center is anymore. We're so off course, I don't know what the course is anymore. I said to my own therapist recently, 'I feel at this level that my life is about death lately. It's not just having to deal with it. It's like, what else is there?'"

Vicarious Traumatization

Vicarious traumatization refers to the disturbance of the therapist's inner experience because of empathic exposure to clients' trauma material. Whereas therapists experience countertransference within the specific and limited relationship of a particular therapy with a particular client, vicarious traumatization floods into the therapist's experience with all her clients and her personal life. It overwhelms "all aspects of the therapist's self, challenging her beliefs about the world, her identity and the realms of spirituality and meaning. The therapist's frame of reference, self-capacities (ability to tolerate and modulate affect), ego resources, and psychological needs and related schemas (for example, safety, esteem, trust, control, intimacy)" are all challenged.

Burnout is a popular term for this state, which is characterized by physical, emotional, and mental exhaustion. Ineffective coping strategies include emotional detachment from the client, cynicism, and rigidity. Studies have identified the factors that lead to burnout in hospice workers and in psychotherapists working with people with HIV. These factors include the non-traditional nature of the work, the idealism of the work, the repetitive formation and termination of relationships, ambiguity, and matched characteristics of the therapist and client.

The notion of vicarious trauma elucidates the intensity of what the therapist is himself exposed to—which parallels in striking ways the impact of other traumas on the person with HIV, including multiple losses of friends and phobic public reactions to HIV and AIDS. This creates more parallel process between the therapist's and client's experience. We can look at these cognitive schemata—regarding safety, control, independence, and alienation—in terms of how HIV may affect the therapist.

In terms of the need for safety, exposure to HIV in treatment may conjure fears of contagion in the therapist's personal life. The therapist's own security may be challenged. How safe is he from infection? What safer sex practices is he following? This can result in rigid abstinence or counterphobic risk-taking. I've heard colleagues describe either reaction.

People with HIV can often express feelings of helplessness and vulnerability against the disease and circumstances surrounding it. The therapist can also begin to wonder about her own power and efficacy. The therapist can slip into feelings of helplessness and despair about the uncontrollable force of the epidemic.

Our clients' independence is often curtailed over the course of HIV. Witnessing this loss may threaten the therapist's feeling of autonomy. There was a period in my own support group for therapists working with HIV in which we all felt terrified and confused about how powerless, dependent, and unsafe we were. Not only were we overwhelmed by the deaths of our clients and friends from HIV, but two members of our group became sick themselves with HIV and died. We surviving members struggled to find our way back to a place of mutual interdependence as we dealt with our shattering losses.

Just as trauma victims experience a profound sense of alienation from others, so, often, do people with HIV. Therapists who work with people with HIV may also experience that alienation. This alienation may be further intensified by other therapists who perceive this work as overwhelming. I frequently hear therapists outside the work comment, "How can you do this work every day?" This comment may feel like a confusing mix of sympathy and marginalization.

In response to all these influences, the therapist's experience parallels that of the client. By understanding his own experience, the therapist will have understanding of his client's experience.

We all need a meaningful frame of reference for life in order to proceed with living. This need is managed by our sense of why things occur. In HIV work, the haunting question can be: Why did this happen to this client and not to me? "Causes," such as "she does IV drugs," or "he had 'promiscuous' sex" can be judgmental and don't fully explain the odds. Sitting with existential randomness can be disconcerting when we wish for more causal order. Yet to risk attributing "cause" can further stigmatize our clients. Conflicting needs to find meaning and to avoid judgment can leave the therapist in a difficult place.

The disturbing exposures to trauma in HIV work can leave therapists with difficulties that spill over into their personal lives. Dimensions of the disturbance may be manifest in dreams, behaviors, and personal relationships.

Here is an example of a powerful HIV-related dream that a colleague shared: "I'm alone on a beach and it's a beautiful day. Family and friends are playing on the beach. I become aware that a tidal wave is forming off the coast. My friends ignore it. I'm not sure if they know it's there. The parents with their children seem aware of it, but they are doing nothing about it. Then I become aware that the tidal wave has shifted its location. It's coming from the land now. We've somehow gotten onto a very narrow peninsula and the tidal wave is coming from the land. I'm panicked and wake up."

Other colleagues talk of losing their sense of control over their own safer sex behavior when they are particularly overwhelmed by overexposure to HIV in this work. This degree of danger to the therapist makes it all the more imperative that we find safeguards against the traumatic hazards of the work.

Multiple Loss

The intimacy possible in this work has two sides: the profound attachment of care and love for the client, and the profound loss when the client dies. The impact of multiple loss for therapists working with HIV deserves ongoing careful attention. Loss is both an inevitable factor in the real relationship and a potential trigger for unconscious and conflictual material from the therapist's own history.

How does the therapist engage enough when at the outset she knows that she'll probably be losing the relationship at some point? How can she do this over and over again? The loss the therapist deals with is unrelenting: not only the losses each client experiences (of autonomy, health, economic security, social network, or mental acuity, for example) but also the cumulative losses of her clients who have died of HIV. These losses don't pace themselves. In a single therapeutic session, these losses can be recapitulated to a devastating degree.

One clinician talked about her hopelessness after sitting with a man with HIV in late stages who was suffering from wasting syndrome.

> I've grown to really like him. He invited me to his home and I saw his odd collection of weird objects. [She laughed.] I thought I was saying goodbye when I visited him at home. Then he showed up at my office last week. I didn't expect him. He's thin as a rail and always out of breath. He was so sad and then the next minute enraged and then laughing as though he'd forgotten he had AIDS at all. It's so hard to witness this kind of cruel dying. He's basically dying of diarrhea. He says he'll shit himself to death. There's no dignity. Sometimes, I wish he'd die and not have to continue to suffer. I feel bad for wishing this. But it's also hard for me to bear it. He's got neuropathy and he sometimes forgets he's sick. I don't. [She wept.]

How can the therapist not be overwhelmed at times! There is no break to grieve one loss when another quickly follows. Another clinician in the support group I facilitate speaks: "There's been a wave of deaths lately among my clients. But I didn't take time to stop until Carlos died. When I learned he died I knew I had to go to his wake. When I went through the door, I couldn't stop crying. I realized I wasn't just crying for Carlos but for the six other guys who've died. I'm glad Ruth [his colleague and fellow support group member] was with me."

The impact of these losses will vary depending on the therapist's ego strengths, character weaknesses, and the circumstances in her life. Deaths of clients may coincide with deaths in a clinician's personal life: of family, colleagues, friends.

One clinician described her desire not to see any more clients with HIV as long as her mother was dying. After her death, she waited six months before taking on any new clients with HIV. At that point, the therapist felt clear enough about her own personal work that she was willing to facilitate a short-term bereavement group.

The other side of this loss for both parties in the therapeutic relationship is the integrity gained through being willing to engage the client in the face of loss. Therapists often experience deep love for clients in this work. It is a particular kind of love expressed within the boundaries of the therapeutic relationship. It is hard to write about it, as any love is. It is deeply felt. It is a reward of the work. The therapist grows through the experience of this love.

This love intensifies our grief when our partner in the clinical relationship dies. This ultimate termination to the therapeutic relationship has a profound impact on the therapist. Celebrating our capacity for attachment and love can sustain us in our survival and ongoing engagement in life.

CARE FOR THE THERAPIST

How do we stay hopeful? How do we deal with our own dread? How do we stay connected and avert our own isolation? How do we avert burnout and not be shattered ourselves in our efforts to relate effectively?

In this work, I have found that the treatment relationship extends beyond my relationship with my client. The holding relationship in this kind of therapy extends beyond the dyad of the clinician and client. I am held by my consultants, my peer supervision group, my ongoing training, and my pursuit of theory in our clinical community. We ask, tell, and pursue each other in order to continue building safe, respectful partnerships.

To manage all these feelings, we need our own means of coping. Just as our patients need support and holding, so do we. First, it is vital to realize our feelings are normal and expectable. It is vital to take our own inventory of feelings about a range of HIV-related issues. Be as clear and realistic about yourself as you can be. Don't shame yourself for what you may not be comfortable with. But do take responsibility for doing the work to overcome your discomfort, whether in supervision, consultation, or personal therapy.

Second, we need to have other places to go with our feelings. Here, consultation is critical for all of us, either in peer groups or with a supervisor. People in private practices can be resourceful by joining together in group supervision or by having individual supervision. I have used both. My peer supervision group is now in its tenth year. I heartily recommend our ritual of combining a meal with our consultation. We are nurtured in body and soul by these meetings!

Therapists in rural settings may need to be more enterprising: monthly meetings and even telephone consultation may be a way to break the isolation, assess traumatization, and get another's perspective in managing boundaries.

In agency settings, managing one's therapeutic boundaries can be bolstered by an open, safe organizational culture. A safe, regular forum for discussions of boundaries and countertransference ensures the therapist time to review his work and continue to monitor the balance of his empathic involvement with his clients.

Your Feelings Are Normal!

At some point in the work, burnout or vicarious traumatization is inevitable. We may be "burned out" many times over the course of doing this work. As with countertransference, feelings of burnout can be instructive. We need to be able to make use of countertransference or symptoms of burnout as ways to check our own capacity to continue in the work. We can also use our affective state as a window into what our clients may be feeling. For example, if you are dreading the session, think of how often the client experiences others' dread of being with him. Or might he feel full of dread and hopelessness himself?

In this work we need to learn about our limits. You may not be able to know yours until you've gone beyond them. This is why it is imperative to have others who can alert you. A therapist who was feeling overwhelmed talks about using his support group: "When I was at the group it was sort of like I was listing the series of disasters and woes and not registering emotionally about what I was saying. I was too burned out. One guy in the group said, 'Your whole life sounds like it's nothing but shattered edges. Maybe you need to do something about that.' That image really broke through. I figured it was time to step back."

Grief Work and Stress Management

Given the ongoing demands of the work and the number of deaths therapists may experience, we need to find the right balance between stress management and grief work to sustain ourselves. The two tasks may appear to be in conflict. In stress management, we need to assess the sources of stress and determine ways in which some stressors can be decreased. One of those may be to avoid the emotional stress of grieving. When we do grief work, anticipating loss and releasing feelings may actually feel more stressful initially, even though the aim of the grief work is cathartic release. There comes a time, however, when the grief work must be done. The assessment of which task to work on takes self-awareness and the feedback of others.

In the support group I co-facilitate for clinic staff working with HIV, we go back and forth between focusing on the need to use our weekly meetings to grieve the deaths of clients and the need to focus on alleviating the stress of staff members. Some weeks, we do an oral version of the Names Project AIDS quilt. Members who had direct relationships with a client who has died tell of their personal experience with the client. Others bear witness to their grief and affirm their loss and their capacity to have connected and mattered. Other weeks, we focus more on stress reduction: for example, we encourage staff members to plan vacations, develop effective ways of dealing with difficult clients, build team spirit, and affirm the value of their work.

COPING STRATEGIES

There are several coping strategies for managing vulnerability to identification and the subsequent risks of burnout in countertransference and vicarious traumatization: (1) behavioral, (2) ego supportive, (3) personal growth, (4) political, (5) spiritual, and (6) cognitive. As you read over the descriptions of these strategies, assess your own. Just as with our clients, we need to assess ourselves for a flexible range of defensive resources. In this work, we are best served by a combination of strategies. Essentially, each strategy offers some way for us to negotiate more perspective and effective distance from the work, allowing us to renew ourselves and to replenish our hope and optimism.

Behavioral Management

There are some basic lessons—wisdom gained by hard experience—that veterans of this work have passed down. Like all pieces of behavioral advice, they may seem to be obvious at first. However, they may be surprisingly difficult to implement. When we are especially challenged in the work, they are a concrete standard against which to compare our work and may be the first rung of a ladder for escaping the burnout predicament.

 • *Limit the number of patients.* One of the lessons that therapists learned early in the epidemic was to limit the number of clients they saw who had HIV. It's important to find a working balance of HIV and non-HIV cases. One therapist describes his quota of HIV cases: "I've settled on 25 percent as a working model, having at one point had probably 50 or 60 percent HIV-related cases and found that was too much. It required me to stop seeing people with HIV for about nine months. The personal impact and the amount of extra work associated with patients with HIV-related illness is enormous."

This may not be possible for clinicians in clinics or hospitals where their job description is specific to HIV patients. One would hope in these cases that extra support would be offered for these staff: support groups, leaves of absence, workshops, additional supervision, and vacation time.

• *Break the isolation.* Private practitioners who work with HIV cases have organized to meet with other therapists in HIV-related organizations, conferences, and in peer support groups. Therapists who are the solitary providers of HIV services in large hospital settings can work to get a more equitable distribution of cases and then create support groups with their peers. Clinicians in rural settings might try to network by phone, computer, or monthly meetings at rotating locations. These groups may or may not be facilitated by experienced professionals. In these groups, the therapist has access to professional, intellectual, and emotional support.

Whether in groups or with dyadic consultation, it is vital that the therapist be able to acknowledge, express, and work through her feelings in a supportive relationship. If her feelings aren't acknowledged and worked through, the therapist may become numb and shut down, which can interfere with the therapist's capacity to empathize with her clients. The goals of the groups should be to normalize the feelings the therapist has in response to doing the work, identify the particular vulnerabilities that may be present, and provide a safe environment where the therapist is free to express and work through emotional reactions that threaten the work.

• *Choose other means of involvement.* Rather than focusing exclusively on HIV clinical work, it's advisable to diversify our practice to include a variety of activities, including teaching, administration, research, supervision, organizing conferences, being an expert witness for public policy hearings, and writing. These activities allow us distance from the exclusive intensity of clinical relationships.

• *Maintain your personal life.* It is important to have a balance in our personal and professional life. It is vital to be aware of and respect our own personal boundaries. Limited weekend and evening work; vacations; spending time with friends and family; an active social life; hobbies such as singing, reading, music, cooking, travel, or home improvements; physical exercise; raising children; and leisure time—all can ensure a balance in life.

Cognitive Strategies

Just as we often cognitively reframe our clients' perceptions to get them out of a corner of their own creation, so we can make use of our rational minds to step back from the emotional intensity of HIV work and to use intellectual strategies for managing our next round of involvement.

• *Clarify your role.* In the role of therapist, it's important to be clear about negotiating the boundaries of the work. As one therapist described her experience: "At first we have an expectable role. When clients get sick, it tends to become less clear. You can feel a pull to be more like a friend. Or maybe you feel more like part of his medical team. It is important to get clear about the role; carve out a niche for yourself. You work at defining the relationship. I'm not there to cure."

• *Distinguish crisis roles from long-term roles.* Initially the pull on the therapist is to get as caught up in the immediate crisis as the client. Over time, the work may expand beyond temporary crisis management. The therapist needs to conceive of involvement in a way that allows for sustained contact over time. Especially now, when different treatments are enabling people to live longer with HIV, the client may have more time to explore questions about the meaning and quality of her continuing life. The therapist needs to be flexible and available to join the client in this exploration.

• *Specialize in aspects of the work.* Different therapists may focus on different tasks that they feel are more manageable. Having a sense of mastery enables the therapist to stay strongly grounded in her sense of providing care. She is less apt to join the patient in hopelessness or panic.

• *Find meaning in the work.* The capacity to conceive of the work as profoundly significant and as having an impact enables therapists to sustain their commitment. Rather than gauging success on some grandiose fantasy of cure, or on being the "best parent," we are better fulfilled by working within our capacity to offer an authentic relationship. The ongoing therapeutic relationship with our patients is our tool for helping them gain more quality in their lives. We must affirm the positive aspects of the work: it enriches and vitalizes our lives. We get personal meaning from working with a critical epidemic and with fundamental human issues. We are energized, and grow in self-esteem and skill through mastery of this front-line work.

Rather than expecting to cure their patients, successful therapists witness and care for their patients. Therapists often describe the process of growth as mutual. Therapists grow in their capacity to sit with loss and to deal with a range of their own feelings: sadness, fear, anger. As one clinician put it: "Having been in the middle of it now for eleven years, a lot of what I feel and learn I am indebted to my patients for. That's the other part that keeps me going. Patients have taught me things to pass on to other patients."

This capacity doesn't happen overnight. It develops over time. There is no short-term workshop solution.

Political and Community Involvement

Commitment to political work for social change can help us feel more empowered in the face of the unrelenting loss of front-line HIV clinical work. Finding a way to have some concrete impact on larger systems can help us achieve a balance with the intensity of the clinical work.

Personal Growth

Our work with such issues as death, loss, drugs, and homophobia triggers the use of a range of intrapsychic defenses that are means of negotiating distance. If these defenses are underdeveloped or overly rigid, we may have difficulty establishing a workable alliance. Instead, we may blur our own boundaries with our client.

Our own therapy may help us identify conflicts and resolve them. We need not be any more alone than we would want our clients to be.

Spiritual Life

Traditional spiritual practices may be resources for therapists to find more grounding. However, loss and death in the HIV pandemic can challenge early, more simple religious beliefs. One therapist described his experience: "To really understand the loss to the community was to challenge any notion of this being a benevolent universe. I then had to consider a spiritual view that incorporated not malevolence but pain. What I need to feel is that however I understand the world, which may change from day to day, I can buy into it."

This therapist expresses the need for an overarching belief system, even if a shifting one, in order to face the uncertainty, pain, and death of the pandemic.

To invoke your strength and skill, I'd like to end with an image, one that comes through powerfully in the writing of Bill Hayes, an HIV-negative gay man. His lover had recently learned that he was no longer only HIV-positive: he had AIDS. They were at the circus watching the acrobats. He looked over at his lover: "He is perched uncomfortably on the hard wooden bench: his future clipped, the years spinning by, his exquisite body falling. And his life strikes me not simply as tragic, but—like the acrobat's leap—sublime, breathtaking: speeded up, a series of complex twists and turns, of beauty and pain, courage and fear, skill and daring, over in a moment. I realize I cannot save him. Nor can I only watch. But I can throw my body into midair with his, gracefully flying."

Our work is like the dexterous art of acrobats. We can throw ourselves in with our clients with HIV. We will not always be graceful. Their dread, our dread—their negative transference and our negative countertransference are not pretty. In our capacity to recover balance is the grace. Then we are graceful. Then we each overcome our dread of the other; we overcome negligence, abuse, fear, and hate. We find our integrity. We join while we can in a caring partnership. In the time we have to survive this epidemic, we all can grow, and deepen our lives together.

NOTES

P. 2, *"to be other than who you are"*: Stark, M. (1994). *Working with resistance.* Northvale, NJ: Aronson.

P. 3, *"presentation, person, and material"*: Saakvitne, K. W. (1995). Trauma and the therapist: How trauma therapy affects and is affected by the therapist. *Developments: The Newsletter of the Center for Women's Development at HRI,* 4(1), 1–4.

P. 3, *This phenomenon is referred to as* countertransference resistance: Alonso, A., & Rutan, S. (in press). Activity/non-activity and the group therapist. *Group.*

P. 5, *Ernest Becker, in his Pulitzer prize–winning book:* Becker, E. (1973). *The denial of death.* New York: Free Press.

P. 7, *the majority used the disease to further marginalize minorities:* Cadwell, S. (1994). Twice removed: The stigma suffered by gay men with AIDS. In S. Cadwell, B. Burnham, & M. Forstein (Eds.), *Therapists on the front line: Psychotherapy with gay men in the age of AIDS.* Washington, DC: American Psychiatric Press.

P. 8, *in the case of syphilis:* Brandt, A. (1988). The syphilis epidemic and its relation to AIDS. *Science, 239,* 375–380.

P. 12, *Other authors have delineated the different, difficult countertransference reactions to psychosis:* Kernberg, O. (1963). Notes on countertransference. *Journal of the American Psychoanalytic Association, 13,* 38–56.

P. 12, *countertransference reactions . . . to suicidality:* Buie, D., & Maltsberger, J. (1974). Countertransference hate in the treatment of suicidal patients. *Archives of General Psychiatry, 30,* 625–633.

P. 12, *countertransference reactions . . . to terminal illness:* Adler, G. (1984). Special problems for the therapist. *International Journal of Psychiatry in Medicine, 16*(2), 91–98.

P. 12, *countertransference reactions . . . to cancer patients:* Weisman, A. (1981). Understanding the cancer patient: The syndrome of caregiver's plight. *Psychiatry, 44,* 161–168.

P. 12, *countertransference reactions . . . to dying patients:* Sanders, C. (1984). Therapists, too, need to grieve. *Death Education, 8,* 27–35.

P. 13, *the countertransference responses of clinicians:* Dunkel, J., & Hatfield, S. (1986). Countertransference issues in working with persons with AIDS. *Social Work, 31*(2), 114–117; Cadwell, S. (1994). Over-identification with HIV clients. *Journal of Gay and Lesbian Psychotherapy, 2*(2), 77–99.

P. 16, *Research suggests that the "real" features of the therapist:* Guy, J., Norcross, J., & Brady, J. (1994, August). *Psychotherapist, heal thyself: Reflections on how psychologists deal with their own distress.* Paper delivered at the annual meeting of the American Psychological Association, Los Angeles.

P. 16, *Contemporary psychoanalytic theories:* Stark, M. (1995, November). *The therapeutic interaction as authentic engagement.* Paper presented at the Boston Institute for Psychotherapy, Boston, MA.

P. 16, *relational theorists:* Mitchell, S. (1988). *Relational concepts in psychoanalysis: An integration.* Cambridge, MA: Harvard University Press; Miller, J. (1990). The corrective emotional experience: Reflections in retrospect. *Psychoanalytic Inquiry, 10,* 372–388.

P. 16, *intersubjectivists:* Stolorow, R., Brandchaft B., & Atwood, G. (1987). *Psychoanalytic treatment: An intersubjective approach* (pp. 1–14). Hillsdale, NJ: Analytic Press.

P. 16, *interpersonalists:* Levenson, E. A. (1991). *The purloined self: Interpersonal perspectives in psychoanalysis.* New York: William Alanson White Institute.

P. 16, *interactive theorists:* Bollas, C. (1987). *The shadow of the object: Psychoanalysis of the unthought known.* New York: Columbia University Press.

P. 18, Vicarious traumatization: McCann, L., & Pearlman, L. (1990). Vicarious traumatization: A contextual model for understanding the effects of trauma on helpers. *Journal of Traumatic Stress, 3*(1), 131–149.

P. 18, *"all aspects of the therapist's self":* Saakvitne, K. (1995). Trauma and the therapist: How trauma therapy affects and is affected by the therapist. *Developments: The Newsletter of the Center for Women's Development at HRI, 4*(1), 1–4; McCann, L., & Pearlman, L. (1990). *Psychological trauma and the adult survivor: Theory, therapy, and transformation.* New York: Brunner/Mazel.

P. 18, *Burnout is a popular term for this state, which is characterized by physical, emotional, and mental exhaustion:* Cherniss, C. (1980). *Professional burnout in human service organizations.* New York: Praeger.

P. 18, *Studies have identified the factors:* Chiriboga, D. A., Jenkins, G., & Bailey, J. (1983). Stress and coping among hospice nurses: Test of an analytic model. *Nursing Research, 32,* 294–298.

P. 25, *coping strategies for managing vulnerability to identification:* Cadwell, S. (1994). Empathic challenges for gay male therapists working with HIV-infected gay men. In S. Cadwell, B. Burnham, & M. Forstein (Eds.), *Therapists on the front line: Psychotherapy with gay men in the age of AIDS.* Washington, DC: American Psychiatric Press.

P. 29, *"He is perched uncomfortably":* Hayes, B. (1995, July 10). About men. *New York Times Sunday Magazine,* p. 16.

2

DISEASE, DISEASE COURSE, AND PSYCHIATRIC MANIFESTATIONS OF HIV

David G. Ostrow

This chapter will focus on the medical and psychological challenges of persons living with HIV infection (PWHIVs). It is based on my experiences as a clinician seeing approximately five hundred PWHIVs since the start of the epidemic and as someone who has been living with HIV infection himself for over fourteen years. Clinicians and researchers are increasingly paying attention to the 10 to 20 percent of PWHIVs whose infection does not appear to progress toward AIDS after ten or more years of infection, otherwise referred to as *non-progressors*, and persons with AIDS (PWAs) who have survived five or more years since their AIDS diagnosis, otherwise referred to as *long-term survivors*. In terms of the neuropsychiatric natural history of HIV infection, it has similarly been observed that the majority of PWHIVs do not experience major dysfunctional episodes, prompting more attention to factors that may confer psychological resilience among the majority of PWHIVs.

Thus, I will discuss in this chapter both vulnerabilities and resources that each individual brings to the experience of living with this virus. Mental health professionals can play important roles in recognizing these individual coping factors and working with each client to minimize the negative impact while maximizing the positive impact that HIV infection can have on the client's life.

THE STAGES OF LIVING WITH HIV INFECTION

When looking at the natural history of HIV infection, it is important to keep in mind that the overwhelming characteristic of this virus is its *variability* in terms of both its structure and its effects on the individual with the virus. This extreme variability means that it is difficult to talk about a uniform disease course with predictable landmarks or signposts. Nevertheless, we can use the general pattern of infection shown in Table 2.1 as a useful guide to the most common patterns of HIV natural history and psychological adaptation to living with HIV, as long as we keep in mind that the picture may vary widely for any individual patient.

It is this variability in HIV's structure and natural history that frustrates scientists trying to develop treatments and vaccines, clinicians trying to predict outcomes to treatments, and PWHIVs trying to gain control over their lives. This frustration then fuels repetitive cycles of hope, denial, and hopelessness, as yesterday's victories turn into today's disappointments, whether it be on the research, clinical, or personal battlegrounds against this ever-changing virus. Thus there is an inherent affective instability that comes with HIV infection and with attempts to gain control over its seemingly inevitable encroachment on our societies, our communities, and our lives.

Despite the individual variability in HIV infection, it is helpful to think of the disease's natural history as encompassing four major stages that roughly parallel the various disease classification systems: initial infection and its accompanying acute HIV infection syndrome; the asymptomatic or "latent" phase of infection; the early symptomatic phase; and AIDS and its defining secondary or "opportunistic" diseases. A complete description of the natural history of HIV infection is beyond the scope of this chapter, but readers are referred to several recent publications that describe the spectrum of HIV infection in more detail.

Acute Syndrome

The acute HIV infection syndrome, marked by the appearance of antibodies to HIV in the blood or seroconversion, encompasses general, neuropathic, and dermatologic symptoms. This stage is being increasingly recognized and is estimated to occur in 50 to 70 percent of individuals between three to six weeks following exposure to the virus. The symptoms of the acute syndrome range in severity from mild to incapacitating and have been likened to acute mononucleosis. In most cases the immune system appears to mount an effective response to this acute infection, with return of CD4 and CD8 cell numbers toward normal and resolution of the clinical symptoms of the acute viral syndrome within one to four weeks. For many persons, this phase of HIV infection will be "silent" or discounted as a flu or cold. However, the acute phase is extremely important in the transmission dynamics of HIV infection, as recent studies have demonstrated that extremely high levels of infectious virus are present in the blood and other bodily fluids during this phase of infection, meaning that the majority of secondary transmissions can easily take place while the individual is unaware of his or her own infection and is continuing to engage in those "risky" sexual and other behaviors that resulted in infection. It has also been suggested that higher circulating levels of virus during the seroconversion stage indicate poorer immune response to the initial infection and may predict more rapid disease progression. (PWHIVs in this group are referred to as *rapid progressors*.)

Asymptomatic or "Latent" Stage

In the vast majority of persons exposed to HIV, the acute stage of primary infection is followed by a prolonged period of clinical latency, usually referred to as the *asymptomatic phase*.

Table 2.1
Common Individual and Family Psychosocial Issues Related to Stage of HIV Infection

Stage in Spectrum of HIV Infection	Time	Developing Psychosocial Issues		
		Infected Individual		*Family*
Exposure.	0 years	*High-risk behaviors*		Possible high-risk behaviors, denial, secrecy, concern, fear
		Denial, fear		
I Testing HIV-Positive		*Crisis reaction*		*Crisis reaction*
		Shock, denial, depression, suicidal thoughts, guilt, withdrawal, anger, relief		Shock, denial, depression, uncertainty
		Disclosure		*Disclosure*
		Fear		Fear
II Symptom-Free Period		*Reestablish equilibrium*		*Reestablish equilibrium*
		Search for meaning, restore self-esteem, try to gain control, uncertainty		Search for meaning, uncertainty
		Changes in lifestyle		*Possible changes in lifestyles*

Developing Psychosocial Issues

Stage in Spectrum of HIV Infection	Time	Infected Individual	Family
III Signs and Symptoms		*Loss of control and independence* Guilt, anger, depression, suicidal thoughts, support reciprocity, disfigurement, treatment decisions, bargaining	*Caregiving* Support reciprocity, treatment decisions, bargaining
IV AIDS	↓	Grief, possible relief at diagnosis, depression	Anticipatory grief, depression
Terminal Stage		*Preparation for death* Depression, acceptance, treatment decisions, assisted suicide	*Preparation for death* Caregiver burnout, final treatment decisions, depression, acceptance, requests for suicide assistance
Death	2–10 years		*Bereavement Recovery*

Source: Adapted from Adelman, M. (1989). Social support and AIDS. *AIDS and Public Policy Journal,* 4(1), pp. 31–39; Kübler-Ross, E. (1987). *AIDS: The Ultimate Challenge.* New York: Macmillan; and Wadland, W. C., & Gleeson, C.J. (1991). A model for psychosocial issues in HIV disease. *The Journal of Family Practice, 33*(1), pp. 82–86.

Although the period of asymptomatic infection varies widely from individual to individual, multiple studies have shown that the average period from HIV infection to diagnosis of AIDS is nine to ten years and that a small proportion of infected individuals are still asymptomatic after ten to fifteen years of infection.

Despite the use of the term *latent* to describe the clinical silence of HIV infection during this phase, the virus itself is actively replicating and slowly destroying the immune system. This is usually monitored by measuring the level of circulating CD4 T-cells, although various measures of actual viral replication are now coming into clinical use. Two particular landmarks during this phase are defined by the decline of CD4 levels to less than 500, when antiretroviral therapy is often initiated, and when they decline to less than 200, when individuals qualify for an AIDS diagnosis and are usually placed on prophylactic treatments against the opportunistic infections that are common at this stage.

Early Symptomatic Stage

Once the immune system has been significantly damaged, PWHIVs often begin to experience symptoms of infection with common opportunistic organisms. The most common characteristics of early symptomatic disease include generalized lymph node enlargement, oral thrush or hairy leukoplakia, shingles (herpes zoster infection), decreased platelet counts, and warts or molluscum contagiosum. Any of these conditions or HIV infection itself can be accompanied by periods of malaise, lethargy, weakness, tendency to bleed, or anorexia.

Although these are usually not serious or debilitating illnesses, they can be painful reminders that HIV is present in the body and continuing to destroy the immune system. Previously these illnesses were classified as "Pre-AIDS" or "AIDS-Related Complex (ARC)." Combination antiretroviral therapy is increasingly being recommended for persons at this stage of infection, as studies have shown its usefulness in slowing viral replication and delaying the further destruction of the immune system that leads to full-blown AIDS.

AIDS

The fourth stage of HIV infection, diagnosed when serious opportunistic diseases or a CD4 cell count of less than 200 occurs, is commonly referred to as AIDS. Treatment at this stage includes both continuation or enhancement of antiretroviral therapy as well as the prophylaxis, diagnosis, and treatment of specific opportunistic diseases as they occur. In addition, the prophylactic treatment to prevent the onset of such common opportunistic infections as *Pneumocystis carinii* pneumonia and *M. avium intracellulare* can have a significant impact on the longevity and quality of life of persons with AIDS (PWAs).

A particularly common AIDS-defining illness among gay men is Kaposi's Sarcoma, which typically manifests itself as purple skin lesions and is thus emblematic of the stigma experienced by gay men with AIDS. Also included in the list of AIDS-defining conditions are the various neurologic diseases, including central nervous system (CNS) involvement leading to dementia. Depending on the type and treatability of secondary diseases that a person with AIDS develops, this stage can last from several months to several years.

MENTAL HEALTH ACROSS THE HIV SPECTRUM

The mental health natural history of HIV infection may also be divided into sequential stages (see Table 2.1), which roughly correspond to the medical phases of retroviral infection previously described. In the first stage, the at-risk person is engaging in sexual or drug use behaviors that place him or her at significant risk for acquiring primary HIV infection. The second stage encompasses the period of time between primary infection (exposure) and the emergence of antibodies to HIV (seroconversion). This period may range from a few weeks to months, usually within six months of exposure. The third stage is known as the *asymptomatic stage*, or that period between when a person first seroconverts and when he or she develops serious symptoms. This period is highly variable, lasting from months to many years, but averaging nine to ten years for adult gay white men.

Although an individual may not experience severe life-threatening disease during this third stage, he or she may experience intermittent symptoms such as night sweats, rashes, or diarrhea. Some may experience more serious physiological symptoms, such as fatigue and weight loss, which can be incapacitating at times.

The fourth stage begins with symptoms of severe immunosuppression or the diagnosis of significant neurological impairment, a life-threatening opportunistic infection, a secondary neoplasm, debilitating wasting syndrome, or a CD4 count below 200. At this point a person is diagnosed as having AIDS according to specific criteria developed by the Centers for Disease Control and Prevention (CDC). During each of these stages, an individual may experience a variety of mental health problems; Table 2.1 indicates which specific problems are more likely to occur at a particular stage of HIV infection, as well as the corresponding family system issues.

Quality of Life

A biopsychosocial model of HIV disease means that mental health, well-being, and cognitive functioning become the ultimate determinants of the quality of life (QOL). Furthermore, many of the proponents of holistic health argue that mental health influences physical health, measured in terms of length of survival, rate of immunological deterioration, and neurological functioning. Thus, if mental disorders are properly detected and treated among HIV-infected individuals, not only would QOL improve but also, quite possibly, immune functioning and length of survival.

This is still an area of considerable debate and controversy; however, several recent studies of gay and bisexual cohorts have suggested that—at least among men in the earlier stages of HIV infection—depression, bereavement, or social isolation can all be associated with faster rates of immunological decline. These results were contradicted, however, by studies of stress or depression effects on immune competency in the same or similar longitudinal cohorts. Thus, although strong arguments can be made for reducing stress or diagnosing and treating depression in order to improve the QOL of persons with HIV infection, the argument that such interventions will alter disease progression remains unproven.

Stress and Coping

As has been found in most chronic illnesses, relationships exist between levels of stress and levels of mental health functioning among PWHIVs, but the resulting levels of distress and psychopathology vary widely among persons suffering equivalent levels of stress. Both coping styles and social support can mediate the relationship between stress and distress, effecting outcomes positively and negatively. In addition, several studies have indicated that familial and prior history of mental illness are additional strong predictors of mental dysfunction among gay and bisexual men, IV drug users, and hemophiliacs with HIV or AIDS. Pre-morbid substance abuse or dependence can also seriously compromise mental health and behavioral functioning at any stage of the HIV spectrum.

Sources of distress for PWHIVs include the knowledge that they carry a lethal infectious virus; have a highly stigmatized disease that the larger society associates with an equally stigmatized lifestyle; may be socially ostracized with significant risk of loss of job, income, housing, family, and other support; and may eventually suffer from a disfiguring, painful, and terminal illness (see Table 2.1). Bisexual and closeted men as well as IV drug users may be at even greater risk of suffering depression and isolation than self-identified gay men, perhaps because self-identified gay men are more connected to supportive networks in their community, whereas bisexual men and IV drug users fear rejection from their social networks and may not readily identify with a supportive community.

In contrast, several studies have demonstrated that specific coping mechanisms—such as active appraisal and adaptation—and supportive social interactions can contribute to well-being and improved QOL for PWHIVs. Conversely, maladaptive coping strategies—such as denial or passive fatalism, use of alcohol or recreational drugs, participation in casual sex, and conflict with one's social network as distraction coping responses—contribute negatively to well-being and have a significant impact on QOL.

Gay and bisexual men as well as IV drug users experience social conflict not only as a result of others' responses to their being infected but also because of societal reactions to their homosexuality or drug abuse. This social conflict may be compounded by fear of eviction from their housing, termination from their place of employment, and loss of their health insurance, all in reaction to their diagnosis. Social conflict has been found to increase the symptoms of depression among men at risk for AIDS. Not surprisingly, social support groups have proven to be effective in ameliorating distress and isolation experienced by PWHIVs. The earliest community support programs, such as Shanti and Gay Mens' Health Crisis, were based on such a social support and coping model.

Intervention Issues for the At-Risk Person

Psychological reactions to the threat of HIV or AIDS are quite varied, but according to my experience can generally be divided into three types. The first are those that are actually exacerbations or recurrences of pre-existing psychopathology, under the stress of HIV or AIDS, but that actually have little to due with the infectious process other than its acting as a source of distress contributing to the recurrence. Second are the types of problems that we will focus on in the rest of this chapter, namely disorders related directly to the stresses involved in having a diagnosis of HIV or AIDS. And third are the neuropsychiatric illnesses that result directly from HIV infection of the CNS, which will be reviewed at the conclusion of this chapter.

Prior to seroconversion, at-risk persons may begin to manifest psychological symptoms from the stress of potentially becoming HIV infected. Such persons have been described as the "worried well." Their psychological distress may take the form of generalized or AIDS-specific anxieties, panic attacks, hypochondriasis, or obsessive-compulsive disorders. In addition, persons at risk for HIV illness (especially gay and bisexual men who are well integrated into the community) may be experiencing the illness or death of friends and lovers, which in turn may cause depression both directly and through the loss of their significant social supports or the threat of their own premature mortality. While observing these reactions, it is important that we account for pre-existing psychiatric disorders (including substance abuse or dependency) that may become exacerbated by the threat of HIV illness but that are not directly caused by HIV.

HIV Antibody Testing

Counseling related to HIV antibody testing is often the first contact HIV-infected persons will have with mental health caregivers. According to the CDC, successful HIV prevention counseling involves four essential components: (1) personalized risk assessment to facilitate a realistic self-perception of risk; (2) identification and discussion of barriers to behavior change, and reinforcement of behavior change already initiated by the client; (3) negotiation between the counselor and the client of a realistic and incremental risk-reduction plan; and (4) establishment of a specific plan to receive test results and post-test counseling.

In addition, prevention requires maintaining the strictest confidentiality in order to develop trust and protect clients from possible discrimination. Of paramount importance is to evaluate all patients for possible adverse behavioral or mental health consequences of testing and to provide psychological therapies aimed at ameliorating those responses. This will often mean referring a patient to one or more community-based AIDS service organizations (ASOs), which provide HIV psychosocial and case management services.

The following ongoing case example illustrates the various mental health concerns that can arise at each stage of treatment of a bisexual male with HIV infection.

STEVE

Steve is a twenty-eight-year-old white bisexual male who comes to see a psychiatrist with the complaint of increasing anxiety, insomnia, poor appetite (with ten-pound weight loss over the past month), and fatigue. The precipitant appears to be his recent break-up with a male lover of five years and the ex-lover's informing Steve that he had tested positive for HIV antibodies. Steve reports frequent nightmares and daytime anxiety attacks, all focusing on fears that he has AIDS and will soon die, alone and disfigured. At times, suicidal thoughts occupy his thinking, and he is unable to concentrate on his work or household chores. He has withdrawn from friends and his female lover, Sarah, for fear that they will notice his illness and react negatively. He was referred for psychiatric evaluation by his internist, who found mildly swollen axillary lymph glands on examination of this otherwise healthy-appearing but extremely anxious patient.

During Steve's first visit, the doctor listens to his concerns and provides reassurance and factual information regarding the natural history of HIV infection, the signs and symptoms of AIDS, and the practical aspects of HIV antibody testing. After discussing Steve's anxiety attacks, she decides to prescribe an anxiolytic (anti-anxiety) medication. She then takes a detailed sexual behavior history, noting Steve's significant potential exposure history and his continuing sexual activities with Sarah. After discussing the pros and cons of HIV antibody testing, she and Steve agree that a test is indicated; blood is drawn for the ELISA and confirmatory Western-blot analyses. The doctor schedules a follow-up appointment for one week later, at which time she will evaluate Steve's response to anxiolytic therapy and the result of his HIV antibody test. She provides him with some written materials about HIV testing and encourages him to call her if he experiences any anxiety attacks or problems with the medication. On leaving her office, Steve informs the doctor that he feels relieved about having finally been tested and about having discussed his fears.

A realistic personalized plan for behavior modification based on the client's own risk behavior history needs to be developed during the pre-test counseling session. It is important that both counselor and client agree on the feasibility of this plan and that they discuss possible barriers to the suggested changes and anticipate reactions to them. Although assessing behavioral risk and planning for behavioral change are of the utmost importance, it is also important that the therapist take into account the psychological needs and state of the person seeking the test.

For at-risk persons requesting testing, there are a number of highly emotionally charged issues: feelings that they may have put themselves or partners at risk for HIV and may actually soon learn that they are HIV-positive; thoughts about the possible consequences of a positive test and fears of having to disclose the result (and related indiscretions) to loved ones; and the associated fears of abandonment. For women, HIV testing often occurs as part of prenatal screening, raising issues of reproductive health, decision making, and the potential loss of the ability to care for their existing or future children.

In anticipation of these fears, the therapist should walk the client through different scenarios. For instance: "What may you feel like and what will you subsequently do if you find out that you are HIV positive? What if you are negative?" A counselor or therapist can and should be as helpful as possible in pointing out behavioral, emotional, societal, legal, and psychological consequences of both scenarios.

Finally, sufficient time should be spent discussing the test procedures, the meaning and limitations of the laboratory findings, and the recommended follow-up procedures for each individual. There are, in addition, many ethical and legal issues that complicate the patient-therapist relationship when HIV testing or treatment is involved. Many states have passed legislation or public health regulations that define the therapist's obligations and the conditions under which patient privacy may be breached for public health considerations. Therapists need to be familiar with their local laws and regulations related to patient confidentiality and HIV testing and discuss their implications with all new at-risk patients.

Seroconversion and Disclosure

Varied and conflicting reports have been made about the impact of testing and disclosure of serostatus for those who are at risk for HIV. Possible impacts include depression, suicidal ideation or suicide attempts, anxiety and somatic preoccupations, an increased sense of isolation, anger, substance abuse or other forms of distraction coping, symptoms of adjustment disorder, and mild transient patterns of psychological distress. Some researchers have reported a sharp rise in anxiety and depression for some individuals at the time of diagnosis of HIV infection, but also found that these states dissipated with time. Specific concerns about AIDS and the long-term impact of being HIV-positive will significantly increase, however, after learning that one is infected; dealing with these "AIDS worries" is often a major goal of therapy for HIV-positive persons. Substance abuse and other forms of maladaptive coping may increase or recur, and issues of informing spouses, sexual partners, and other significant persons are frequently central to therapy in the post-disclosure period.

Steve returns for his post-test counseling appointment, at which time he reports a significant decrease in his anxiety, with no incapacitating attacks or suicidal ideation during the past week. However, he reports significant increased anxiety this morning, focusing on his reaction to an expected positive test result. He appears somewhat relieved when told that his test was indeed positive but that he is in the earliest stage of infection.

Steve's anxiety returns when the issue of informing his girlfriend, Sarah, about his HIV seropositivity is raised. She has always been aware of his bisexuality, and Steve expects her to be supportive of him, but he feels extreme embarrassment and guilt over the thought that he might have infected her. The doctor reassures Steve and counsels him about the importance of HIV testing for Sarah and any other unprotected sexual contacts he might have had in the past year. The doctor and Steve agree on the need to continue the anxiolytic therapy and weekly psychotherapy with her, focusing on his anxiety and AIDS-specific worries. As Steve expresses a preference for seeing a gay physician specializing in HIV/AIDS care, he is referred to the infectious disease practitioner with whom the psychiatrist works most closely; she also provides him with a list of local ASOs.

Social Support and Interventions for Recently Seropositive Persons

In addition to the psychological impact of HIV infection, there are also obvious social effects, both positive and negative. Researchers have speculated on the occurrence of depression and suicidal ideation at the time of HIV antibody testing and again at the time of an AIDS diagnosis. Most clinicians believe that recently diagnosed HIV-positive persons need to be watched closely for suicidality. Philip Marzuk and colleagues reported the relative risk for suicide in men between the ages of twenty and fifty-nine to be thirty-six times greater in those with AIDS than in men without the diagnosis; however, Samuel Perry and colleagues found that the increased risk for suicide dissipated two months after diagnosis. Less reassuring, Perry found that suicidal ideation persisted after notification for 15 percent of both seropositive and seronegative gay men.

Regardless of the initial psychological reaction at the time of a seropositive test notification, it is important to assess suicide potential and begin appropriate intervention if indicated. The usual risk factors for serious suicide potential also apply to the recently diagnosed HIV-positive patient, including pre-existing affective illness, prior suicidality, substance abuse, social isolation and conflict, extreme hopelessness, and impulsivity. These issues may be difficult to assess during the immediate post-test counseling period, as the patient may be in a state of acute shock.

Therefore, after the clinician has paid immediate attention to the acute psychological reaction, he or she should arrange a follow-up session, at which time further assessment and initiation of appropriate treatment can take place. Individual psychotherapy and social support group interventions are often sufficient to reduce suicidal ideation. However, if serious suicidality persists, it may be necessary to consider more intense intervention, including possible inpatient treatment.

Issues for Seropositive Persons

During Stages II and III (Table 2.1), patients may experience a wide range of intermittent physiological symptoms, such as thrush, diarrhea, or night sweats. These symptoms vary in both magnitude and frequency among all HIV-positive individuals, but will generally not be serious or meet the criteria for AIDS until several to ten or more years after the initial infection. For those who experience minor symptoms, the symptoms serve as frequent reminders that they are indeed ill; for those who do not experience symptoms or are unaware that their symptoms are HIV-related, the lack of symptoms may add to the denial that they are infected.

Psychological reactions, such as depression, may take the form of sadness, hopelessness, or anticipatory grief. Some authors have reported difficulty differentiating between depression that is a reaction to HIV infection, demoralization, and hopelessness, and symptoms of HIV infection itself, which may be similar to depression, such as difficulty sleeping, poor concentration, and fatigue. In addition, multiple AIDS-related bereavements may be related to increased levels of hopelessness and depression, as well as increased rates of immune suppression and development of HIV-related symptoms.

Depression: Prevalence, Diagnosis, and Treatment

Steve returns quarterly after the resolution of his initial anxiety attacks at the time of his HIV diagnosis. He has done well for the past four years, both in terms of physical and mental health. He has continued working as a massage therapist, has stayed active in his support group, and has not needed any antiretroviral or prophylactic medications. His CD4 T-cell counts have fluctuated between 1,000 and 600, but more recently have been in the 500–650 range. When seen on the fifth anniversary of his initial positive antibody test, he complains of poor appetite, loss of interest in social activities, feeling depressed, being frequently tired and unable to get out of bed, and occasionally being tearful. He reports first noticing these symptoms after Tim, one of the long-term members of his support group and Steve's "buddy" when he first joined the group, died from an opportunistic infection. Aside from fatigue, Steve denies difficulties in his work as a massage therapist, but does complain of occasional forgetfulness, which is unusual for him.

The psychiatrist and Steve decide that even if his depressive symptoms are in reaction to Tim's death, a trial of an antidepressant that may restore his energy, concentration, and mood is warranted given the degree of discomfort he is suffering. He is started on a low dose of an activating antidepressant, and he reports an immediate improvement in sleep, appetite, and energy levels. Over the next several weeks, his dosage is gradually increased as his mood returns to normal. He is kept on a maintenance dose of the antidepressant for six months, meanwhile continuing psychotherapy focusing on the issues of loss and of coping with his own physical deterioration and that of close friends. Steve eventually volunteers to be a "buddy" for someone else in the group and volunteers one evening per week in the HIV clinic of the local medical center.

This case illustrates a common difficulty in the management of depressive symptoms in an otherwise asymptomatic person with a CD4 count below 500. Although it is highly unlikely that the symptoms are organic in origin, it may be extremely difficult to differentiate between symptoms that are reactive to HIV-related losses and those of "pseudo-depression" resulting directly from HIV infection of the brain. The situation is made even more difficult if typical vegetative signs and symptoms are not present, yet the person appears to be significantly impaired in work or social performance.

The field is still divided over whether or not to be aggressive in treatment of what may be reactive or subsyndromal depression in such patients. Although prospective cohort studies of largely asymptomatic gay men have indicated low current rates of major depression, clinicians frequently see varying levels of depression in HIV-infected patient populations. Many have also described the effects in PWHIVs of living with a chronic disease. Several of the symptoms of depression seen with HIV infection are similar to those seen with other chronic diseases, such as cancer, heart disease, or Alzheimer's disease. Although PWHIVs may share some of the same concerns—such as the prospect of debilitating disease, loss of financial resources, or early death—HIV-related conditions additionally elicit fear and stigma from the community at large. African Americans with HIV infection may be at even greater risk of depression and suicide than their white counterparts. Susan Cochran and Vicky Mays found that one-third to almost one-half of HIV-positive African-American gay or bisexual men reported elevated levels of depression symptoms, compared to 10 to 20 percent of white gay or bisexual men in most studies. Given the theorized contributions of social stigma and isolation to distress related to HIV infection, it is likely that racial or ethnic minority PWHIVs in general are at increased risk of depression. This problem will become even more evident as the distribution of new infections and disease continues to increasingly affect minority populations.

Depression occurring in PWHIVs can be treated with an increasingly wide spectrum of antidepressants, regardless of the underlying cause, as long as the medications are given in judicious doses and are matched carefully in terms of the patient's symptoms and the medication's activity and side-effect profile (see Table 2.2). Furthermore, there appear to be no untoward immunological effects of at least acute antidepressant treatment in HIV infection. In fact, one recent study of HIV-infected gay and bisexual men suggests that depressed individuals suffer more accelerated deterioration of their immune systems than do non-depressed individuals, although this finding remains controversial, and the converse—that treatment of depression may lead to slower progression of immunodeficiency in HIV—has not been demonstrated. The therapist's emphasis should be on maximizing the QOL, and aggressive treatment of depression in PWHIVs has been shown to markedly improve their QOL and preference for life-sustaining treatments.

Anxiety: Differential Diagnosis and Treatment

Most persons with adverse reactions to their initial HIV diagnosis will experience a decrease in anxiety symptoms upon acceptance into psychosocial treatment; some, as in the case study, respond well to a combination of acceptance, reassurance, and brief anxiolytic therapy.

However, a careful evaluation of anxiety symptoms is necessary before beginning treatment, in order to determine the

Table 2.2
Traditional and Nontraditional Antidepressants Used Across Spectrum of HIV Disease

Antidepressant	Product Name	Type	Rate of Response	Stage Recommended	Side Effect Profile
Imipramine		Tricyclic	Medium[a]	Early stages	Anticholinergic, sedative, weight gain, constipation
Desipramine		Tricyclic	Medium[a]	Early stages	Anticholinergic, activating, weight loss
Fluoxetine	(Prozac)	Serotonin, reuptake blocker	Medium[a]	All	Sexual dysfunction, insomnia, nausea
Sertraline	(Zoloft)	Serotonin reuptake blocker	Fast[b]	All	Sexual dysfunction, insomnia, nausea
Venlafaxine	(Effexor)	Combined norepinephrine and serotonin reuptake blocker	Medium[a]	Not known, presumably all	Activating, hypertension, nausea, weight loss
Bupropion	(Wellbutrin)	Dopamine and norepinephrine stimulation	Medium[a]	All, but particularly useful in anergic/fatigue patients	Lowers seizure threshold, activating

Antidepressant	Product Name	Type	Rate of Response	Stage Recommended	Side Effect Profile
Dextroamphetamine or Methylphenidate	(Ritalin)	Psychostimulant	Fast[b]	Late, especially if fatigue and/or concentration problems	Activating, "nervousness," insomnia, psychosis (rare)
Testosterone		Androgen hormone	Medium	Late, especially if accompanied by hypogonadism or weight loss	Hair loss, irritability

Note: [a]Medium = significant response within two to six weeks. [b]Fast = significant response within two weeks.

underlying causes and type of disorder. The differential diagnosis of anxiety in HIV-infected patients is similar to that for any person facing a life-threatening chronic illness—complicated by concerns about loss of social support due to the stigma of AIDS and HIV-transmitting lifestyles. In addition, it is also necessary to assess possible underlying medical disorders (such as hyperthyroidism), excess caffeine consumption, stimulant drug usage or withdrawal, and medications used in the treatment of HIV or AIDS that can also have anxiety-producing side effects. When evaluating any patient presenting with excess anxiety, the clinician should also consider possible depression or panic disorder, both of which may present with prominent anxiety symptoms. Given the relatively high degree of overlap between anxiety, depression, and somatic symptoms frequently observed in PWHIVs, diagnoses of "subsyndromal" anxiety or "mixed anxiety-depression" may be relatively common.

Supportive or cognitive psychotherapy is the first-line treatment for anxiety, and often includes referral to ASOs offering support group services. Counseling of a patient's partners, close friends, and family members can often be of benefit in relieving social conflict or fears of abandonment. The clinician should consider anxiolytic treatment if the anxiety is severe and disabling or is accompanied by panic attacks, or if there is a diagnosis of generalized anxiety disorder or posttraumatic stress disorder. There is an increasingly wide spectrum of anxiolytic medications available, and the less addictive non-benzodiazepine medications should be considered for all patients not previously treated chronically with a benzodiazepine compound, as well as for those who can be successfully tapered off of benzodiazepines.

Neuropsychology

Both anxiety and depression can be accompanied by mild cognitive deficits, such as poor concentration or short-term memory. For the person with HIV infection, these symptoms can themselves be stressful, as they may be experienced as indicators of early HIV brain involvement. If the cognitive symptoms are mild and in keeping with the degree of affective dysfunction, the patient should be counseled that the symptoms will probably disappear when the anxiety or depression is adequately treated. However, if the cognitive symptoms appear out of proportion to the degree of affective involvement or they do not respond to adequate antidepressant or anxiolytic treatment, then a neuropsychological evaluation is indicated, even in patients with a CD4 count of over 500.

In terms of HIV and mental functioning, it is not clear if significant CNS involvement precedes the development of full-blown AIDS. In part, this controversy reflects our lack of knowledge about the highly variable natural history of HIV infection of the central nervous system (CNS) and the source and course of specific pathological developments in HIV-related cognitive and motor disease. Further complicating the picture are the myriad factors that may affect the neuropsychological functioning of PWHIVs—prescribed and recreational drug side effects, the stresses of living with HIV and its manifest social consequences, nutritional deficiencies, CNS opportunistic infections and neoplasms, and altered affective states.

Again, careful assessment, which may include formal neuropsychological testing, and treatment of any underlying conditions that may be contributing to cognitive dysfunction are essential before a diagnosis of HIV-associated cognitive-motor syndrome is made. A list of the most common signs and symptoms of CNS infection at the various stages of development of HIV-related cognitive-motor dysfunction is given in Table 2.3. A list of neuropsychiatric side effects of drugs commonly used over the course of HIV disease appears as an appendix to this book. Psychostimulant treatment has been shown to be particularly useful in ameliorating mixed affective and cognitive symptoms in persons with later-stage HIV illness.

Table 2.3
Signs and Symptoms of HIV-Related CNS Infection

Early cognitive impairments
  Short-term memory deficits; "forgetfulness" rather than amnesia
  Decreased concentration and attention
  Confusion and disorientation
  Difficulty following other speakers, especially when multiple
    sensory inputs are present
  Overall intellectual ability generally well preserved until late
  Visuospatial perception deficits (rare)

Changes in personality and behavior
  Apathy, decreased interest
  Impaired judgment
  Erratic or hypomanic behavior
  Social withdrawal
  Rigidity of thinking
  Later: speech impairment, slowing, dysarthria, hypophonia

Psychotic symptoms
  Hallucinations
  Suspiciousness and delusions
  Agitation and inappropriate behavior
  Full mania, particularly in AIDS and possibly exacerbated
    by antivirals

Motor symptoms
  Ataxia
  Loss of coordination
  Weakness, especially in distal extremities
  Tremors

Table 2.3
Signs and Symptoms of HIV-Related CNS Infection (*continued*)

Generalized systemic symptoms
  Fatigue
  Sleep changes, including hypersomnia
  Anorexia, weight loss
  Enuresis
  Hypersensitivity to medications, alcohol, and substances of abuse

Cognitive symptoms associated with advanced dementia
  Global cognitive impairment
  Rudimentary social functioning
  Disorientation
  Psychomotor retardation, decreased spontaneity
  Agitation, "sundowning," that is, nighttime delusions,
    agitation, and so on
  Mutism, vacant stare
  Coma

Motor symptoms associated with advanced dementia
  Ataxia
  Spastic weakness
  Paraplegia, quadraparesis
  Hyperreflexia, myoclonus
  Seizures
  Bladder and bowel incontinence

SYMPTOMATIC INFECTION, AIDS, AND TERMINAL ILLNESS

After almost ten years of living and working with HIV infection, Steve learns that his CD4 cell count has gone below 200, qualifying him for the diagnosis of AIDS according to current Centers for Disease Control and Prevention (CDC) criteria. Through his work with the therapist and the support group, he has prepared himself for this eventuality. This has included writing a living will and formally designating his long-term female partner as the person responsible for medical and financial decisions were he to become incapacitated. When next seen, he is somewhat sad, having just retired from work and applied for SSI disability and Medicaid coverage. The doctor discusses the plans he has made for this, the fourth and final stage of his HIV illness. In response to questions about suicidal ideation, Steve states that he has decided to end his life if and when he becomes mentally incapacitated. The doctor suggests a group counseling session with Steve, his long-term partner, Sarah, his support "buddy," and other members of his immediate support network. That session is very emotional, but provides an opportunity for Steve to make his terminal care preferences known to his support network and for them to reaffirm their support for him.

Grief over receiving a diagnosis of AIDS may begin with an acute response of shock and denial, which may then be followed by guilt, anger, or sadness. This is frequently followed by a transitional state during which individuals may alternate between anger, guilt, self-pity, anxiety, and denial. These feelings can be particularly distressing and confusing, and can be accompanied by changes in self-esteem and identity and by considerations of suicide. New symptoms or events may precipitate new crises for the individual. This has caused some to describe the uncertainty of HIV illness as an "emotional roller coaster." Many will find reinforcement for their denial through recurring reports in the press and popular media about the "myth of HIV" being the cause of AIDS, while others will be forced to acknowledge the life-threatening nature of AIDS when hearing media accounts of disappointments in antiviral drug development.

Inevitably, issues of loss re-emerge at the time of an AIDS diagnosis and complicate the management of end-of-life issues. Psychological treatment must usually be refocused on helping clients adapt to changes in their levels of mental and physical functioning and deal with other issues: associated fears of debilitation and dependency on others, managing pain, maximizing quality of life, and terminal care preferences. It may be particularly difficult for psychotherapists who have worked with patients across multiple stages of HIV infection to discuss those patients' fears and wishes about terminal care, especially plans for assisted suicide. The involvement of spiritual and palliative care can be extremely important for both improving the QOL of the terminal patient and preventing depression and burnout among mental health caregivers.

Assisted Suicide

Among the most difficult issues confronting the caregiver of patients in the terminal phase is that of requests for assistance in termination of life. While the term *assisted suicide* is often used, we are talking about a range of assisted activities that include terminating life-support systems, stopping nutritional support, terminating anti-HIV treatment regimens, and the actual assistance in ending life. All of these activities and the role(s) that caregivers are increasingly asked to play in them raise important legal and ethical questions, which are discussed in Chapter Nine.

While there are no right or wrong answers to these questions, each caregiver must ask himself or herself whether or not the activity is a reasonable extension of patients' autonomy and ability to exercise control over even the terminal phase of their illness. If the answer is no, is there a treatable mental illness, such as depression, that needs to be addressed in therapy? If the answer is yes but you are unable to agree to your patient's request because of your own ethical principles, then it may be necessary to refer your patient to someone else who is able to assist her. Whatever the reason, persons with end-stage AIDS are increasingly turning to planned suicide, with or without the assistance of their caregivers, and we need to be aware of this inevitable issue.

I recommend that therapists discuss this issue early on and make sure that each patient's wishes for terminal care are put into a written document before she is so ill that the medical system is making those choices for the patient. In most states, this is easily done with a medical power of attorney and the designation of individuals as executors of that power of attorney who are in agreement with the patient's terminal care wishes.

Consideration in this chapter of the complex interrelations among the various goals in treating PWHIVs—physical health, immunocompetence, mental health, social and functional well-being, and overall quality of life—and the accompanying case study, have emphasized the importance of an integrated biopsychosocial treatment approach. Given the central role of QOL issues in the treatment of any person living with HIV, I have emphasized the coordinating role of the mental health care provider. An integrated holistic or biopsychosocial treatment approach works best when it is applied to the full range of problems experienced by HIV-infected persons and includes all the diverse elements of health care required.

For this reason, many communities have established central HIV/AIDS care coordinating organizations, which, in turn, either provide or contract for comprehensive HIV case management services. The complex and multidisciplinary nature of coordinated biopsychosocial HIV care—frequently involving not only medical and mental health services but also a host of education and support services for patients and their families—dictates the use of a case management model of care whenever possible.

The establishment of interdisciplinary care teams, AIDS task forces, and HIV case management systems does not automatically solve the major problems inherent in the delivery of such care for PWHIVs. For example, programs that provide comprehensive long-term care need to minimize actions that will isolate patients from mainstream society, while maximizing the availability of specialized services. The intense stigma and discrimination to which HIV-infected patients are still subject require both extraordinary attention to the confidentiality of medical records and adequate communication among the diverse care team members.

The prevalence of dual or triple diagnosis patients—usually a combination of a functional mental health disorder, a substance use disorder, and organic illness—means that already limited treatment facilities for such patients are oftentimes unavailable, and specific efforts have to be made to create appropriate treatment options. (For further discussion of the issues of treating dual diagnosis patients, the reader is referred to Chapter Eight of this book.)

The occurrence of cognitive deficits in late-stage HIV illness means that patients may have difficulty with the complicated diagnostic and treatment regimens made necessary by the nature of their illness. The close involvement of ASOs able to provide in-home assistance, support "buddies," and transportation can frequently make outpatient treatment possible across the full spectrum of HIV infection.

The daily stresses of working in the HIV/AIDS health care arena, combined with the experience of seeing relatively young patients deteriorate and die despite one's best efforts, is a formula for burnout. Any viable HIV/AIDS treatment program must, therefore, provide adequate education, emotional support, and counseling not only for patients but also for those who care for them. With such support, mental health caregivers can contribute enormously to the compassionate care of all persons living with HIV infection, improving the quality of life of their patients while setting a leadership example for the practice of holistic health care.

NOTES

P. 33, *Clinicians and researchers are increasingly paying attention:* Remien, R. H., Rabkin, J. G., Williams, J. B. W., & Katoff, L. (1992). Coping strategies and health beliefs of AIDS long-term survivors. *Psychology and Health, 6,* 331–345.

P. 33, *In terms of the neuropsychiatric natural history of HIV infection:* Ostrow, D. G., Joseph, J., Monjan, A., Kessler, R., Emmons, C., Phair, J., Fox, R., Kingsley, L., Dudley, J., Chmiel, J., & VanRaden, M. (1986). Psychosocial aspects of AIDS risk. *Psychopharmacology Bulletin, 22,* 678–683.

P. 34, *When looking at the natural history of HIV infection:* Clement, M., & Hollander, H. (1992). Natural history and management of the seropositive patient. In M. A. Sande & P. A. Volberding (Eds.), *The medical management of AIDS* (3rd ed., pp. 87–96). Philadelphia: Saunders.

P. 34, *Thus there is an inherent affective instability:* Nichols, S. E. (1985). Psychosocial reactions of persons with the acquired immunodeficiency syndrome. *Annals of Internal Medicine, 103,* 765–767.

P. 34, *A complete description of the natural history of HIV infection:* Fauci, A. S., & Lane, H. C. (1994). Human immunodeficiency virus (HIV) disease: AIDS and related disorders. In K. J. Isselbacher, E. Braunwald, J. D. Wilson, J. B. Martin, A. S. Fauci, & D. L. Kasper (Eds.), *Harrison's principles of internal medicine* (13th ed., pp. 1567–1618). New York: McGraw-Hill.

P. 35, *readers are referred to several recent publications:* Clement, M., & Hollander, H. (1992). Natural history and management of the seropositive patient. In M. A. Sande & P. A. Volberding (Eds.), *The medical management of AIDS* (3rd ed., pp. 87–96). Philadelphia: Saunders; Atkinson, J. H., & Grant, I. (1994). Natural history of neuropsychiatric manifestations of HIV disease. In L. S. Zegans & T. J. Coates (Eds.), *Psychiatric manifestations of HIV disease. The Psychiatric Clinics of North America, 17*(1), 17–34.

P. 35, *The symptoms of the acute syndrome:* Fauci, A. S., & Lane, H. C. (1994). Human immunodeficiency virus (HIV) disease: AIDS and related disorders. In K. J. Isselbacher, E. Braunwald, J. D. Wilson, J. B. Martin, A. S.

Fauci, & D. L. Kasper (Eds.), *Harrison's principles of internal medicine* (13th ed., pp. 1567–1618). New York: McGraw-Hill.

P. 35, *In most cases the immune system appears to mount:* Pantaleo, G. (1993). The immunopathogenesis of human immunodeficiency virus infection. *New England Journal of Medicine, 328,* 327.

P. 35, *However, the acute phase is extremely important in the transmission dynamics:* Clark, S. J., Saag, M. S., Decker, W. D., Campbell-Hill, S., Roberson, J. L., Veldkamp, M. S., Kappes, J. C., Hahn, B. H., & Shaw, G. M. (1991). High titers of cytopathogenic virus in plasma of patients with symptomatic primary HIV-1 infection. *New England Journal of Medicine, 324,* 954–960; Daar, E. S., Moudgil, T., Meyer, R. D., & Ho, D. D. (1991). Transient high levels of viremia in patients with primary human immunodeficiency virus type 1 infection. *New England Journal of Medicine, 324,* 961–964.

P. 35, *the majority of secondary transmissions can easily take place:* Jacquez, J. A., Koopman, J. S., Simon, C. P., & Longini, I. M., Jr. (1994). Role of the primary infection in epidemics of HIV infection in gay cohorts. *Journal of Acquired Immune Deficiency Syndromes, 7,* 1169–1184.

P. 35, *It has also been suggested that higher circulating levels of virus:* Fauci, A. S., & Lane, H. C. (1994). Human immunodeficiency virus (HIV) disease: AIDS and related disorders. In K. J. Isselbacher, E. Braunwald, J. D. Wilson, J. B. Martin, A. S. Fauci, & D. L. Kasper (Eds.), *Harrison's principles of internal medicine* (13th ed., pp. 1567–1618). New York: McGraw-Hill.

P. 38, *Although the period of asymptomatic infection varies widely:* Bacchetti, P., & Moss, A. R. (1989). Incubation period of AIDS in San Francisco. *Nature, 338,* 251–253.

P. 38, *Two particular landmarks during this phase:* Centers for Disease Control and Prevention. (1992). 1993 revised classification system for HIV infection and expanded surveillance case definition for AIDS among adolescents and adults. *Morbidity and Mortality Weekly Report, 41,* 1–19.

P. 38, *The most common characteristics of early symptomatic disease:* Fauci, A. S., & Lane, H. C. (1994). Human immunodeficiency virus (HIV) disease: AIDS and related disorders. In K. J. Isselbacher, E. Braunwald, J. D. Wilson, J. B. Martin, A. S. Fauci, & D. L. Kasper (Eds.), *Harrison's principles of internal medicine* (13th ed., pp. 1567–1618). New York: McGraw-Hill.

P. 38, *Combination antiretroviral therapy is increasingly being recommended:* Schooley, R. (1992). Antiretroviral chemotherapy. In Wormser, G. P. (Ed.), *AIDS and other manifestations of HIV infection* (2nd ed., pp. 609–624). New York: Raven Press.

P. 39, *Treatment at this stage includes both continuation or enhancement:* Fauci, A. S., & Lane, H. C. (1994). Human immunodeficiency virus (HIV) disease: AIDS and related disorders. In K. J. Isselbacher, E. Braunwald, J. D. Wilson, J. B. Martin, A. S. Fauci, & D. L. Kasper (Eds.), *Harrison's principles of internal medicine* (13th ed., pp. 1567–1618). New York: McGraw-Hill.

P. 40, *During each of these stages, an individual may experience a variety of mental health problems:* Ostrow, D. G. (1990). *Psychiatric aspects of human immunodeficiency virus infection.* Kalamazoo, MI: Scope.

P. 40, *A biopsychosocial model of HIV disease:* Ostrow, D. G. (1992). Alternative and complementary therapies. In D. G. Ostrow & P. Wren, (Eds.), *Mental health aspects of HIV/AIDS: Curriculum modules* (module 9, pp. 287–362). Michigan: Comprehensive HIV and AIDS Mental Health Education Project (CHAMHEP), University of Michigan.

P. 40, *Furthermore, many of the proponents of holistic health argue:* Temoshok, L. (1991). Malignant melanoma, AIDS, and the complex search for psychosocial mechanisms. *Advances, 7,* 20–28.

P. 41, *This is still an area of considerable debate and controversy:* Burack, J. H., Barrett, R. D., Stall, M. A., Chesney, M., Ekstrand, M. L., & Coates, T. (1993). Depressive symptoms and CD4 lymphocyte decline among HIV-infected men. *Journal of the American Medical Association, 270,* 2568–2573; Caumartin, S., Joseph, J., & Chmiel, J. (1991, June). *Premorbid psychosocial factors associated with differentiated survival time in AIDS patients.* Paper presented at seventh international AIDS conference, Florence, Italy.

P. 41, *These results were contradicted:* Kessler, R., Foster, C., Joseph, J., Ostrow, D. G., Wortman, C., Phair, J., & Chmiel, J. (1991). Stressful life events and symptom onset in HIV infection. *American Journal of Psychiatry, 148,* 733–738; Williams, J. B. W., Rabkin, J. G., Remien, R. H., Gorman, J. M., Ehrhardt, A. A. (1991). Multidisciplinary baseline assessment of homosexual men with and without human immunodeficiency virus infection. *Archives of General Psychiatry, 48,* 124–130; Perry, S., Fishman, B., Jacobsberg, L., & Francis, A. (1992). Relationships over one year between lymphocyte subsets and psychosocial variables among adults with infection by human immunodeficiency virus. *Archives of General Psychiatry, 49,* 396–401; Lyketsos, C. G., Hoover, D. R., Guccione, M., Senterfitt, W., Morgenstern, H. (1993). Depressive symptoms as predictors of medical outcomes in HIV infection. *Journal of the American Medical Association, 270,* 2563–2567.

P. 41, *As has been found in most chronic illnesses:* Folkman, S., Chesney, M., Pollack, L., & Coates, T. (1993). Stress, control, coping and depressive mood in human immunodeficiency virus-positive and -negative gay men in San Francisco. *Journal of Nervous and Mental Disorders, 181,* 409–416; Lackner, J., Joseph, J., Ostrow, D. G., Kessler, R., Eshleman, S., Wortman, C.,

O'Brien, K., Phair, J., & Chmiel, J. (1993). A longitudinal study of psychological distress in a cohort of gay men: Effects of social support and coping strategies. *Journal of Nervous and Mental Disorders, 181*, 4–12.

P. 41, *Both coping styles and social support can mediate the relationship:* O'Brien, K., Wortman, C., Kessler, R., & Joseph, J. (1993). Social relationships of men at risk for AIDS. *Social Science and Medicine, 36*, 1161–1167.

P. 41, *In addition, several studies have indicated:* Atkinson, H., Grant, I., Kennedy, C. J., Richman, D. D., Spector, S. A., & McCutchan, J. A. (1988). Prevalence of psychiatric disorders among men infected with human immunodeficiency virus. *Archives of General Psychiatry, 45*, 859–864; O'Dowd, M. A., Biderman, D. J., & McKegney, F. P. (1993). Incidence of suicidality in AIDS and HIV-positive persons attending a psychiatry outpatient program. *Psychosomatics, 34*, 33–40; Perkins, D. O., Stern, R. A., Golden, R. N., Murphy, C., Naftolowitz, D., & Evans, D. L. (1994). Mood disorders in HIV infection: Prevalence and risk factors in a nonepicenter of the AIDS epidemic. *American Journal of Psychiatry, 151*, 233–236; Perry, S., Jacobsberg, L., Card, C. A., Ashman, T., Frances, A., & Fishman, B. (1993). Severity of psychiatric symptoms after HIV testing. *American Journal of Psychiatry, 150*, 775–779; Wickland, B. M., & Jackson, M. A. (1992). Coping with AIDS in hemophilia. In P. I. Ahmed (Ed.), *Living and dying with AIDS* (pp. 255–268). New York: Plenum.

P. 41, *Sources of distress for PWHIVs include:* Thompson, S. C., Nanni, C., & Levine, A. (1996). The stressors and stress of being HIV-positive. *AIDS Care, 8*(1), 5–14.

P. 41, *Bisexual and closeted men as well as IV drug users:* Dew, M. A., Ragni, M. V., & Nimorwica, P. (1990). Infection with human immunodeficiency virus and vulnerability to psychiatric distress. *Archives of General Psychiatry, 47*, 737–744.

P. 42, *In contrast, several studies have demonstrated:* Halman, L. J., Ostrow, D. G., Eshleman, S., Caumartin, S., & Joseph, J. (1994, July). *Structure of coping in a gay cohort at risk for AIDS.* Paper presented at AIDS' Impact: Second International Conference on Biopsychosocial Aspects of HIV Infection, Brighton, England; Hays, R. B., Turner, H., & Coates, T. (1992). Social support, AIDS-related symptoms and depression among gay men. *Journal of Consulting and Clinical Psychology, 60*, 463–469; Wolf, T. M., Galson, P. M., Morse, E. V., Simon, P. M., Gaumer, R. H., Dralie, P. W., & Williams, M. H. (1991). Relationship of coping style to affective state and perceived social support in asymptomatic and symptomatic HIV-infected persons: Implications for clinical management. *Journal of Clinical Psychiatry, 52*, 171–173.

P. 42, *Conversely, maladaptive coping strategies:* Miller, D. (1990). Diagnosis and treatment of acute psychological problems related to HIV infection and disease. In D. G. Ostrow (Ed.), *Behavioral aspects of AIDS*. New York: Plenum.

P. 42, *Not surprisingly, social support groups have proven to be effective:* Kelly, J. A., Murphy, D. A., Bahr, G. R., Kalichman, S. C., & Bernstein, B. (1993). Outcome of cognitive-behavioral and support group brief therapies for depressed, HIV-infected persons. *American Journal of Psychiatry, 150,* 1671–1686.

P. 43, *Such persons have been described as the "worried well":* Faulstich, M. E. (1987). Psychiatric aspects of AIDS. *American Journal of Psychiatry, 144,* 551–555. Jenike, M., & Pato, C. (1986). Disabling fear of AIDS responsive to imipramine. *Psychosomatics, 27,* 143–144; Morin, S. F., Charles, K. A., & Malyon, A. K. (1984). The psychological impact of AIDS on gay men. *American Psychologist, 39,* 1288–1293.

P. 43, *While observing these reactions, it is important that we account:* Perry, S., Jacobson, L., Fishman, B., Frances, A., Bobo, J., & Jacobsberg, B. K. (1990). Psychiatric diagnosis before serological testing for the human immunodeficiency virus. *American Journal of Psychiatry, 147,* 89–93.

P. 43, *According to the CDC:* Centers for Disease Control and Prevention. (1993). Technical guidance on HIV counseling. *Morbidity and Mortality Weekly Report, 42,* 11–17.

P. 45, *For women, HIV testing often occurs as part of prenatal screening:* See Chapter Six in this volume.

P. 46, *There are, in addition, many ethical and legal issues:* Wren, P. (1993). Legal and ethical issues. In D. G. Ostrow & P. Wren (Eds.), *Mental health aspects of HIV/AIDS: Curriculum modules* (module 8, pp. 227–286). Ann Arbor: University of Michigan; the reader is also referred to Chapter Nine of this volume.

P. 46, *Varied and conflicting reports have been made:* Ostrow, D. G. (1990). *Psychiatric aspects of human immunodeficiency virus infection*. Kalamazoo, MI: Scope.

P. 46, *Some researchers have reported a sharp rise in anxiety:* Ostrow, D. G., Leite, M. C., Lackner, J., & Eshleman, S. (1992, June). *Time course, mental health, and social support changes after learning HIV serostatus in the Chicago MACS/CCS cohort*. Paper presented at the Neuroscience of HIV Satellite Meeting, Amsterdam; Holland, J., & Tross, S. (1985). The psychosocial and neuropsychiatric sequelae of the acquired immunodeficiency syndrome and related disorders. *Annals of Internal Medicine, 103,* 760–764; Jacobsen, P. B., Perry. S. W., & Hirsch, D. A. (1990). Responses to HIV antibody testing: Behavioral and psychological responses to HIV antibody testing. *Journal of Consulting and Clinical Psychology, 58,* 31–37; Kelly, J. A., Murphy, D. A., Bahr, G. R., Koob, J., Morgan, M., Kalichman, S. C., Stevenson, L. Y., Brasfield, T. L., Bernstein, B., & St. Lawrence, J. (1993). Factors associated with severity of depression and high-risk behavior among persons diagnosed with immunodeficiency virus (HIV) infection. *Health Psychology, 12,* 215–219; Kelly, J. A., & St. Lawrence, J. (1988). *The AIDS health crisis: Psychological and social interventions.* New York: Plenum.

P. 46, *Substance abuse and other forms of maladaptive coping:* Montgomery, S. M., & Ostrow, D. G. (in press). Pre- and post-test counseling: Achieving behavior change and mental health. In J. Dilley & R. Marks (Eds.), *Face to face* (2nd ed). San Francisco: AIDS Health Project.

P. 47, *Researchers have speculated on the occurrence of depression and suicidal ideation:* Ostrow, D. G., Leite, M. C., Lackner, J., & Eshleman, S. (1992, June). *Time course, mental health, and social support changes after learning HIV serostatus in the Chicago MACS/CCS cohort.* Paper presented at the Neuroscience of HIV Satellite Meeting, Amsterdam; Perry, S., Jacobsberg, L., & Fishman, B. (1990). Suicidal ideation and HIV testing. *Journal of the American Medical Association, 263,* 679–682; Beckett, A., & Shenson, D. (1993). Suicide risk in patients with human immunodeficiency virus infection and acquired immunodeficiency syndrome. *Harvard Review of Psychiatry, 1,* 27–35.

P. 47, *Philip Marzuk and colleagues reported:* Marzuk, P. M., Tierney, H., Tardiff, K., Gross, E. M., Morgan, E. B., Hsu, M. A., & Mann, J. (1988). Increased risk of suicide in persons with AIDS. *Journal of the American Medical Association, 259,* 1333–1337.

P. 47, *Samuel Perry and colleagues found that the increased risk:* Perry, S., Jacobsberg, L., Card, C. A., Ashman, T., Frances, A., & Fishman, B. (1993). Severity of psychiatric symptoms after HIV testing. *American Journal of Psychiatry, 150,* 775–779; Perry, S., Jacobsberg, L., & Fishman, B. (1990). Suicidal ideation and HIV testing. *Journal of the American Medical Association, 263,* 679–682.

P. 48, *These issues may be difficult to assess:* Ostrow, D. G. (1990). Psychiatric aspects of human immunodeficiency virus infection. Kalamazoo, MI: Scope.

P. 48, *For those who experience minor symptoms:* Ostrow, D. G., Grant, I., & Atkinson, H. (1991). Assessment and management of AIDS patients with neuropsychiatric disturbances. *Journal of Clinical Psychiatry, 49,* 14–22.

P. 48, *Some authors have reported difficulty differentiating:* Kalichman, S. C., Sikkema, K. J., & Somlai, A. (1995). Assessing persons with human immunodeficiency virus (HIV) infection using the Beck Depression Inventory: Disease processes and other potential confounds. *Journal of Personality Assessment, 64*, 86–100.

P. 49, *In addition, multiple AIDS-related bereavements:* Kessler, R., Foster, C., Joseph, J., Ostrow, D. G., Wortman, C., Phair, J., & Chmiel, J. (1991). Stressful life events and symptom onset in HIV infection. *American Journal of Psychiatry, 148*, 733–738; Martin, J. L. (1988). Psychological consequences of AIDS-related bereavement among gay men. *Journal of Consulting and Clinical Psychology, 58*, 856–862; Neugebauer, R., Rabkin, J. G., Williams, J. B. W., Remien, R. H., Goetz, R., & Gorman, J. M. (1992). Bereavement reactions among homosexual men experiencing multiple losses in the AIDS epidemic. *American Journal of Psychiatry, 149*, 1374–1379; Rabkin, J. G., Williams, J. B. W., Neugebauer, R., Remien, R. H., & Goetz, R. (1990). Maintenance of hope in HIV-spectrum homosexual men. *American Journal of Psychiatry, 147*, 1322–1326; Martin, J. L., & Dean, L. (1993). Effects of AIDS-related bereavement and HIV-related illness on psychological distress among gay men: A seven-year longitudinal study. *Journal of Consulting and Clinical Psychology, 60*(1), 94–103.

P. 50, *The situation is made even more difficult if typical vegetative signs and symptoms:* Hintz, S., Kuck, J., Peterkin, J. J., Volk, D. M., & Zisook S. (1990). Depression in the context of human immunodeficiency virus infection: Implications for treatment. *Journal of Clinical Psychiatry, 51*, 497–501.

P. 50, *Although prospective cohort studies of largely asymptomatic gay men:* Williams, J. B. W., Rabkin, J. G., Remien, R. H., Gorman, J. M., Ehrhardt, A. A. (1991). Multidisciplinary baseline assessment of homosexual men with and without human immunodeficiency virus infection. *Archives of General Psychiatry, 48*, 124–130; Markowitz, J., Rabkin, J. G., & Perry, S. (1994). Treating depression in HIV-positive patients. *AIDS, 8*, 403–412; Bornstein, R. A., Pace, P., Rosenberger, P., Nasrallah, H., Para, M., Whitacre, C., & Fass, R. (1993). Depression and neuropsychological performance in asymptomatic HIV infection. *American Journal of Psychiatry, 150*, 922–927.

P. 50, *Although PWHIVs may share some of the same concerns:* Holland, J., & Tross, S. (1985). The psychosocial and neuropsychiatric sequelae of the acquired immunodeficiency syndrome and related disorders. *Annals of Internal Medicine, 103*, 760–764; Faulstich, M. E. (1987). Psychiatric aspects of AIDS. *American Journal of Psychiatry, 144*, 551–555; Kelly, J. A., Murphy, D. A., Bahr, G. R., Koob, J., Morgan, M., Kalichman, S. C., Stevenson, L. Y., Brasfield, T. L., Bernstein, B., & St. Lawrence, J. (1993). Factors associated with severity of depression and high-risk behavior among persons diagnosed with immunodeficiency virus (HIV) infection. *Health Psychology, 12*, 215–219.

P. 50, *Susan Cochran and Vicky Mays found:* Cochran, S., & Mays, V. (1994). Depressive distress among homosexually active African-American men and women. *American Journal of Psychiatry, 151,* 524–529; Kalichman, S. C., & Sikkema, K. J. (1994). Psychological sequelae of HIV infection and AIDS: Review of empirical findings. *Clinical Psychology Review, 14,* 611–632; Markowitz, J., Rabkin, J. G., & Perry, S. (1994). Treating depression in HIV-positive patients. *AIDS, 8,* 403–412.

P. 51, *Depression occurring in PWHIVs can be treated:* Fernandez, F., Adams, F., & Levy, J. K. (1988). Cognitive impairment due to AIDS-Related Complex and its response to psychostimulants. *Psychosomatics, 29,* 38–46; Markowitz, J., Rabkin, J. G., & Perry, S. (1994). Treating depression in HIV-positive patients. *AIDS, 8,* 403–412; Rabkin, J. G., Rabkin, R., Harrison, W., & Wagner, G. (1994). Imipramine effects on mood and enumerative measures of immune status in depressed patients with HIV illness. *American Journal of Psychiatry, 151,* 516–523; Rabkin, J. G., Rabkin, R., & Wagner, G. (1994). Fluoxetine effects on mood and immune status in depressed patients with HIV illness. *Journal of Clinical Psychiatry, 55,* 92–97.

P. 51, *Furthermore, there appear to be no untoward immunological effects:* Rabkin, J. G., Rabkin, R., Harrison, W., & Wagner, G. (1994). Imipramine effects on mood and enumerative measures of immune status in depressed patients with HIV illness. *American Journal of Psychiatry, 151,* 516–523; Rabkin, J. G., Rabkin, R., & Wagner, G. (1994). Fluoxetine effects on mood and immune status in depressed patients with HIV illness. *Journal of Clinical Psychiatry, 55,* 92–97.

P. 51, *In fact, one recent study of HIV-infected gay and bisexual men:* Burack, J. H., Barrett, R. D., Stall, M. A., Chesney, M., Ekstrand, M. L., & Coates, T. (1993). Depressive symptoms and CD4 lymphocyte decline among HIV-infected men. *Journal of the American Medical Association, 270,* 2568–2573; Kessler, R., Foster, C., Joseph, J., Ostrow, D. G., Wortman, C., Phair, J., & Chmiel, J. (1991). Stressful life events and symptom onset in HIV infection. *American Journal of Psychiatry, 148,* 733–738; Lyketsos, C. G., Hoover, D. R., Guccione, M., Senterfitt, W., & Morgenstern, H. (1993). Depressive symptoms as predictors of medical outcomes in HIV infection. *Journal of the American Medical Association, 270,* 2563–2567; Perry, S., Fishman, B., Jacobsberg, L., & Francis, A. (1992). Relationships over one year between lymphocyte subsets and psychosocial variables among adults with infection by human immunodeficiency virus. *Archives of General Psychiatry, 49,* 396–401.

P. 51, *The therapist's emphasis should be on maximizing the QOL:* Fogel, B. S., & Mor, V. (1993). Depressed mood and care preferences in patients with AIDS. *General Hospital Psychiatry, 15,* 203–207.

P. 54, *Given the relatively high degree of overlap between anxiety, depression, and somatic symptoms:* Hintz, S., Kuck, J., Peterkin, J. J., Volk, D. M., & Zisook, S. (1990). Depression in the context of human immunodeficiency virus infection: Implications for treatment. *Journal of Clinical Psychiatry, 51,* 497–501.

P. 54, *There is an increasingly wide spectrum of anxiolytic medications available:* Fernandez, F. (1989). Anxiety and the neuropsychiatry of AIDS. *Journal of Clinical Psychiatry, 50*(11), 9–14.

P. 55, *However, if the cognitive symptoms appear out of proportion:* Hinkin, C. H., van Gorp, W. G., Satz, P., Weisman, J. D., Thommes, J., & Buckinham, S. (1992). Depressed mood and its relationship to neuropsychological test performance in HIV-1 seropositive individuals. *Journal of Clinical and Experimental Neuropsychology, 14*(2), 289–297.

P. 55, *In terms of HIV and mental functioning:* Grant, I., Atkinson, H., Hesselink, J. R., Kennedy, C. J., Richman, D. D., Spector, S. A., & McCutchan, J. A. (1987). Evidence for early central nervous system involvement in the acquired immunodeficiency virus (HIV) infections. *Annals of Internal Medicine, 107,* 823–836; Levy, R. M., & Bredesen, D. E. (1988). Central nervous system dysfunction in acquired immunodeficiency syndrome. *AIDS, 1,* 13–17; McArthur, J. C., Cohen, B. A., Farzedegan, H., Cornblath, D. R., Selnes, O. A., Ostrow, D. G., Johnson, R. T., Phair, J., & Polk, B. F. (1988). Cerebrospinal fluid abnormalities in homosexual men with and without neuropsychiatric findings. *Annals of Neurology, 23*(suppl.), S34–S37; Ostrow, D. G. (1990). Psychiatric aspects of human immunodeficiency virus infection. Kalamazoo, MI: Scope.

P. 55, *Psychostimulant treatment has been shown to be particularly useful:* Fernandez, F., Adams, F., & Levy, J. K. (1988). Cognitive impairment due to AIDS-Related Complex and its response to psychostimulants. *Psychosomatics, 29,* 38–46.

P. 59, *This has caused some to describe the uncertainty of HIV illness:* Nichols, S. E. (1985). Psychosocial reactions of persons with the acquired immunodeficiency syndrome. *Annals of Internal Medicine, 103,* 765–767.

P. 59, *The involvement of spiritual and palliative care can be extremely important:* Hall, B. A. (1994). Ways of maintaining hope in HIV disease. *Research Nursing and Health, 17*(4), 283–293; Peri, T. A.-C. (1995). Promoting spirituality in persons with acquired immunodeficiency syndrome: A nursing intervention. *Holistic Nurse Practitioner, 10*(1), 68–76; Slome, L., Moulton, C., Huffine, R., Groter, R., & Abrams, D. (1992). Physicians' attitudes toward assisted suicide in AIDS. *AIDS, 5,* 712–718; Maj, M. (1991). Psychological problems of families and healthworkers dealing with people infected with human immunodeficiency virus-1. *Acta Psychiatrica Scandinavia, 83,* 161–168.

P. 60, *The complex and multidisciplinary nature of coordinated biopsychosocial HIV care:* Tucker, C. (1993). Supportive psychosocial interventions. In D. G. Ostrow and P. Wren (Eds.), *Mental health aspects of HIV/AIDS: Curriculum modules* (module 10, pp. 363–406). Ann Arbor: Comprehensive HIV and AIDS Mental Health Education Project (CHAMHEP), University of Michigan.

P. 62, *With such support, mental health caregivers can contribute . . . living with HIV infection:* Folkman, S., Chesney, M., & Christopher-Richards, A. (1994). Stress and coping among caregiving partners of men with AIDS. *Psychiatric Clinics of North America, 17,* 35–53; Bennett, L., Miller, D., & Ross, M. W. (Eds.). (1995). *Health workers and AIDS: Research, intervention and current issues in burnout and response.* London: Harwood Academic; the reader is also referred to the discussion of transference and countertransference issues in Chapter One of this book.

3

TREATING PEDIATRIC AND ADOLESCENT HIV

Roberta Ann Olson, Heather Huszti, and Jeffrey T. Parsons

Most children with HIV infection were infected while in the womb. With treatments for HIV/AIDS increasing in number, many of these children are surviving into their teenage years. Because of increasing rates of survival, the clinician may establish a long-term relationship with the child and his family that can focus on anticipating normal developmental issues, coping with a chronic medical illness, and preventing the spread of HIV. This chapter will focus on HIV-related assessment, treatment, and prevention strategies for infants, school-age children, adolescents, and their family members or caretakers. We have chosen to take a developmental perspective that addresses issues throughout the child's life span.

Each of the authors has a unique set of experiences in the treatment of children, adolescents, and families who are struggling to cope with a diagnosis of HIV-positive or AIDS. All of the authors have learned that when faced with a child with a chronic but eventually terminal illness, it's easy to focus on the illness and forget about all of the normal developmental issues children also face. Therefore, it is important that we be familiar with the normal cognitive, emotional, and social issues of both childhood and adolescence.

INFANCY AND PRESCHOOL

The majority of infants and preteen children with HIV infection were infected in utero. Women of childbearing age are most often infected as a result of IV-drug use or by having sex with an infected partner. HIV is then passed to the fetus as she develops. Therefore, the demographics of HIV infection in women of childbearing age and children are closely matched. Pediatric AIDS occurs disproportionately in Black (50 percent of cases) and Hispanic (25 percent) children. Cases occur disproportionately in poor urban areas. Many of the parents of infected children are involved in current or past drug use. A small minority of the cases are due to the mother's infection from blood or blood products or as a result of direct transmission to the child. Anonymous testing of heelstick samples of newborns in several states suggests that there are 1.5 cases of HIV per 1,000 children born. Transmission rates from an HIV-positive mother to her unborn child are generally 25 to 30 percent. Whereas children with HIV infection in the early 1980s usually died in the first several years of life, young children are now increasingly surviving into school age and adolescence. In fact, in one study, 49.5 percent of children infected in utero survived to the age of nine.

Of course, the only rule of the HIV epidemic is that the disease is constantly changing. For instance, in 1994, it was announced that an intensive treatment protocol using AZT in pregnancy could reduce the rate of transmission in utero to 8.5 percent. We may therefore start to see a decrease in the number of children born with HIV infection.

Clinicians working with children infected with HIV in hospitals, clinics, state-funded agencies, or private practices must be attuned to issues that stem both from the actual HIV infection as well as those related to the child's background. When looking at the demographics of HIV infection, it becomes very clear that the majority of children with HIV/AIDS are dealing with many difficult issues. In addition to the complications associated with growing up in poor urban areas, these children are quite likely to have biological parents who are ill themselves and dealing with their own medical care and complications. In some cases, the biological parents are unable to care for the child, and the child may have an alternate caretaker. Quite frequently, the primary caretaker is the child's grandmother, who may also be caring for the child's mother or father.

Family life for low-income HIV-positive children can often be chaotic. Given the involvement of extended family members and the numerous long-term issues that eventually need to be decided, it is usually most beneficial to work with the child's entire family or social system. Chapter Seven in this volume provides additional information on working with couples and families.

ADAM

Adam was a four-year-old Black male who was first referred to us by his infectious-disease physician. Adam's mother, who had abused IV drugs in the past, was dying. His physician requested assistance in helping Adam to understand that his mother would die soon, to be able to experience his grief, and to begin to adjust to a new living arrangement with his grandmother. Adam was an active, normal four-year-old who was adjusting to life in public housing as well as to his mother's illness. He was facing moving from his current neighborhood to another town to be with his grandmother. Numerous issues were addressed with Adam throughout the course of treatment, some of which were related to his HIV infection, some related to the loss of a parent, the move to another town, and the separation from his friends in the housing project preschool. In sessions, Adam often moved quickly from one problem to another, requiring a thorough understanding of all of his many issues.

You will quickly discover that when working with an HIV-infected infant, the majority of any therapeutic interventions are likely to take place with the adult parents or other caretakers of the child. There are myriad psychosocial issues that families must face. Immediate daily concerns, such as getting to doctors' appointments, finding services for the family's needs, and surviving day to day, must be dealt with so that the caretakers have the time and energy to deal with longer-term psychosocial issues. We have found it very useful to work with all other professionals involved with the family whenever possible. These professionals might include social workers, state or private agencies, and physicians and other health care providers. When circumstances permit, it is very helpful to have group meetings with all of these professionals to discuss the family and coordinate the services and interventions needed by the child and her family.

Impact of the Diagnosis

In some cases, the infant's diagnosis with HIV infection or AIDS may be the first time the mother and other family members have learned of the mother's HIV status.

MARY AND RONNIE

Mary had repeatedly brought her young son, Ronnie, to his pediatrician because of respiratory infections and a failure to gain weight. Her pediatrician was confused about what was causing Ronnie's illnesses. He finally suggested an HIV antibody test to rule out any possibility of this disease. Both he and Mary were amazed when the test came back positive. He then told Mary that she too would need to be tested. Mary's test was also positive. Although Mary had not known that she had engaged in any high-risk behavior, it turned out that a man she had dated briefly before her marriage was HIV infected. In therapy Mary and her husband had to deal with their feelings of distress about Ronnie's diagnosis. In addition, Mary had to learn to deal with her feelings of guilt over "infecting" her child. While helping Mary and her husband make plans for Ronnie's and her own treatment, we also helped Mary examine her prior knowledge and understand that she had made reasonable choices based on the knowledge she had at the time. Once Mary could accept the fact that she had not knowingly caused her or her child's HIV infection, she was better able to enjoy her time with Ronnie and her husband.

On hearing the diagnosis of HIV infection, parents must reevaluate their expectations and dreams for their child as well as for themselves. Often, the family believes that the child will immediately die. Although this can occur, you can help the family understand that children with HIV can live into adolescence, and perhaps beyond. Family members may need help in thinking about HIV infection as a chronic illness that is treatable for a number of years rather than as an immediately fatal one. Given the increasing life expectancy, families need to make plans based on the child's surviving for a number of years. In order to achieve this goal, it can be crucial for the clinician to help family members access their own feelings of hope for all family members. Hope need not be unrealistic; instead it can be a sustaining force for family members during times of crisis.

SUSAN

Susan, a nineteen-year-old mother, was told she was HIV-positive while carrying her second child. She was unaware that her boyfriend had a past history of IV-drug use. Susan experienced significant depression and feelings of guilt and anger. A family conference was held in which the father, Jimmy, the maternal grandmother, and two paternal aunts attended. Each family member talked about the pending birth and their hopes for this child to be a normal and healthy child. Susan's diagnosis of HIV infection left each family member with the fear that the child would die before her first birthday. When family members began to understand that the child might not be infected, and even if she were, she could live a decade or longer, their perspective changed. Each family member began to look at the possibility that the child could grow up, attend school, and find joy in her life. The family also began to hope for continued improvements in treatment for HIV. The child, Shandi, was born, was HIV infected, and is now eight years old. Even as the family has had to deal with difficult times, such as Susan's death, they also continue to find moments of joy in achievable goals, such as Shandi's first day of school.

In other cases, the mother knew her HIV status prior to her pregnancy. Even knowing the chances of infecting her unborn child, the mother chose to continue the pregnancy hoping that her child would not be infected. In some cases, the mother had other children who were not infected. In both of these scenarios, the child's status may come as a shock to the mother who believed her child would not be infected. The mother may need to deal with her feelings of grief and loss. As mentioned previously, when mothers take AZT during pregnancy the transmission rate has been significantly lowered. Thus the mother may have expected that her cooperation with the treatment would spare her child from HIV infection. In this case the mother may experience feelings of anger or bewilderment that the treatment did not work.

For both the mother who was unaware of her HIV status prior to the child's birth as well as for the mother who was aware, there may be intense feelings of guilt for "giving" the child HIV. Seropositive fathers may also experience feelings of guilt and shame. Feelings of anger toward the parent who was initially infected are common. In cases where the father remains uninfected, he may experience anger at the mother. In each case, family therapy may be extremely helpful to allow all family members to sort out their feelings and to begin to plan for the future.

In all of the scenarios we have described here, it can be helpful to ask the family to discuss what their expectations had been for the pregnancy and the child's life. The disparity between this description and the current reality can help the clinician understand what types of issues the family might be experiencing.

Family Assessment

It is important to do a careful assessment of the child's family. We often find it helpful to use a genogram as a first step in providing an accurate representation of who the family includes. A genogram can also be used to identify the family members who are most involved in the child's care and should be included in any family therapy sessions. The reader is referred to Chapter Seven in this volume for a more thorough discussion of family assessment and intervention.

Infant Assessment

HIV can infect the central nervous system directly. As a consequence, children with HIV infection often experience impaired brain function. The decline in the function of the immune system, which is a key feature of HIV infection, can also cause brain dysfunction. In addition, many of the diseases children contract due to their damaged immune system can also cause brain injury.

Because many women of childbearing age are infected with HIV through drug use, many children who are infected with HIV during their mother's pregnancy are also exposed to drugs. The effects of prenatal drug exposure alone can cause brain dysfunction.

One study compared three groups of infants. The first group of infants was HIV infected but had not been exposed to drugs during the prenatal period. The second group was HIV infected and had been exposed to drugs during the prenatal period. The third group had been exposed to drugs during the prenatal period and was seroreverters—they had HIV antibodies at birth, but lost them by eighteen months. Children who were HIV infected performed significantly lower on the Bayley Scales of Infant Development compared to the other group. Children who were both HIV infected and had been prenatally exposed to drugs had the lowest scores of any other combination on both the psychomotor and mental scales. Thus, exposure to both drugs and HIV infection may put infants at an even greater risk for experiencing impaired cognitive and motor functions. As all clinicians are aware, an adequate assessment of infant functioning must take into account whether the child was exposed to drugs (such as crack cocaine) while the mother was pregnant.

Children with HIV infection who have brain impairments generally first experience problems in attention and concentration, verbal expression, motor coordination, and language skills. Generally, these children appear to have a diffuse dementia. This constellation of symptoms has been referred to as AIDS Dementia Complex (ADC). Severe symptoms, such as memory loss and a decrease in overall intellectual functioning, are generally seen only in the late stages of AIDS.

In infancy and the preschool years, problems with cognitive functioning are usually seen as delays in achieving normal developmental milestones. In several studies, infants with HIV infection had more developmental delays than other children. Studies have estimated that as many as 40 percent to 90 percent of children with HIV infection may have some type of cognitive dysfunction. In general, more children have problems with cognitive and motor skills as their disease progresses to later stages.

Psychological Assessment

Given the deficits that infants and children can experience as a result of their infection with HIV, psychological assessment is essential. These tests serve several functions. Initially, they can provide a baseline measure of the infant's functioning, so that subsequent problems can be identified and compared to baseline functioning. This assessment can also be used to help parents or guardians understand the child's current abilities and capabilities. It is useful to assess what expectations the parent has for the child's behavior. Often the parent assumes that the child who is

HIV infected will achieve developmental milestones at the same time as HIV-negative children. Although this may be the case, it is also possible that the infant infected with HIV will be developmentally delayed. Thus, it is important to help parents understand the child's true capabilities and help them to develop plans for working with the child's deficits.

Assessment in infancy should include an assessment of the infant's cognitive development, attention, memory, social competence, and temperament. The use of standardized tests allows for a comparison of the child's abilities to that of other children. Currently there are no recognized standard batteries used to assess infants and children with HIV infection. However, the following instruments have been used in a variety of studies of infants and children with HIV infection and are well-recognized measures.

The Bayley Scales of Infant Development are a good choice because they allow for the assessment of both cognitive and motor development. The Bayley Scales include norms for children from birth to two years. In addition, the Peabody Developmental Motor Scales can be used with children over six months through six years. For children older than two years and younger than eight, the McCarthy Scales of Children's Abilities can be used to assess cognitive development. The Peabody Picture Vocabulary Test-Revised can be used to assess language capabilities in children over two years through adulthood. The Stanford-Binet Intelligence Scale IV can be used with children over the age of two through adulthood. The child's adaptive and social behavior can be assessed through scales such as the Vineland Adaptive Behavior Scale, which measures a wide range of domains, such as communication (receptive, expressive, and written), daily living skills, socialization, motor skills, and maladaptive behaviors, throughout the life span. The Achenbach Child Behavior Checklist can be used with children two years and older to assess both internalizing and externalizing behaviors.

It is also important to assess the infant's home environment. The home environment and the stimulation a child receives in that environment have been shown to be better predictors of the child's future cognitive abilities than other traditional infant assessments. One multicultural standardized instrument is the Home Observation for Measurement of the Environment (HOME). This instrument is completed during a home visit.

As previously mentioned, cognitive deficits in infants and preschool children with HIV infection become more pronounced as the disease progresses. We therefore recommend repeated assessments. It is helpful to choose instruments that can be compared across a wide range of ages. When comparing results from different tests, it can be difficult to determine whether the child's abilities have truly changed or if the results are a function of differences in the instruments used, especially when there are subtle declines in scores.

Because changes in cognitive functioning can indicate a progression in HIV disease or the beginning of a treatable infection, any changes noted in neuropsychological functioning should be pointed out to the caretakers. Ideally, you will have a direct relationship with the infant's health care provider and can alert the medical personnel directly after receiving the parent's permission to do so. It is important for medical staff to be aware of any changes, as medical treatment for disease progression can be helpful in reducing these deficits. For instance, one study of children with symptoms from their HIV infection found that after six months of Zidovudine (AZT), their adaptive behaviors and cognitive abilities increased.

Other Treatment Issues

For preschool children who are experiencing anxiety or behavioral symptoms, adjunctive play therapy may be helpful. Through the use of play therapy, mental health professionals may be able to elicit issues of concern to the child. In younger children, we have generally found their fears and concerns to revolve around medical issues. HIV-positive children often undergo repeated medical procedures including injections, IVs, and the taking of blood for various routine tests. We often start by allowing children to safely manipulate specific medical instruments. The goal of this type of play is to help children become more familiar with these medical tools, thus decreasing anxiety and developing a sense of mastery. Specific techniques have included using syringes (without the needle) to paint, or more specific role-playing, such as giving a doll a shot. It is often helpful to allow children to play the role of the perceived powerful health care provider. During this play, the mental health counselor can ask the child how the doll is feeling and what the doll can do to feel better. The mental health counselor can also ask the child how the doctor or nurse is feeling. Sometimes children perceive the doctor or nurse to enjoy "hurting" the child. In these cases, it is important to work with the child to increase her understanding of the benefits of her treatment.

We have found that for those children who are experiencing behavioral distress associated with medical procedures, behavioral treatments are useful. Children can be taught specific coping techniques, such as deep breathing or distraction. These techniques can be practiced during play with the therapist. The child's parents can also be taught the techniques so that the child can practice at home.

MITCHELL

Mitchell was a two-year-old child with HIV infection. He was large for his age, and fought all procedures to the extent that he needed to be placed in restraints. The therapist was called in to help Mitchell adjust to his shots and blood drawing. The therapist worked with Mitchell and his mother to develop a game of holding out his finger, the behavior necessary for the blood drawing, and staying as still as he possibly could. Mitchell and his mother practiced this game at home repeatedly. Mitchell enjoyed the game and his behavior in the clinic rapidly improved. In fact, his mother reported that he held out his finger and stood still whenever a doctor was shown on the television at home.

In addition to having the child engage in behavioral rehearsal, it can also be useful to have the child role play the doctor or nurse. The child can be in control as she "instructs" the doll on how best to cope with the medical procedure. Role-play with a doll allows the child to recognize that distress (moving away, not holding still) can interfere with the procedure and make it last longer. Through practice with a doll, the child learns how to cope more effectively with a medical procedure and reduce the amount of time and pain associated with needles or other painful procedures.

Parental Issues

When working with the infected infant or preschool child, we must be aware of the dual nature of death and dying issues in this age group. As already discussed, HIV infection in infants and preschool children is usually a result of the mother's IV-drug use or unprotected sex with an infected partner. Mothers must face the dual issues of responsibility for the infection of their child and a personal diagnosis of a terminal illness. Issues of guilt, anger, and fear are common reactions to a diagnosis of a terminal illness. Depression, overwhelming stress, and suicidal ideation are common concerns for seropositive mothers. It is important to assess the mother's level of depression and suicidal ideation. Common brief diagnostic screening tools such as the Beck Depression Inventory or the *DSM-IV* diagnostic criteria contain items regarding physical symptoms of depression. These vegetative signs, such as feelings of fatigue, weight loss, muscle aches, diarrhea, and neurological disturbances (headaches, memory loss), are common symptoms of HIV that may overlap with a diagnosis of depression. A more accurate method of assessing depression focuses on cognitive and emotional indicators of depression, such as guilt, hopelessness, and helplessness.

Treatment of depression may include antidepressant medications and individual or group therapy. An essential aspect of the treatment of depression and the reduction of the risk of suicide is to help the mother experience a sense of control of her life and that of her child. If the mother is able to feel bonded, responsible, and involved in the care of the child, she can experience decreased feelings of helplessness and an increased sense of control. The diagnosis of HIV/AIDS is often thought to lead to a quick death. In fact, children often survive longer than their parents. Mothers are burdened with the knowledge of a terminal illness and the responsibility for planning for their family's future. It is important for the clinician to help the mother focus on issues of how she can gain control of her life by providing for her child while she can and making plans for herself and her child to receive care from a relative, friend, nonprofit organization, or governmental agency when the disease progresses. Many intermediate steps need to be discussed and evaluated, including the use of home health care nurses, help with shopping and food preparation, and assistance with transportation to medical appointments. Longer-term issues of foster care or family care will need to be addressed.

Mothers often feel overwhelmed by their illness and are physically or emotionally unable to cope with the needs of a chronically ill child. Early intervention using health care professionals, social worker, and child-care workers is essential in aiding a parent to care for her seropositive child. Early intervention also allows time to help the parent identify individuals or organizations that can provide assistance.

A final issue to consider in the treatment of seropositive mothers is the realization that IV-drug use and crack cocaine use are highly correlated with HIV infection. It is essential to evaluate the history and possibility of continuing drug use. Inpatient drug treatment, outpatient follow-up, and medications must be considered. It is not possible to expect active drug users to be able to care for a child with significant medical needs. Some mothers are unable to stop using drugs. Some infants have been abandoned or removed from the home; these children are typically placed with family members or foster parents. Common experiences of foster parents or family members include anger at the mother or father and fear and depression regarding the child's illness and limited future. You must therefore help caretakers to explore their feelings toward the parents and child. Providing a safe place to express anger and sadness is important for the mental health of the caretakers. Foster parents or other caretakers will need to be given accurate information about the child's illness, treatment options, and life expectancy. The provision of hope and faith are essential for the caretaker and the child. The young child and caretakers must learn to cope with the knowledge that the parent is addicted to drugs and as a result of this illness cannot care for the child.

Children's Concepts of Death and Dying

As children grow older it becomes essential to help them understand their disease and to focus on issues of coping with the illness and infection control. It is important to take into consideration the child's level of cognitive development when explaining his illness and coping strategies to deal with the chronic and eventually terminal illness. We have found that the child's level of cognitive development is a better indicator of the level of understanding of death than chronological age.

Many adults erroneously believe that discussions of illness and death will unnecessarily upset the child and interfere with the few happy years the child may have left. Joseph Spinetta has provided an excellent review of adult concerns and the needs of children to be told about their terminal illness and impending death. Mindy's story is typical of the concerns of many parents of dying children.

MINDY

Mindy, an attractive five-year-old, had been infected through a blood transfusion two years before. During the past two years, Mindy had many bacterial infections and experienced weight loss and lowered energy. The medications often made her feel sick. Mindy, like many other children, was afraid of shots, IVs, and having blood drawn. The initial consultation was to help Mindy cope with painful procedures. During the private interview with the mother it was discovered that Mindy had not been told of her diagnosis nor that she had a terminal illness. Instead the mother told Mindy that she was going to get better. At each hospitalization, Mindy became sicker and weaker. During her last hospitalization she began to repeat "I want a bath," and refused to respond to questions or comfort from her mother or the staff. When the therapist talked with Mindy, she revealed that she did not believe she would get better and was afraid her mother would be mad at her if she revealed her fear of dying. Her desire to take a bath would require the IV to be removed. It became apparent that she was telling her mother and the staff that she wanted treatment to stop. When Mindy was able to tell her mother that she knew she was going to die and that she wanted to go home, the mother agreed. The IV was removed. Mindy had a bubble bath at the hospital. Her mood dramatically changed. She laughed and talked with her mother and the staff. Mindy's mother was able to talk about death, her belief in God, and who would be in heaven to take care of Mindy when she died. Mindy was sent home, and she died a short time later at home with her mother by her side.

PRESCHOOL CHILDREN

Children in the preoperational stage of development (two to five years) tend to view death as temporary and reversible. We have found that young children view the dead as possibly having some biological functioning, including sensations of hunger, hearing, sight, or feelings of pain. Children may view death as similar to sleeping. Illness and death may be seen as a punishment for bad behavior. Children's misperceptions are often exacerbated by adults' discomfort and subsequent use of euphemisms for death ("God took your mother," "Your mother just went to sleep and now she is at peace").

Clinicians need to directly assess children's understanding of illness and death. An assessment may include: What does *dead* mean? Can dead people come back to life again or not? Where do dead people go? Can dead people get hungry? If you gave a dead person a shot, would it hurt him?

It is important to understand the child's conceptions of death. For instance, if the child believes the parent can still experience hunger or pain, he will be extremely upset to be told that his parent's casket will be closed and covered with dirt. Young children need to be reassured that a dead person no longer experiences bodily sensations. It is important for the clinician to explain to the child that people die from an illness and not as a punishment for bad thoughts or behaviors. Children can be helped to understand and feel less fearful through the use of direct conversations, reassurances from family members, play, and books about death.

SCHOOL-AGE CHILDREN

This section covers issues that are specific to school-age children, ages six to twelve years old. Generally these are children who have been infected perinatally (in their mother's womb) and have thus been infected all of their lives. There are a smaller number of children who have been infected by blood transfusions or through the use of blood products (such as factor concentrate in the case of children with hemophilia).

Assessment of School-Age Children

In school-age children there are some additional manifestations of neurologic disease progression in addition to those discussed in the previous assessment section. The school-age child may develop an attention deficit disorder, or previous attention problems may worsen. Emotional lability may increase, and conduct disorders can also be seen. As HIV disease progresses, apathy, cognitive impairment, reduced speech, global memory problems, and motor dysfunction often occur.

Although longitudinal assessment is important, it can be difficult to determine whether changes are due to further deterioration in the child, to a change in assessment instruments as the child grows older, or to practice effects from repeated testing. It is also important to remember that HIV-positive children fatigue easily and should not be exposed to unnecessary testing.

Given these issues, there are several important considerations in performing assessments. As discussed earlier, it is helpful to choose screening instruments that can be used with a wide age range to allow direct comparisons over time. Testing frequency should be limited to reduce practice effects. Testing instruments should be limited to reduce the child's fatigue. It may be necessary to administer the tests in several short sessions. As the child becomes more symptomatic and her abilities decrease, it may be necessary to become more liberal in the administration of the tests, by relaxing timing requirements or allowing for additional cues, for example. Although scores obtained with this testing cannot be compared with normative samples, the results will give an indication of the child's current abilities and functioning. This information can be useful in helping parents and schools develop reasonable expectations for the child and adjust to her disabilities.

Several functional domains should be assessed in school-age children. The goal of assessing the child with HIV infection is twofold. One goal is to assess the progression of the disease. Often changes in neuropsychological functioning are the first signs of disease progression. The second goal is to assess the child's capabilities and to determine ways that the child can maximize his functional abilities. For instance, testing might identify problems with encoding verbal instructions but also show an ability to learn from written instructions. Thus the examiner can help the school and family to produce written cues for the child.

A comprehensive assessment of the HIV-infected child includes assessment of the child's general intellectual abilities, memory and learning ability, attention, visuospatial abilities, motor functioning, and adaptive behavior. Of course, abbreviated batteries can also be administered depending on the needs of the child, the child's degree of fatigue, and the examiner's comfort and expertise.

A commonly used standardized measure of general intelligence is the Weschler Intelligence Scale for Children-III, which can be used with children from six to sixteen years old. Memory and learning skills can be assessed with the Rey Auditory Verbal Learning Test, which can be used with children older than six. Attention skills can be assessed with tests such as the Trail-Making Test. Visuospatial abilities can be evaluated by the Beery Visual Motor Integration Test. The Grooved Pegboard assesses motor functioning in children over the age of five. The most common assessment instrument for adaptive behavior is the Vineland Adaptive Behavior Scales, used for children from birth to nineteen years of age. Children's behavioral problems can be assessed through the Achenbach Behavior Checklist, which can be used with children ages two to sixteen years.

Disclosure

There are many issues related to disclosure when working with school-age children infected with HIV and their families. These issues include disclosing the diagnosis to the child, revealing the HIV status of other family members, and deciding who else should be told of the child's diagnosis.

In beginning a therapeutic relationship with a child with HIV infection, it is important to determine whether the child knows of his diagnosis, and who in the family and social support system knows. Deciding to disclose this information to the child can be a painful decision for the family members. As a result, children are often not told. In one survey of adults with HIV infection attending an HIV clinic who had children older than four years of age, 55 percent reported that their child knew of the parents' diagnosis, and 35 percent said their child did not know. One of the main worries of the parents was that their child would face discrimination if people knew of the parent's HIV infection. Because discrimination against persons with HIV infection still occurs, this must be a consideration in deciding about disclosure issues.

PHILLIP

One family decided to tell the school officials in their small, rural town about the HIV status of their son, Phillip. Unfortunately, confidentiality was breached, and a teacher from another school system learned of his HIV status. The fourteen-year-old played on his school's basketball team. Soon, teams from other schools were being called anonymously and told that an HIV-positive boy was playing basketball. Schools began canceling games. The team decided to stand behind Phillip and reaffirmed their commitment to have him on their team. The family and school system appealed to the state school and athletic board, who were not helpful in combating this situation. After much soul searching, this private family decided to go public with their story. After a front page story appeared in the largest newspaper in the state, the public supported Phillip and his team.

The decision to disclose is complex. Every family is different, and the right course of action in disclosure differs as well. The therapist can help families weigh the alternatives and make a decision. It is important to consider the child's developmental level, which may be lower than the child's physical age might indicate. The therapist can explore with the child what she thinks is causing her symptoms, how the child views the causality of illness (how do people get sick?), and her general knowledge about

HIV/AIDS. There has been previous work done in construct-ing developmental schemata for children's understanding of ill-ness that detail questions to ask and how to determine the developmental level of understanding.

It is also important to assess the effects on the child and the family members of keeping the "secret" of the diagnosis. The clinician and parents must consider the fact that children often attempt to come up with explanations to bits and pieces of infor-mation they overhear. These "explanations" may be much more frightening than the actual truth. The therapist can also assess what the child has been told. In some cases, children are told that they do not have HIV infection by well-meaning parents who do not want their children to worry. However, this lie can have far-reaching effects when the truth is later learned. It is impor-tant that children be secure that the information they are told is true; that way, when the child is told there is nothing to worry about, she can be secure that this is indeed the case.

The therapist, family, and medical staff should also understand that disclosure is a process. Telling a child one time is not suffi-cient. Information needs to be given over time in a develop-mentally appropriate manner. As the child's developmental level increases, and as the child requests information, additional infor-mation should be given. For instance, as children mature, they will need increasingly specific information about the prevention of the transmission of HIV. Families should also be aware that it will take time for the child to work through the myriad emo-tional reactions disclosure might bring. Parents can be reminded of their own reactions and how long it took them to adjust. Chil-dren can experience anger, depression, grief, and loss. Support-ive therapeutic interventions can help with these reactions. It is important for the child to find a way to understand that although the illness cannot be changed, there are ways to cope with it and live a positive and happy life.

School systems may differ in their policies regarding the admission of HIV-infected children. Most HIV-infected chil-dren have been integrated into the school system. However, in the past, some school systems and their surrounding population have protested the child's attendance. Education of school personnel and the public may be helpful in reducing negative effects. Some pediatric AIDS treatment centers have designed school programs for this purpose; others have worked with their state health departments or state departments of education to develop education for school personnel.

When children with HIV infection are integrated into public schools, they face additional problems with regular attendance. Weakness and fatigue associated with HIV infection as well as repeated infections and illnesses may cause the child to miss a great deal of school. Missing significant amounts of school may make it difficult for the child to keep up with his studies. Additionally, missed school may interfere with the child's social relationships. Children with HIV infection may already experience intense feelings of isolation, due to having a disease that can cause extreme societal rejection. Missed school may add to this sense of isolation.

School-age children with HIV infection may experience delayed growth rates. Because HIV infection can have direct neurological effects, children can also experience learning disabilities. Children, parents, medical staff, and school personnel need to be aware of the likelihood of learning disabilities and work together to design appropriate educational programs.

Concepts of Death and Dying

Children in the concrete operational stage of development (six to twelve years old) develop a more accurate and complex sense of death. Research has found that children between the ages of six and eight have gained a sense of death as irreversible and universal. School-age children understand that the dead do not experience bodily sensations. Primary issues for children of grade school age include fear of abandonment and fear of the unknown. When working with these children, it is helpful to ask them what they think about death. What happens to dead people? How do people feel when they die? What would make it less scary for a kid if he were dying? Are you religious? Why does God let children die? It is essential to first understand how the child views death before trying to provide the child with more accurate information or to reduce the child's fear of death.

Children are profoundly affected by the loss of a primary caretaker. You must understand the impact on cognitive and emotional development of children experiencing the loss of a parent. School-age children interpret the death of a parent in an egocentric manner. Typical concerns of a child include "Who will take care of me?" Medically ill children can experience intense fears of abandonment, vulnerability, and loss.

It is very important that you allow the child to express her feelings of loss, sadness, and vulnerability. Children need to be given concrete information about future living arrangements and changes in school or neighborhood. If the child is going to live with relatives or foster parents, it may be helpful for the child to meet and get to know the family before the death of the parent. If the parent is hospitalized or placed in a hospice, the child should be able to visit the setting prior to the parent's placement. Helping the child to anticipate and prepare for the loss of a parent can be aided by having the child talk to other children with similar experiences, conducting family sessions where death and dying are discussed, and providing the child with reading material appropriate for her cognitive development.

ADOLESCENTS

It is difficult to determine an accurate estimate of the prevalence of HIV infection among adolescents. As of December 1994, a total of 1,304 males and 661 females between the ages of thirteen and nineteen were diagnosed with AIDS. However, this figure underestimates the number of adolescents infected with HIV. Given the length of time between initial infection and an AIDS-related diagnosis, it can be assumed that the majority of the twenty- to twenty-nine-year-olds with AIDS (approximately 19 percent of all AIDS cases, 14,112 females and 67,533 males) were infected during their adolescent years. HIV/AIDS risk among adolescents differs substantially according to gender, ethnicity, and geographic region.

Adolescent males, adolescents of color, and inner-city adolescents appear to be at greatest risk. Further data suggest that HIV infections are increasing most rapidly among adolescents. Approximately one in four new seroconversions in the United States occurs among those under the age of twenty-two. Prevalence rates for other STDs (such as chlamydia and gonorrhea) among adolescents are also on the increase, suggesting even greater need for prevention efforts.

Risk Behaviors

Although adolescents constitute a relatively small percentage of all reported cases of AIDS, they represent a difficult cohort in terms of HIV risk behaviors. Adolescence is a developmental period characterized by feelings of invulnerability and immunity to the dangerous consequences of the adolescent's own risk-taking behaviors. Among seronegative adolescents, this egocentrism may put them at risk for HIV infection through their own cognitive minimization of personal susceptibility. Studies have shown that only 15 to 39 percent of adolescents reported a change toward using safer sexual behaviors as a result of their increased concern about contracting HIV. This same egocentrism among HIV-infected adolescents, however, may lead to perceptions that sexual intercourse will not transmit HIV, with the result that they may engage in unsafe intercourse and infect their sexual partners.

Sexual contact and IV-drug use, behaviors which are likely to transmit HIV, are commonly initiated during the adolescent years. Due to the increasing frequency of adolescent experimentation with sexual behaviors and drug use, related increases in adolescent HIV cases can be expected. By the age of twenty, more than 80 percent of males and 75 percent of females have engaged in sexual intercourse. Adolescents begin having sexual intercourse, on average, at age sixteen, and approximately 30 percent of males and 20 percent of females have had their first act of intercourse before the age of fifteen.

Numerous research endeavors have supported the finding that sexual risk-taking is highest among adolescents and young adults, compared to older adults. Adolescents engage in sexual activity with multiple partners. In a study of adolescents (ages fourteen to nineteen) attending teen health clinics, 40 percent of females and 69 percent of males reported more than one sexual partner in the past year. A study of eighteen- and nineteen-year-old college students found that 32 percent reported more than five life-time sexual partners.

Although adolescents know the facts about HIV transmission, they continue to have intercourse without using a condom. Further, those adolescents with the highest number of sexual partners are the least likely to self-report condom use. Numerous studies of adolescents have shown that 21 to 37 percent rarely or never used condoms. In addition, 64 percent of college students had not used a condom during their last episode of intercourse. The higher percentage of individuals who did not use condoms at last intercourse makes sense, as condom use among adolescents appears to decline once a partner is perceived to be "safe."

Both of these sexual risk-taking behaviors (having multiple partners and failing to use condoms) place the adolescent at risk for HIV transmission. Likewise, they place the HIV-infected adolescent at risk for transmitting the virus to a sexual partner.

Prevention Issues

As clinicians, we can provide needed clinical and research-based consultations to public and private schools. Schools offer an excellent opportunity to educate adolescents, regardless of their serostatus, about HIV and AIDS. However, one-time presentations or lectures are not likely to have a lasting impact.

HIV/AIDS education should be an ongoing process that increases in sophistication as the adolescent's own cognitive skills mature. School-based HIV/AIDS education programs are often opposed based on the argument that giving adolescents information will encourage them to be sexually active. A comprehensive review of twenty-three school-based HIV/AIDS education programs found the opposite to be true: adolescents receiving HIV/AIDS education were less likely to engage in sex. Sexually active adolescents who received this education were more likely to decrease their frequency of sexual activity and practice safer sex. This review of existing school-based programs suggested the following elements for a successful program:

- A narrow, specific focus
- Instruction regarding social influences and pressures
- Age-appropriate and experience-appropriate reinforcement of values and norms against unprotected sexual intercourse
- Skill-building activities

School-based education has some potential problems that require consideration. Some schools may not provide adequate training for personnel. Others may limit what is discussed. For example, although 75 percent of school-based sex education programs mention condoms, only 9 percent include specific instruction in condom use. Research has shown that for teenagers to use condoms, they must have faith in their technical ability to use condoms in the correct way. When educating adolescents who are HIV infected, as well as those who are not, it is essential to include specific information about the accurate use of condoms.

The use of small group discussions and peer counselors is especially effective when working with adolescents, as peer opinions can be especially persuasive for this age group. Clinicians can also challenge students to problem-solve reasons why people might use a condom and why they might not. It is also helpful to allow adolescents an opportunity to develop refusal skills for when partners insist on intercourse or intercourse without a condom. Skill-building exercises using role-playing can be very useful in developing these skills.

School-based programs also fail to reach a particular cohort in greater need of education, the adolescent dropout. Adolescent dropouts tend to engage in more unsafe sexual and drug-use behaviors, placing them at risk for contracting or transmitting HIV. These teens are not easily accessed for prevention, yet efforts should be made to provide dropouts with both primary and secondary HIV prevention information. *Secondary prevention* refers to the prevention of the further spread of HIV from an infected individual to uninfected individuals.

Runaway youth are another group who cannot be accessed through the school setting. Prevention efforts aimed at residential shelters can be successful. One study reported an increase in consistent condom use and a decrease in high-risk sexual behavior following education, skills training, and counseling sessions in runaway shelters.

Specific Secondary Prevention Issues for Seropositive Adolescents

Although it is important to prevent seronegative youth from becoming infected with HIV, it is equally important to help individuals with HIV infection to keep from further spreading the virus. Seropositive adolescents benefit from many of the same prevention efforts aimed at HIV-negative youth. Basic education and information, skill-building, and values clarification exercises are essential. It is vital to remember that adolescents who are HIV-positive are still adolescents. Their basic developmental needs to take risks, develop their identity, maintain autonomy, assert their independence, and think egocentrically remain paramount. Clinically, HIV-infected adolescents require the same considerations as noninfected youth. They need support and guidance in decision-making and skill-building exercises to promote their self-efficacy. In addition, issues regarding their emerging sexuality and desire for sexual activity must be addressed. Because parents may or may not have the desire or ability to deal with these issues, the clinician has an opportunity to play an influential role.

In working with HIV-infected adolescents regarding sexuality, you must recognize that although teenage sexual experimentation is usually viewed negatively by adults, it provides the potential for desirable developmental outcomes. Sexual behavior and related sexual issues are strongly related to the development of independence and assist the adolescent in the development of their identity and sense of self. However, these same benefits can be obtained through the practice of safer sexual behaviors. Clinicians working with HIV-positive youth should be aware of their own beliefs regarding teen sexuality and recognize that abstinence-based treatment plans are not appropriate for all adolescents.

HIV prevention efforts for HIV-negative youth are often aimed at getting adolescents to realize that their behaviors place them at risk for becoming infected. Thus the focus is on self-protection. With the HIV-positive adolescent, however, one of the major issues to address is the protection of others. Many of the same variables found to be predictive of self-protection with regard to HIV prevention (self-efficacy, perceived advantages, communication skills, and so on) are essential for the protection of others.

PHILIP, BENJAMIN, ANDRE, AND RICKY

Philip, Benjamin, Andre, and Ricky ranged in age from fourteen to sixteen years old; all four were HIV infected. They came to a weekend-long retreat designed to address issues faced by HIV-positive teenagers. The retreat took place on a local college campus. In one session, the young men discussed their decisions about becoming romantically involved. Benjamin and Andre talked about not allowing themselves to become attracted to anyone, because they felt that it was impossible that anyone would like them if they knew of their status, but that they needed to disclose their status to anyone they wanted to date. Philip and Ricky talked about not telling people about their status. The young men got into a lively debate and discussed what their obligation was to protect others from becoming infected. During the debate, I (JTP) helped them to think about their values and determine what types of decisions they wanted to make. As the young men debated amongst themselves, they clearly decided that they did not want to put anyone else in the same situation they found themselves. Once this decision had been made, we proceeded with skills-based communication exercises in which the young men practiced how and when to disclose their status, how to turn down sexual overtures, and how to discuss and insist on condom use.

Adaptation and coping among HIV-positive adolescents can and should be addressed in a clinical setting. With the increasing life expectancy of HIV-infected individuals, the coping strategies used by seropositive youth may dramatically affect their quality of life. Patterns of adaptation may have an impact on compliance with safer sex recommendations, and are thus essential for secondary HIV prevention among infected adolescents. Adolescents who tend to use denial and avoidance coping mechanisms may be more likely to avoid using condoms and disclosing their HIV status. The clinician can assess what the adolescent thinks about HIV, how she deals with it on a day-to-day basis, and how she deals with reminders of HIV. If necessary, the clinician can help the adolescent find more positive ways to cope with her illness and develop proactive plans to deal with situations that might spread HIV infection.

The issue of distress among HIV-infected youth should be addressed in the clinical setting. Interventions that focus on peer-based social support might reduce their distress by reducing feelings of isolation. These adolescents may also need to find "meaning" in their HIV disease through cognitive restructuring and to use problem-focused coping strategies aimed at specific, attainable goals (such as establishing intimate friendships or adopting healthy lifestyles). These coping strategies were rated "most useful" by a cohort of HIV-infected adolescents.

During the same retreat, the young men spent a great deal of time talking with each other about their own experiences with the disease. The young men all remarked that it was very helpful to meet others with similar experiences. As they talked, they discussed their initial shock when diagnosed, their anger, and their strategies for making their lives more positive. During their discussion, I helped them identify specific behaviors they had used to improve their lives and discussed how each of them could adopt strategies that the others had used. At the end of the retreat, the young men exchanged addresses and phone numbers and made plans to meet again in a month's time.

Drug and Alcohol Use

Drug and alcohol use among adolescents, despite recent decreases in illicit drug use, remains quite high. Drug and alcohol use are associated with other risk-taking behaviors, including unprotected sexual behaviors. One study of adolescents found that 64 percent reported engaging in sexual intercourse after drinking alcohol. These same sexually active adolescents also indicated that they were less likely to use condoms after consuming alcohol.

Among HIV-infected adolescents, additional problems resulting from drug and alcohol use emerge. A study of adolescents with hemophilia and HIV-infection found that 37 percent of the sexually active youth reported that they used alcohol at least half the time they had engaged in sexual activity. Clearly, those who use drugs or alcohol are less likely to be concerned about practicing safer sex or transmitting HIV to a sexual partner. In addition, the use of alcohol and other drugs can further negatively affect the health status of a person with HIV infection or an AIDS-related diagnosis. Clinicians should assess alcohol and drug use behaviors among their HIV-positive adolescent clients. In addition, the health and transmission risks resulting from such use should be discussed. Prevention programs for infected youth should recognize that adolescents may exhibit multiple risk behaviors (for example, alcohol or drug use and unprotected sexual behavior) that require intervention on multiple levels.

Issues for Sexual Minority Youth

It is important for the clinician to recognize that sexual identity and sexual orientation may remain unsettled issues during the adolescent years. A variety of forms of sexual activity resulting from curiosity, opportunity, or familial and peer pressure may occur, regardless of the adolescent's true attractions or identity. Gay, lesbian, bisexual, transgendered, or sexually confused adolescents face the same HIV/AIDS-related issues as their heterosexual counterparts. In addition, however, they encounter unique issues that tend to remain ignored by the general population.

Recent studies of HIV infection and sexual behaviors among young gay men have indicated that, contrary to their older counterparts, gay youth are at great risk for HIV infection. Various studies have identified high seroincidence rates among these youth—18 percent among gay men ages eighteen to twenty-nine; 9 percent among gay men ages seventeen to twenty-two; 9 percent among gay men ages eighteen to twenty-four; and 21 percent among African-American gay men ages eighteen to twenty-two. These high incidence rates result from high rates of unprotected sexual activity among young gay men. One study of young gay men (ages eighteen to twenty-five) from three cities found that 43 percent reported engaging in unprotected anal intercourse during the past six months. Another study of adolescent gay and bisexual males identified 63 percent to be at "extreme risk" for HIV transmission from either unprotected anal intercourse or IV-drug use. Part of the reason for the increased engagement in unsafe sex among young gay adolescents may be because they are most likely to learn about homosexuality via sexual encounters and thus may not know about the risk of HIV without prior education.

Many gay teens perceive AIDS and HIV to be problems only for older gay men. They may feel that having unprotected sex with other young gay men is "safe." It is also possible, given the egocentrism of youth and their associated feelings of invulnerability, that even knowing the risks of HIV, adolescents feel that it "can't happen to me."

Because adolescence is a time of experimentation with regard to sexuality and sexual behavior, young gay men are likely to have multiple sex partners and be willing to engage in a variety of sexual behaviors (many of which may potentially transmit HIV). Their inexperience, and the lack of specific education targeted at gay youth, may result in an inability to negotiate safer sex practices with a partner, or they may not know how to make safer sex behaviors enjoyable. In addition, "coming out" issues among gay youth are associated with greater emotional distress. This distress could result in problems with self-esteem and self-efficacy and reduce the gay teenager's motivation to engage in safer sexual behaviors. Additional problems exist for HIV-infected gay youth. Homophobia and social stigma, as well as familial and peer conflicts associated with homosexuality, may prevent infected gay teenagers from seeking out support services.

DALE

Dale, a seventeen-year-old, was struggling with issues of his sexuality. He had recently tested HIV-positive. He had become HIV-positive after one homosexual encounter with an older male. Initially Dale expressed a great deal of anger toward the man who had infected him, and stated that he saw no need to use safer sex, because others hadn't protected him. As the therapist explored Dale's life, Dale disclosed that his family did not know of his homosexual feelings and his related fears that they would reject him. His one experience with an older man had been a quick affair. Dale perceived the outcome—his HIV-positive status—as punishment for his homosexual feelings. The therapist helped Dale express these perceptions and evaluate their validity. As Dale came to terms with his own feelings, and the legitimate nature of these feelings, he began to feel better about himself. As his self-esteem improved, so did his commitment to using safer sexual behaviors to protect others. Eventually Dale became a peer counselor for other young gay men.

Few programs that specifically address the HIV/AIDS needs of gay, bisexual, or sexually confused adolescents have been designed, implemented, or evaluated. One successful program in Minnesota used individual risk-reduction counseling sessions, followed by peer-based educational sessions. These efforts, combined with referrals to counseling, drug, alcohol, and other health services, were found to decrease unprotected anal sex among young gay and bisexual males. Results from a study of intensive, multisession, small-group interventions for gay youth (ages fourteen to nineteen) found that attending a greater number of sessions resulted in greater positive changes in HIV risk behaviors.

Psychosocial programs for HIV-infected gay youth need to address the same secondary prevention issues discussed previously, as well as psychosocial issues related to homophobia, stigma, coming out, self-esteem, and social support. Creative efforts will be necessary to gain access to HIV-infected homosexual or bisexual adolescents. Typically, school systems will not address the needs of gay youth. Building ties with community-based support services within the gay community, as well as creating "hangouts" for gay teens, will be necessary to provide support for this particular cohort.

Finally, it is important to note that for infected gay and bisexual youth, disclosure of HIV status may also involve the disclosure of sexual orientation. The decision to come out is a difficult one and one that can be made only by the individual. Disclosure of sexual orientation can bring discrimination and rejection from family and friends. Because disclosure of homosexuality or bisexuality can be so sensitive, many youths who have experienced homosexual encounters may be fearful of seeking HIV testing, fearing that this testing would require them to disclose their homosexuality. It would be helpful for communities to develop outreach educational programs for gay and bisexual youth to educate them about their emerging sexuality, provide support, and provide HIV risk–reduction services.

"It was the best of times, it was the worst of times." Charles Dickens's sentiments are shared by most mental health professionals who work with children and families affected by HIV and AIDS. Witnessing and experiencing the premature death of a child is devastating for all involved. All of the authors have experienced great sadness at the death of children and adolescents with whom we have worked. At the same time, the threat of early death can also sharpen and heighten all experiences. It can also clarify one's perceptions of what is truly important in life.

In the film *Starman,* the alien visitor to the earth said, "What I love most about your people is that when things are at their worst, you are at your best." All of the authors have been privy to this sentiment as well. Children and families often show their best and most impressive sides while struggling with the complications of HIV infection. As professionals we have been continually awed by the families with whom we have had the honor to work. We have been reminded that life is precious and that even tremendous travails can be faced with wisdom, wit, and courage. Although working with these children has been challenging with associated sadness, it has ultimately been the most rewarding work of our careers, both professionally and personally.

NOTES

P. 74, *disproportionately in Black (50 percent of cases):* Boland, M., & Oleske, J. (1995). The health care needs of infants and children: An epidemiological perspective. In N. Boyd-Franklin, G. L. Steiner, & M. Boland (Eds.), *Children, families, and HIV/AIDS: Psychosocial and therapeutic issues.* New York: Guilford Press.

P. 74, *there are 1.5 cases of HIV per 1,000 children born:* Boland, M., & Oleske, J. (1995). The health care needs of infants and children: An epidemiological perspective. In N. Boyd-Franklin, G. L. Steiner, & M. Boland (Eds.), *Children, families, and HIV/AIDS: Psychosocial and therapeutic issues.* New York: Guilford Press.

P. 74, *Transmission rates from an HIV-positive mother to her unborn child:* Boland, M., & Oleske, J. (1995). The health care needs of infants and children: An epidemiological perspective. In N. Boyd-Franklin, G. L. Steiner, & M. Boland (Eds.), *Children, families, and HIV/AIDS: Psychosocial and therapeutic issues.* New York: Guilford Press.

P. 74, *49.5 percent of children infected in utero:* Tovo, P., de Martino, M., Gabiano, C., Cappello, N., D'Elia, R., Loy, A., Plebani, A., Zuccotti, G. V., Dallacasa, P., Ferraris, G., Caselli, D., Fundaro, C., D'Argenio, P., Galli, L., Principi, N., Stegagno, M., Ruga, E., Palomba, E., and the Italian Register for HIV Infection in Children. (1992). Prognostic factors and survival in children with perinatal HIV-1 infection. *Lancet, 339,* 1249–1253.

P. 74, *it was announced that an intensive treatment protocol:* Centers for Disease Control and Prevention (CDC). (1994). Recommendations for the use of Zidovudine to reduce perinatal transmission of human immunodeficiency virus. *Morbidity and Mortality Weekly Report, 43*(RR-12), 1–5.

P. 79, *many of the diseases children contract:* Belman, A., & Dickson, D. W. (1992). Neurologic aspects. In M. Stuber (Ed.), *Children and AIDS.* Washington, DC: American Psychiatric Press.

P. 79, *are also exposed to drugs:* Gabiano, C., Tovo, P., de Martino, M., Galli, L., Giaquinto, C., Loy, A., Schoeller, M. C., Giovannini, M., Ferranti, G., Rancilio, L., Caselli, D., Segni, G., Liuadiotti, S., Conte, A., Rizzi, M., Viggiano, D., Mazza, A., Ferrazin, A., Tozzi, A. E., & Capello, N. (1992). Mother-to-child transmission of human immunodeficiency virus type 1: Risk of infection and correlates of transmission. *Pediatrics, 90,* 369–374.

P. 79, *prenatal drug exposure alone can cause brain dysfunction:* Mellins, C., Levenson, R., Zawadzki, R., Kairam, R., & Weston, M. (1994). Effects of pediatric HIV infection and prenatal drug exposure on mental and psychomotor development. *Journal of Pediatric Psychology, 19,* 617–628.

P. 79, *One study compared three groups of infants:* Mellins, C., Levenson, R.,

Zawadzki, R., Kairam, R., & Weston, M. (1994). Effects of pediatric HIV infection and prenatal drug exposure on mental and psychomotor development. *Journal of Pediatric Psychology, 19,* 617–628.

P. 79, *Bayley Scales of Infant Development:* Bayley, N. (1969). *Manual for the Bayley Scales of Infant Development.* New York: Psychological Corporation.

P. 80, *AIDS Dementia Complex (ADC):* Price, R., Sidtis, J., & Rosenblum, M. (1988). The brain in AIDS: Central nervous system HIV-1 infection and AIDS Dementia Complex. *Science, 239,* 586–592.

P. 80, *delays in achieving normal developmental milestones:* Hanna, J., & Mintz, M. (1995). Neurological and neurodevelopmental functioning in pediatric HIV infection. In N. Boyd-Franklin, G. L. Steiner, & M. Boland (Eds.), *Children, families, and HIV/AIDS: Psychosocial and therapeutic issues.* New York: Guilford Press.

P. 80, *In several studies, infants with HIV infection:* Hittleman, J. (1992). Neurodevelopmental aspects of HIV infection. In P. Kozlowski, D. Sider, P. Vietz, & H. Wisniewski (Eds.), *Brain and behavior in HIV infection.* Basel, Switzerland: Karger.

P. 80, *40 percent to 90 percent of children with HIV infection:* Hanna, J., & Mintz, M. (1995). Neurological and neurodevelopmental functioning in pediatric HIV infection. In N. Boyd-Franklin, G. L. Steiner, & M. Boland (Eds.), *Children, families, and HIV/AIDS: Psychosocial and therapeutic issues.* New York: Guilford Press; Hittleman, J. (1992). Neurodevelopmental aspects of HIV infection. In P. Kozlowski, D. Sider, P. Vietz, & H. Wisniewski (Eds.), *Brain and behavior in HIV infection.* Basel, Switzerland: Karger; Koch, T., Jeremy, R., Lewis, E., et al. (1989, June). *Developmental abnormalities in uninfected infants born to HIV infected mothers.* Abstract presented at the 5th International AIDS Conference, San Francisco.

P. 80, *more children have problems with cognitive and motor skills:* Price, R. W., Sidtis, J., & Rosenblum, M. (1988). The brain in AIDS: Central nervous system HIV-1 infection and AIDS Dementia Complex. *Science, 239,* 586–592.

P. 81, *The Bayley Scales of Infant Development are a good choice:* Bayley, N. (1969). *Manual for the Bayley Scales of Infant Development.* New York: Psychological Corporation.

P. 81, *Peabody Developmental Motor Scales-Revised:* Folio, M., & Fewell, R. (1983). *Peabody Developmental Motor Scales.* Austin, TX: DLM.

P. 81, *McCarthy Scales of Children's Abilities:* McCarthy, D. (1972). *McCarthy Scales of Children's Abilities.* San Antonio, TX: Psychological Corporation.

P. 81, *Peabody Picture Vocabulary Test:* Dunn, L., & Dunn, L. (1981). *Peabody Picture Vocabulary Test-Revised.* Circle Pines, MN: AGS.

P. 81, *Stanford-Binet Intelligence Scale IV:* Thorndike, R., Hagen, E., & Sattler, J. (1986). *Stanford-Binet Intelligence Scale* (4th ed.). Chicago, IL: Riverside Publishing.

P. 81, *Vineland Adaptive Behavior Scale:* Sparrow, S. S., Balla, D. A., & Cicchetti, D. V. (1984). *Vineland Adaptive Behavior Scales.* Circle Pines, MN: AGS.

P. 81, *Achenbach Child Behavior Checklist:* Achenbach, T., & Edelbrock, C. (1983). *Manual for the child behavior checklist and revised child behavior profile.* Burlington: University of Vermont.

P. 81, *The home environment and the stimulation a child receives in that environment:* Bradley, R., Caldwell, B., Rock, S., Ramey, C. T., Barnard, K. E., Gray, C., Gottfried, A. W., Siegel, L., & Johnson, D. L. (1989). Home environment and cognitive development in the first three years of life: A collaborative study involving six sites and three ethnic groups in North America. *Developmental Psychology, 25,* 217–235.

P. 82, *Home Observation for Measurement of the Environment (HOME):* Caldwell, B., & Bradley, R. (1984). *Home Observation for Measurement of the Environment.* Little Rock: University of Arkansas.

P. 82, *after six months of Zidovudine (AZT):* Wolters, P., Brouwers, P., Moss, H. A., & Pizzo, P. A. (1994). Adaptive behavior of children with symptomatic HIV infection before and after Zidovudine therapy. *Journal of Pediatric Psychology, 19,* 47–61.

P. 82, *adjunctive play therapy may be helpful:* Levenson, R., & Mellins, C. A. (1992). Pediatric HIV disease: What psychologists need to know. *Professional Psychology: Research and Practice, 23,* 410–415.

P. 83, *children who are experiencing behavioral distress associated with medical procedures:* Elliott, C., & Olson, R. A. (1983). The management of children's behavioral distress in response to painful medical treatments for burn injuries. *Journal of Behavior Therapy, 21,* 675–683; Jay, S., Elliott, C., & Ozolins, M. (1985). Behavioral management of children's distress during painful medical procedures. *Behavior Research and Therapy, 19,* 205–215.

P. 84, *Beck Depression Inventory:* Beck, A. (1972). *Depression: Causes and treatment.* Philadelphia: University of Pennsylvania Press.

P. 84, *DSM-IV:* American Psychiatric Association (1994). *Diagnostic and statistical manual of mental disorders* (4th ed.). Washington, DC: Author.

P. 85, *such as guilt, hopelessness, and helplessness:* Kalichman, S. C. (1995). *Understanding AIDS: A guide for mental health professionals.* Washington, DC: American Psychological Association.

P. 86, *Joseph Spinetta has provided an excellent review:* Spinetta, J. (1982). Psychosocial issues in childhood cancer: How the professional can help. In M. Wolraich & D. Routh. (Eds.), *Advances in developmental and behavioral pediatrics* (Vol. 3). Greenwich, CT: JAI Press.

P. 87, *young children view the dead as possibly having some biological functioning:* Olson, R. A. (1980, November). *Children's conceptions of life, animism and death*. Paper presented at the meeting of the Oklahoma Psychological Association, Oklahoma City, OK.

P. 88, *punishment for bad behavior:* Jay, S., Elliott, C., & Ozolins, M. (1985). Behavioral management of children's distress during painful medical procedures. *Behavior Research and Therapy, 19,* 205–215.

P. 89, *and conduct disorders can also be seen:* Belman, A. (1990). AIDS and pediatric neurology. *Neurologic Clinics, 8,* 571–603; Loveland, K., & Stehbens, J. (1990). Early neurodevelopmental signs of HIV infection in children and adolescents. In P. D. Kozloski (Ed.), *The brain in pediatric AIDS.* Farmington, CT: Karger.

P. 89, *As HIV disease progresses, apathy:* Belman, A., & Dickson, D. (1992). Neurologic aspects. In M. L. Stuber (Ed.), *Children and AIDS.* Washington, DC: American Psychiatric Press.

P. 89, *to assess the child's capabilities and to determine ways:* Watkins, J., Brouwers, P., & Huntzinger, R. (1992). Neuropsychological assessment. In M. L. Stuber (Ed.), *Children and AIDS.* Washington, DC: American Psychiatric Press.

P. 90, *A comprehensive assessment of the HIV-infected child includes:* Watkins, J., Brouwers, P., & Huntzinger, R. (1992). Neuropsychological assessment. In M. L. Stuber (Ed.), *Children and AIDS.* Washington, DC: American Psychiatric Press.

P. 90, *Weschler Intelligence Scale for Children-III:* Glasser, A. J., & Zimmerman, I. L. (1967). *Weschler Intelligence Scale for Children-III.* New York: Grune & Stratton.

P. 90, *Rey Auditory Verbal Learning Test:* Rey, A. (1964). *L'ecamen clinique nen psychologie.* Paris: Universaire de France.

P. 90, *Trail-Making Test:* Reitan, R., & Davidson, L. A. (1974). *Clinical neuropsychology: Current status and applications.* New York: Winston/Wiley.

P. 90, *Beery Visual Motor Integration Test:* Beery, K., & Dickson, D. (1992). *Developmental test of visual-motor integration.* Chicago: Fillet.

P. 90, *Grooved Pegboard:* Love, H. (1963). Clinical neuropsychology. *Medical Clinics of North America, 26,* 592–600.

P. 90, *Vineland Adaptive Behavior Scales:* Sparrow, S., Balla, D., & Cicchetti, D. (1984). *Vineland Adaptive Behavior Scales.* Circle Pine, MN: AGS.

P. 90, *Achenbach Behavior Checklist:* Achenbach, T., & Edelbrock, C. (1983). *Manual for the child behavior checklist and revised child behavior profile.* Burlington: University of Vermont.

P. 90, *These issues include disclosing the diagnosis:* Pollack, S., & Thompson, C. L. (1995). The HIV-infected child in therapy. In N. Boyd-Franklin, G. L. Steiner, & M. Boland (Eds.), *Children, families, and HIV/AIDS: Psychosocial and therapeutic issues.* New York: Guilford Press.

P. 90, *survey of adults with HIV infection attending an HIV clinic:* Niebuhr, V., Hughes, J., & Pollard, R. (1994). Parents with human immunodeficiency virus infection: Perceptions of their children's emotional needs. *Pediatrics, 93,* 421–426.

P. 92, *previous work done in constructing developmental schemata:* Bibace, R., & Walsh, M. (1981). Children's conceptions of illness. In R. Bibace, & M. Walsh (Eds.), *Children's conceptions of health, illness, and bodily functions.* San Francisco: Jossey-Bass.

P. 92, *disclosure is a process:* Pollack, S., & Boland, M. G. (1990). Children and HIV infection. *New Jersey Psychologist, 40,* 17–21.

P. 93, *may experience delayed growth rates:* Gertner, J., Kaufman, F., Donfield, S., Sleeper, L., Shapiro, A., Howard, C., Gomperts, E., & Hilgartner, M. (1994). Delayed somatic growth and pubertal development in human immunodeficiency virus–infected hemophiliac boys: Hemophilia growth and development study. *The Journal of Pediatrics, 124,* 896–902.

P. 93, *children can also experience learning disabilities:* Watkins, J., Brouwers, P., & Huntzinger, R. (1992). Neuropsychological assessment. In M. L. Stuber (Ed.), *Children and AIDS.* Washington, DC: American Psychiatric Press.

P. 93, *Research has found that children between the ages of six and eight:* Crisp, J., Ungerer, J., & Goodnow, J. (1996). The impact of experience on children's understanding of illness. *Journal of Pediatric Psychology, 21,* 57–72; Spinetta, J. (1974). The dying child's awareness of death: A review. *Psychological Bulletin, 81,* 256–260.

P. 94, *As of December 1994, a total of 1,304 males and 661 females:* Centers for Disease Control and Prevention (CDC). (1995). *HIV/AIDS Surveillance Report, 6*(2), 16.

P. 95, *14,112 females and 67,533 males:* Centers for Disease Control and Prevention (CDC). (1995). *HIV/AIDS Surveillance Report, 6*(2), 16.

P. 95, *infected during their adolescent years:* Hein, K. (1990). Lessons from New York City on HIV/AIDS in adolescents. *New York State Journal of Medicine, 90,* 143–145; Kalichman, S. C. (1995). *Understanding AIDS: A guide for mental health professionals.* Washington, DC: American Psychological Association.

P. 95, *Adolescent males, adolescents of color:* Gayle, H., & D'Angelo, L. J. (1991). Epidemiology of AIDS and HIV in adolescents. *Pediatric Infectious Disease Journal, 10,* 322–328; Vermund, S., Hein, K., Gayle, H., Carey, J., Thomas, P., & Drucker, E. (1989). AIDS among adolescents. *American Journal of Diseases in Children, 143,* 1220–1225.

P. 95, *Approximately one in four new seroconversions:* Rosenberg, P., Biggar, R., & Goedert, J. (1994). Declining age of HIV infection in the United States. *New England Journal of Medicine, 330,* 789–790.

P. 95, *Prevalence rates for other STDs:* Werner, M., & Biro, F. (1990). Contraception and sexually transmitted diseases in adolescent females. *Adolescent Pediatric Gynecology, 3,* 127–136.

P. 95, *Adolescence is a developmental period characterized by feelings of invulnerability:* Elkind, D. (1985). Egocentrism redux. *Developmental Review, 5,* 218–226; Hein, K. (1989). AIDS in adolescence: Exploring the challenge. *Journal of Adolescent Health Care, 10,* 10–35.

P. 95, *only 15 to 39 percent of adolescents reported a change:* Goodman, E., & Cohall, A. (1989). AIDS and adolescents: Knowledge, attitudes, beliefs, and behaviors in a New York City adolescent minority population. *Pediatrics, 84,* 36–42; Hingson, R., Strunin, L., & Berlin, B. (1989). AIDS transmission: Changes in knowledge and behaviors among adolescents, 1986 to 1988. *Pediatrics, 85,* 24–29; Hingson, R., Strunin, L., Berlin, B., & Heeren, T. (1990). Beliefs about AIDS, use of alcohol and drugs, and unprotected sex among Massachusetts adolescents. *American Journal of Public Health, 80,* 295–299.

P. 95, *commonly initiated during the adolescent years:* Kandel, D., & Logan, J. (1984). Patterns of drug use from adolescence to young adulthood: Periods of risk for initiation, continued use, and discontinuation. *American Journal of Public Health, 74,* 660–660; Bartlett, J., Keller, S., Eckholdt, H., & Schleifer, S. J. (1995). HIV-relevant issues in adolescents. In N. Boyd-Franklin, G. L. Steiner, & M. Boland (Eds.), *Children, families, and HIV/AIDS: Psychosocial and therapeutic issues.* New York: Guilford Press.

P. 95, *related increases in adolescent HIV cases can be expected:* Bartlett, J., Keller, S., Eckholdt, H., & Schleifer, S. J. (1995). HIV-relevant issues in adolescents. In N. Boyd-Franklin, G. L. Steiner, & M. Boland (Eds.), *Children, families, and HIV/AIDS: Psychosocial and therapeutic issues.* New York: Guilford Press.

P. 95, *By the age of twenty:* Centers for Disease Control and Prevention (CDC). (1992). Sexual behavior among high school students—United States, 1990. *Morbidity and Mortality Weekly Report, 40,* 885–888.

P. 96, *Adolescents begin having sexual intercourse:* Kalichman, S. C. (1995). *Understanding AIDS: A guide for mental health professionals.* Washington, DC:

American Psychological Association; Sonstein, F., Pleck, J., & Ku, L. (1989). Condom use and AIDS awareness among adolescent males. *Family Planning Perspectives, 21,* 152–158.

P. 96, *sexual risk-taking is highest among adolescents and young adults:* Boyer, C., & Kegeles, S. (1991). AIDS risk and prevention among adolescents. *Social Science Medicine, 33,* 11–23; Anderson, J., Kann, L., Holtzman, D., Arday, S., Truman, B., & Kolbe, L. (1990). HIV/AIDS knowledge and sexual behavior among high school students. *Family Planning Perspectives, 22,* 252–255; Hingson, R., Wenger, N., Greenberg, J., Hilborne, L., Kusseling, F., Mangotich, M., & Shapiro, M. F. (1992). Effect of HIV antibody testing and AIDS education on communication about HIV risk and sexual behavior. *Annals of Internal Medicine, 117,* 905–911.

P. 96, *In a study of adolescents (ages fourteen to nineteen):* Kegeles, S., Adler, N., & Irwin, C. (1988). Sexually active adolescents and condoms: Changes over one year in knowledge, attitudes and use. *American Journal of Public Health, 78,* 460–461.

P. 96, *A study of eighteen- and nineteen-year-old college students:* Rimburg, H., & Lewis, R. (1994). Older adolescents and AIDS: Correlates of self-reported safer sex practices. *Journal of Research on Adolescence, 4,* 453–464.

P. 96, *least likely to self-report condom use:* DiClemente, R., Durbin, M., Siegel, D., Krasnovsky, F., Lazarus, N., & Comacho, T. (1992). Determinants of condom use among junior high school students in a minority, inner-city school district. *Pediatrics, 89,* 197–201.

P. 96, *21 to 37 percent rarely or never used condoms:* Hingson, R., Wenger, N., Greenberg, J., Hilborne, L., Kusseling, F., Mangotich, M., & Shapiro, M. F. (1992). Effect of HIV antibody testing and AIDS education on communication about HIV risk and sexual behavior. *Annals of Internal Medicine, 117,* 905–911; Hingson, R., Strunin, L., Berlin, B., & Heeren, T. (1990). Beliefs about AIDS, use of alcohol and drugs, and unprotected sex among Massachusetts adolescents. *American Journal of Public Health, 80,* 295–299.

P. 96, *condom use among adolescents appears to decline:* Ku, L., Sonestein, F., & Pleck, J. (1994). The dynamics of young men's condom use during and across relationships. *Family Planning Perspectives, 26,* 246–251.

P. 97, *A comprehensive review of twenty-three school-based HIV/AIDS education programs:* Kirby, D., Short, L., Collins, J., Rugg, D., Kolbe, L., Howard, M., Miller, B., Sonenstein, F., & Zabin, L. (1994). School-based programs to reduce sexual risk behaviors: A review of effectiveness. *Public Health Reports, 109,* 339–360.

P. 97, *the following elements for a successful program:* Kirby, D., Short, L., Collins, J., Rugg, D., Kolbe, L., Howard, M., Miller, B., Sonenstein, F., & Zabin,

L. (1994). School-based programs to reduce sexual risk behaviors: A review of effectiveness. *Public Health Reports, 109,* 339–360.

P. 97, *although 75 percent of school-based sex education programs mention condoms:* Marsigalio, E., & Mott, F. L. (1986). The impact of sex education on sexual activity. *Family Planning Perspectives, 18,* 151–162.

P. 97, *for teenagers to use condoms:* Jemmott, J., Jemmott, L., & Gong, G. (1992). Reductions in HIV risk-associated sexual behaviors among Black male adolescents: Effects of an AIDS prevention intervention. *American Journal of Public Health, 82,* 372–377.

P. 98, *Adolescent dropouts tend to engage:* Centers for Disease Control and Prevention (CDC). (1994). Sexual behaviors and drug use among youth in dropout-prevention programs. *Morbidity and Mortality Weekly Report, 43,* 873–876.

P. 98, *increase in consistent condom use and a decrease in high-risk sexual behavior:* Rotheram-Borus, M. J., Koopman, C., Haignere, C., & Davies, M. (1991). Reducing HIV sexual risk behaviors among runaway adolescents. *Journal of the American Medical Association, 266,* 1237–1241.

P. 98, *developmental needs to take risks, develop their identity:* Baumrind, D. (1987). A developmental perspective on adolescent risk taking in contemporary America. In C. E. Irwin (Ed.), *Adolescent social behavior and health.* New Directions for Child Development, no. 37. San Francisco: Jossey-Bass; Shedler, J., & Block, J. (1990). Adolescent drug use and psychological health: A longitudinal study. *American Psychologist, 45,* 612–630.

P. 99, *Sexual behavior and related sexual issues:* Moore, S., Rosenthal, D., & Boldero, J. (1993). Predicting AIDS-preventive behaviour among adolescents. In D. J. Terry, C. Gallois, & M. McCamish (Eds.), *The theory of reasoned action: Its application to AIDS-preventive behaviour.* New York: Pergamon.

P. 101, *"most useful" by a cohort of HIV-infected adolescents:* Brown, L., Schultz, J., & Gragg, R. (1995). HIV-infected adolescents with hemophilia: Adaptation and coping. *Pediatrics, 96,* 459–463.

P. 101, *Drug and alcohol use among adolescents:* Siegel, A., Cousins, J., Rubovits, D., Parsons, J., Lavery, B., & Crowley, C. (1994). Adolescents' perceptions of the benefits and risks of their own risk taking. *Journal of Emotional and Behavioral Disorders, 2,* 89–98.

P. 101, *unprotected sexual behaviors:* Siegel, A., Cousins, J., Rubovits, D., Parsons, J., Lavery, B., & Crowley, C. (1994). Adolescents' perceptions of the benefits and risks of their own risk taking. *Journal of Emotional and Behavioral Disorders, 2,* 89–98; Bartlett, J., Keller, S., Eckholdt, H., & Schleifer, S. (1995). HIV-relevant issues in adolescents. In N. Boyd-Franklin, G. L.

Steiner, & M. Boland (Eds.), *Children, families, and HIV/AIDS: Psychosocial and therapeutic issues.* New York: Guilford Press.

P. 101, *reported engaging in sexual intercourse after drinking alcohol:* Hingson, R., Strunin, L., Berlin, B., & Heeren, T. (1990). Beliefs about AIDS, use of alcohol and drugs, and unprotected sex among Massachusetts adolescents. *American Journal of Public Health, 80,* 295–299.

P. 101, *A study of adolescents with hemophilia and HIV infection:* Brown, L., Schultz, J., & Gragg, R. (1995). HIV-infected adolescents with hemophilia: Adaptation and coping. *Pediatrics, 96,* 459–463.

P. 102, *the health status of a person with HIV infection or an AIDS-related diagnosis:* Hein, K. (1990). Lessons from New York City on HIV/AIDS in adolescents. *New York State Journal of Medicine, 90,* 143–145.

P. 102, *A variety of forms of sexual activity:* Savin-Williams, R. (1995). Lesbian, gay male, and bisexual adolescents. In A. R. D'Augelli & C. Patterson (Eds.), *Lesbian, gay, and bisexual identities over the lifespan.* New York: Oxford University Press.

P. 102, *Various studies have identified high seroincidence rates:* Osmond, D., Page, K., Wiley, J., Garrett, K., Sheppard, H. W., Moss, A. R., Shrager, L., & Winkelstein, W. (1994). HIV infection in homosexual and bisexual men 18–29 years of age: The San Francisco young men's health study. *American Journal of Public Health, 84,* 1933–1937; Lemp, G., Hirozawa, A., Givertz, D., Nieri, G. N., Anderson, L., Lindegren, M. L., Janssen, R. S., Katz, M. (1994). Seroprevalence of HIV and risk behaviors among young homosexual and bisexual men: The San Francisco/Berkeley young men's survey. *Journal of the American Medical Association, 272,* 449–454; Dean, L., & Meyer, I. (1995). HIV prevalence and sexual behavior in a cohort of New York City gay men (aged 18–24). *Journal of Acquired Immune Deficiency Syndrome, 8,* 208–211.

P. 102, *43 percent reported engaging in unprotected anal intercourse:* Hays, R., Kegeles, S., & Coates, T. (1990). High HIV risk-taking among young gay men. *AIDS, 4,* 901–907.

P. 102, *Another study of adolescent gay and bisexual males:* Remafedi, G. (1994). Predictors of unprotected intercourse among gay and bisexual youth: Knowledge, beliefs, and behavior. *Pediatrics, 94,* 163–168.

P. 103, *may not know about the risk of HIV without prior education:* Paroski, T. (1987). Health care delivery and concerns of gay and lesbian adolescents. *Journal of Adolescent Health Care, 8,* 188–192.

P. 103, *perceive AIDS and HIV to be problems only for older gay men:* Remafedi, G. (1994). Predictors of unprotected intercourse among gay and bisexual youth: Knowledge, beliefs, and behavior. *Pediatrics, 94,* 163–168.

P. 103, *adolescents feel that it "can't happen to me":* Elkind, D. (1967). Egocentrism in adolescence. *Child Development, 38,* 1025–1034; Hays, R., Kegeles, S., & Coates, T. (1990). High HIV risk-taking among young gay men. *AIDS, 4,* 901–907.

P. 103, *"coming out" issues among gay youth:* Savin-Williams, R. (1995). Lesbian, gay male, and bisexual adolescents. In A. R. D'Augelli & C. Patterson (Eds.), *Lesbian, gay, and bisexual identities over the lifespan.* New York: Oxford University Press.

P. 103, *reduce the gay teenager's motivation to engage in safer sexual behaviors:* Gonsoriek, J. (1989). Mental health issues of gay and lesbian adolescents. *Journal of Adolescent Medicine, 9,* 114–122.

P. 103, *may prevent infected gay teenagers from seeking out support services:* Grossman, A. (1994). Homophobia: A cofactor of HIV disease in gay and lesbian youth. *Journal of the Association of Nurses in AIDS Care, 5,* 39–43.

P. 104, *One successful program in Minnesota:* Remafedi, G. (1994). Cognitive and behavioral adaptations to HIV/AIDS among gay and bisexual adolescents. *Journal of Adolescent Health, 15,* 142–148.

P. 104, *a study of intensive, multisession, small-group interventions:* Rotheram-Borus, M., Koopman, C., Haignere, C., Davies, M. (1991). Reducing HIV sexual risk behaviors among runaway adolescents. *Journal of the American Medical Association, 266,* 1237–1241.

4

TREATING GAY MEN WITH HIV

Michael F. O'Connor

The specter of a potentially fatal illness is enough to foster enormous distress in the strongest of us. Some individuals will use such an event to grow and change. Others will be chronically overwhelmed by the diagnosis, possibly falling into a stance of stubborn hopelessness, anger, and victimization. Still others will land somewhere between these two extremes, adapting as best they can to what is typically the most challenging event of their lives.

As a psychologist, I have worked since the early eighties with HIV and with gay men. When I entered clinical training, the disease had not yet been discovered. Now I, like many others, cannot imagine my current reality, work or play, without it. And I have been profoundly affected by the lives I have shared with this disease. These individuals have certainly left me richer.

There are many important things to understand in treating gay men. HIV provides a new and formidable wrinkle, but it is only a part of the larger cultural fabric surrounding this group.

In my early work with HIV among gay men, I assumed that the previously mentioned range of reactions pretty much covered what I would be up against. I knew the work would be difficult, but felt certain that I had the ability to understand and respond to such reactions. So it struck me as odd at first that the men in my practice were not afraid of sickness and dying so much as of the reactions of the world to their disease. They could face their demise fairly steadily, but their families only with enormous trepidation. I was amazed at the incredible strength they exhibited in the face of terrifying circumstances; I was troubled by what their interpersonal anxiety might reflect. It quickly became clear that for most gay men, HIV is their worst nightmare come true not only for obvious medical reasons but for even more immediate social and psychological ones. The difficulty of adjustment to a serious, and likely fatal, illness is complicated by several factors related not to death and dying so much as to living and the struggle for identity and acceptance. The gay man dealing with concerns about HIV often faces a battle he has fought for years—the battle over intolerance.

There are many wonderful people both inside and outside the gay community who are willing and able to help, and certainly have done so. But the HIV epidemic reflects all that is wrong with our culture's notions of morality, illness, and minority status, as well as the incredible depth of human compassion and strength in the face of adversity. If we are to help gay men in the struggle against this disease, we must attend carefully to the psychological and social effects as well as to the physiological effects of the virus on the individual.

It is impossible to treat a gay man for HIV-related psychological concerns without understanding the broad-ranging impact an HIV-positive diagnosis is likely to have, beyond that typically associated with serious illness.

Perhaps no modern minority group remains more fully repudiated, nor held in lower esteem in this culture than are gay men, with the possible exception of pederasts. And in the average person's mind, pederasts are often erroneously associated with homosexuality. Research has even shown that lesbian women tend to be viewed more positively than gay men. The reasons for this fact are at once fascinating and elusive, having as much to do with values related to masculinity, femininity, and power perhaps as with the behavior of the individuals in question. So it is not homosexuality per se that accounts for the repudiation of the gay man by segments of this society, but something more: a matter of evolved patterns of dominance, an evolutionary response to the unknown, a Freudian response to the too familiar—whatever. As the mental health provider preparing to approach the gay man with HIV concerns, one must become familiar with the likely enormity of an experience of chronic prejudice and oppression, trauma either witnessed or experienced, and ongoing marginality. Only then can the overlay of loss, bereavement, and the ravages of a deadly illness begin to be addressed. Only then can the therapist experience the necessary empathic response.

Gay men have usually been faced with social obstacles from an early age. Many, though not all, have had experiences of discrimination and marginality even before grammar school, and almost certainly in the latency period of development. Stories abound of boys who were picked last for sports teams, called "sissies," teased or ridiculed by peers and, in not a few cases, assaulted. This results from the apparent difference evident in their behavior and manner, in many cases. Gay men as children are often noticed as different, less "boy-like," and as having interests that are atypical for the majority of boys. Those who are more sex-role typical are at the very least likely to witness what happens to those who are not.

Consequently, most gay men as children have been the victim or witness of discrimination—on the playground, in the community, and even in the family living room. Other minority-group children might return to their family home with a sense of sameness, even belonging, in the company of their relatives and neighbors. Whatever else their reality may contain in the way of hardship, they are not without company in their minority status. Gay men, on the other hand, may learn from an early age that they are different from virtually all those around them. They are also likely to learn in childhood that their difference is neither positive nor speakable.

A recent study showed that 58 percent of gay men reported some form of victimization related to their sexual orientation in the previous year, and 78 percent had been victimized as a result of anti-gay bias sometime during the period beginning at age six-teen. These findings did not include verbal threats. When the latter are included, fully 88 percent of the men surveyed reported such an event since the age of sixteen. This experience of oppression and marginality—of being a "minority of one" who is then identified with a stigmatized group—sets the stage for many of the most important issues to arise in psychotherapy with the gay man, especially in therapy related to HIV.

In this chapter, we will review the impact of this enculturation and its connection to treatment concerns and objectives. We will also examine our culture's reaction to HIV and the consequent doubling of impact this creates for the gay man. We will then explore assessment and treatment objectives and strategies, as they relate to each phase of illness. The chapter concludes with a discussion of termination issues and provider concerns.

HIV, STIGMA, AND THE HISTORICAL CONTEXT

HIV disease was first identified as Acquired Immune Deficiency Syndrome (AIDS) in 1981. The disease has also been called the "gay cancer" or "gay plague," and, by the medical establishment, "Gay-Related Immune Deficiency (GRID). It is important to establish that in the United States, the disease was linked to homosexuality from the very start of its examination by both medical and media sources. This was not the case in Africa, where transmission of the virus primarily occurred through het-erosexual contact. In the early 1980s, the disease was also asso-ciated with hemophiliacs, Haitians, and IV-drug users, and discussions of the disease through the late 1980s typically focused on treating members of these and other groups (women and adolescents, for example). In retrospect, we can say that such an orientation to the disease may have in part served a defensive function for those trying to understand it. Reflecting a pre-dictable response of the public to a new and devastating scourge,

HIV disease was conveniently seen as circumscribed by minority group status. Thus, although HIV disease was a worrisome (if distant) reality, most individuals who were not members of these groups felt insulated from its devastation. It couldn't happen to them.

However, it has now become clear that the group to which one belongs is not the best predictor of disease incidence. Rather, it is behavior, and perhaps fate—not affiliation—that are responsible for the spread of the virus. Nonetheless, in the minds of many, the connection between minority status and HIV remains as strong as ever.

Cultural Values

Gregory Herek, a social psychologist, has studied the sources of both homophobia and AIDS phobia. He has noted that illness and stigma historically have often been linked and that disease is in large part a social construction. He points out that cholera, an epidemic in this country in the early nineteenth century, was broadly seen as the result of moral failings, in part because it affected the poor in larger numbers, and the poor were already marginalized by society. Herek also notes that the conflict between moralism and pragmatism was evident in that era, as it was to be in the AIDS epidemic.

The moralistic perspective focuses on the moral evaluation of behavior and outcome, and from this proposes a course of action. Prayer, banishment, and exorcism are possible alternatives in the moralistic view of how to grapple with disease, as is abstinence and social conscientiousness. The latter alternatives may have obvious benefit to a society. But it is surely as true that many people can be unfairly harmed by an analysis and action plan based on moral teachings as opposed to medical fact.

The pragmatic approach to disease would therefore argue for factual underpinnings to proposed actions, and for solutions that are intended to say little about the moral characterization of the disease, speaking instead to its pragmatic resolution through prevention and medical treatment, for example. Herek has noted that the pragmatic perspective is still influenced by the culture from which it derives, and may therefore carry a moral message. Thus the framing of HIV disease, as it was first examined, was representative of the cultural values from which it derived, according to this analysis.

Herek goes on to show that depending on how a disease is seen to originate—by way of behavior as opposed to fate, for example—victims of the disease are frequently defined in terms of innocence and guilt. The media, the medical establishment, and the government responded in just such terms to the emergence of AIDS. Media interest in the disease increased enormously once heterosexual partners of infected individuals were identified, whereas prior to this time, media coverage in the mainstream press was minimal. Ronald Reagan did not mention AIDS publicly until 1987, six years after the disease was first identified, and his secretary of Health and Human Services, Margaret Heckler, was quoted in 1985 as having an interest in stopping the disease "before it affects the heterosexual population and the general population." Initial scientific investigations focused on sexual behaviors and drug use ("poppers," for example) among gay men, in particular, thereby framing the disease as behaviorally related, but only relative to certain groups.

We now know, of course, that heterosexuals are also at risk on the basis of behavior. One could argue that the scientific community responded to the obvious sources of the disease first. Yet the disease was known to be heterosexually transmitted in Africa and Haiti, where sexual behavior was also a consideration, and where poppers were not in popular use. Was it more interesting or compelling for investigators to consider extreme sexual behavior and drug use, as opposed to the more the mundane transmission routes shared by other sexually transmitted diseases? Herek would argue that the culturally biased morality of the era

Influenced both the framing and the initial direction of investigators.

Deserving the Disease

HIV disease, like other sexually transmitted diseases, is commonly associated with sexual behavior and therefore, to a greater or lesser extent, with controversial behavior. Persons with HIV disease have been discriminated against from the beginning of the epidemic; in the minds of many Americans, these individuals somehow deserved the illness that struck them. Members of the Christian Right were among the first to publicly pronounce this conclusion. Such action is consistent with the moralist view previously described and with accepted theories about stigma and its development.

However, the notion of moral failing consistently met its match with the infected hemophiliac, who, though innocent of an identifiable behavioral or character transgression, seemed also to receive comparatively little attention. And even among this group, as with other groups that are atypical in some way, the experience of HIV-related discrimination was not and still is not unknown. Perhaps the conflict between moralist and pragmatic perspectives was best exemplified in the early debate about hemophiliacs and HIV. Many who felt most strongly that the disease was deserved had trouble arguing that case concerning this group of individuals.

In any case, HIV disease was a terrific tool for anyone who wanted or needed a reason to discriminate against gays, blacks, or drug users. Once again, disease became an opportunity to further ostracize and definitively separate those already marginalized from "the rest of us."

In concert with medical science, the media fueled public attention early on with a focus on gay men's drug use and sexual behavior. Promiscuity was of particular interest, even though it is now clear that it is not the number of partners but the risks taken and, of course, the partner's serostatus that accounts for viral transmission. The focus on number of sexual partners, extreme sexual behavior, and drug use and abuse served to exacerbate existing negative stereotypes about gay men.

For gay men themselves, the disease and accompanying public comment and coverage, warnings, and proscriptions served to reinforce an already common problem with healthy self-esteem. The timing could hardly have been worse. Gays and lesbians had witnessed enormous changes in their level of freedom from the previous decade. After the Stonewall riots of 1969, up to and including the emergence of gay pride celebrations in most major cities in the 1970s and early 1980s, gays and lesbians were beginning to experience personal pride and social integration in a way never before achieved. Legal hurdles, to equal housing and job protection for example, were overcome in many communities by way of local referenda. A large number of gays and lesbians began the painful and glorious process of "coming out" in a context of camaraderie and optimism, and with increasing support from non-gays.

But the 1980s were by many standards a decade of excess. This was certainly the case for many gays as well as for drug users, baby boomers, and financial opportunists. The economy was booming and people were spending, especially for the latest and the greatest. The pervasive morality that characterized this era is reflected in caricature by *Dynasty*, one of the most popular television shows of that time. If the 1970s ushered in a permissive "me" generation, then the 1980s funded the movement. But while broad segments of the population of the country were indulging themselves in one way or another, a deadly virus was establishing a foothold. When the disease was identified, many hopes and dreams were put on hold or cruelly crushed. It was easy for a gay man to think "I knew it was too good to be true."

As Owen, forty-four, put it: "We were like kids in a candy store. The possibility of openly approaching another man for a date, to flirt in public, to be surrounded by other men like us, was overwhelming. And we ate it up. A typical weekend night started at the bars and ended at the baths. Sex was free and very, very easy. I think most of us knew this was extreme behavior. But it was very exciting, and we had been denied so long."

Stigma and HIV

The stigma associated with HIV emanates from several sources. We have discussed the historical link between illness and stigma. HIV is a viral, contagious illness. It is most frequently sexually transmitted. Perhaps most important, however, is its association with gay men and other marginalized groups. HIV stigma is in many respects an extension of the stigma of homosexuality. Gays have frequently been seen as mysterious, dangerous, mentally abnormal, and even contagious. These ascriptions have been associated with other stigmatized groups. Enter a disease that is in fact contagious, and the leap from stereotypical to emblematic is an easy one. Hence, the reality of HIV infection for many gay men is a validation of the stereotype of being "ill." A history of psychiatric musings that defend this now well refuted notion is well known to most gays.

American psychiatry has been particularly damaging to the cause of truth and clarity about what gay men are or are not, having claimed at various times that homosexuality is perverse, reflects paranoia or narcissism, and can and should be corrected. Modern research with unbiased samples proved these conclusions erroneous. Yet despite the ultimate conclusions of the American Psychological Association and the American Psychiatric Association that homosexuality does not constitute psychopathology, and despite the fact that such treatments have not been proven to be effective, practitioners still offer "conversion" therapies designed to change sexual orientation. Most gay men are aware of the availability of such "treatments." An unfortunate number of people have been victimized by providers of these treatments, only to be told that the failure was theirs when the treatment didn't take. To encounter a disease that seems to strike gay men specifically is yet another terrific blow to whatever fragile peace the individual may have come to regarding his sexual orientation. Likewise, the media and medical establishment's framing of the disease with such a slant added salt to the wound.

In addition to the very real effects of the disease in the gay community, it is fair to speculate that the agenda of those who would deny equal rights to gays and lesbians was furthered by the growing presence of HIV in the gay community. In any case, many of the hard-won battles for gay rights were countered in the late 1980s and early 1990s by centralized efforts to reverse legislation and rekindle hatred toward gays. This, with the community on its sickbed.

HIV and Identity

These events and their consequences can prove overwhelming to the gay man grappling with HIV. Considerations of HIV and its meaning raise the familiar questions of self-worth and identity, and existential concerns. HIV infection is likely to cause a reevaluation of these concerns whether or not they were previously laid to rest. Because many gay men have adapted to a stigmatized role by way of a combination of confrontation, assimilation, and denial, those conflicts that have been denied (for example, sick versus healthy, sexually aberrant versus sexually OK, able to integrate with society versus needing to hide away) quickly come up for reexamination.

It is easy for the gay man in this context to assume that HIV disease is evidence of all that is wrong with him and his sexual orientation. The experience of marginality and oppression from childhood is easily reinforced. In addition, the issue of "concealability," a factor in the experience of stigma, is raised. HIV-infected individuals may spend years in an asymptomatic phase during which the disease is not visibly obvious to others. This experience often recapitulates the gay man's earlier struggle with sexual orientation and "coming out." Indeed, many of the issues are the same. Whom to tell, when, and "what then" are common concerns for the HIV-infected individual, and are unfortunately all too familiar.

DAVID

David was a successful vice president for a computer-related start-up company when he contacted me for an initial appointment. His business had prospered, to no small extent due to his diligence, and he was well respected for his business acumen. The HIV-positive diagnosis was like a body-blow. The stress of the illness pressed him to be more authentic at work with his boss and managers, yet he feared their reaction to his sexual orientation and his illness. In treatment, he began almost immediately to examine long-held feelings of inadequacy, of being different in some shameful way. The pain he'd experienced in childhood was palpable.

As a child, he had constantly sought his parents' attention and interest. He was a clever, pleasing, and adult-oriented child. His mother would alternately reinforce his affections and show disdain for his dependent or nonmasculine traits. He was held at a distance by his father and brother, who were clearly more alike and therefore aligned. He had learned to adopt a funny, pleasing persona that asked little of anyone and disclosed little of himself in the process. Under the circumstances, his old defenses were both rekindled and useless.

People with AIDS have been shown to be more negatively evaluated than people with other diseases. The gay man with HIV must decide whether to be honest about his illness with others— "discredited" in Goffman's terms—or "discreditable," that is, hidden. But one who is hidden must constantly cope with the risk of discovery. Even those who opt to expose the truth of their illness to others are often reinforced for hiding the intensity, or the ugly details, of dealing with it. They are reinforced to make a "good adjustment" to the illness, at least publicly.

This strategy is likely to cue up emotional responses from the past, as in David's case. It is not unusual for a gay man, infected or otherwise, to need a review of the traumatic events of his developmental history in the course of psychotherapeutic treatment. That history is likely to include experiences of teasing, denigration, and disappointment from parents, adults, and peers, and of marginality and oppression, whether witnessed or experienced. Additionally, he will likely suffer or witness marginality and oppression in an ongoing way as it is exemplified in the cultural debate or by more personal experience. Now there is a new reason, this one with deadly consequences.

THERAPEUTIC OPPORTUNITY

Despite the horror of HIV disease, the affected individual is faced with enormous opportunities for growth. This notion is important, among other reasons because it provides propulsion for the therapeutic work. Most men can understand this point, but for many, the therapist's framing of opportunity is all-important.

Naturally, this must be accomplished with great sensitivity. The individual in shock from a recent diagnosis, or deep in grieving for a lost loved one or for his own former capacities, will not be ready for such an interpretation. At some point in therapy, most men will have the capacity to see the changes they have made or are making, however. These effects may fuel optimism and offer respite and hope, and should therefore be identified by the therapist, if the client has not already noticed. These changes also help to create a positive focus for the provider and act as a counterforce to the many difficult realities of treating HIV disease.

The client has the opportunity to

- Become more authentic
- Improve self-esteem and its foundation in the self

- Resolve old conflicts—with self, family, and others
- Decrease isolation and increase a sense of belonging
- Learn to accept help
- Learn to be imperfect
- Explore and experience emotion
- Live more fully in the moment
- Stop procrastinating—to act on wishes
- Come to terms with his sexual orientation
- Review existential and spiritual issues

STUART

Stuart was a medical doctor by profession, and a friend of mine. He worked in the emergency room as a trauma physician, in part, as he said, "because you only see the patient once." Stuart could tell you the incidence rate of tuberculosis in the homeless, the number of stitches a wound would require, the exact distance from Paris to New York, and any of a long list of learned facts about the world.

But in his presence one felt dwarfed by his intelligence and stymied by his absolute control over emotion. This was not a man who cried in his beer. Over the course of sixteen months from diagnosis, he went from the literally mad scientist, searching for every new piece of information he could get his hands on related to HIV, to a nature lover who took long walks, read poetry, and even cried. Somehow the disease had allowed a softer side of him to emerge. His friends were startled and sometimes unsettled by his behavior, yet all agreed he had never seemed so much at peace with himself.

Some would argue that a central goal of psychotherapy is to increase the individual's capacity for authenticity. By *authenticity* I mean the pragmatic joining of real self and persona in as seamless a way as possible. From a psychodynamic perspective, authenticity reflects the need to integrate all aspects of oneself, including those considered unbecoming or dangerous, in order to achieve mental health.

Living authentically, one is, as much as possible, the same on the outside as on the inside. For most of us, the many needs and goals in our lives collude at times to prevent an authentic presentation in public, and perhaps even in private. We are likely to create a persona that meets our needs in specific environments, such as work, social settings, and so on. We don't tell the police officer who stopped us for speeding to take a leap, nor do we tell our boss that his arrogance is beyond comprehension. The persona is necessary and pragmatic both culturally and socially, but personally may cause enormous stress as one attempts to shelter disavowed aspects of self from prying eyes.

Often, these considerations are relatively unconflicted, and the individual is able to balance the need for social tact and pragmatism with the need to project a true and consistent identity. Sometimes, however, confusion results—about values, direction, commitment, and the like. And at other times, the authentic self is almost completely separated from consciousness, and the individual lives an existence devoid of emotional connection to self and, therefore, to others.

For the gay man, disavowal of sexual orientation is likely to occur at the very least in the early stages of sexual identity development. We know, for example, that most gay men do not self-identify as gay until their late teens or early twenties. This is often true despite their having had a long-term awareness of same-sex sexual attraction, and their disavowal may persist even after same-sex sexual contact. Many gay men do not begin to integrate their sexual identity, which typically includes "coming out," until much later.

This experience of covering and later exposing oneself cuts both ways, relative to HIV. The individual may well know how to hide, but he may also know the value of opening up to and joining with others. For the individual who has not yet integrated his sexual identity into his self-image, HIV infection represents a double crisis. For those in the midst of such integration, various courses are possible. The disease may speed the process of sexual identity integration, as the individual risks disclosure in order to get much-needed support. Infection may drive the individual back into the closet, confirming that to be gay is at worst wrong, and at best unworkable.

We cannot overestimate the importance of the strategy chosen. In particular, those who choose to avoid the issue entirely are at significant risk for emotional disturbance, as we shall soon discuss. There is also the possibility that HIV, and even imminent death, can free a person to engage in behaviors and realize dreams that were heretofore unimaginable. So much of what the individual experiences depends on the meaning ascribed to infection, and on the developmental stage, and the disease stage, at which he is diagnosed.

ASSESSMENT AND TREATMENT

For the purposes of assessment and treatment, it is convenient to separate HIV-affected individuals into four categories, as follows:

1. Those who are uninfected, but are affected by the disease in other ways, commonly known as the "worried well"

2. Those who have recently discovered seroconversion

3. Those who have known of their infection for a time but remain largely asymptomatic

4. Those who are in the midst of experiencing the usually progressive symptoms and infections resulting from significant immunosuppression, including those with AIDS

Naturally, an individual may discover his infection only after the immune system is largely compromised and physical symptoms are upon him. Others may know of their infection almost immediately after infection. Still others may be infected for many years without significant symptoms.

Luckily, much has been discovered about how to assess and treat individuals in these stages, which will be reviewed in the remainder of this chapter. However, it is important to understand that new treatments are allowing individuals to live longer and, increasingly, to be effectively treated for previously debilitating symptoms. Pentamidine has enormously reduced risk for *Pneumocystis carinii* pneumonia (PCP), for example, and AZT and other antiretroviral drugs have allowed patients to extend the asymptomatic period significantly. Protease inhibitors and so-called "combinant therapies" hold promise for eliminating viral presence in the body, and even restoration of the immune system in some cases. The playing field is constantly changing, and it is crucial that clinicians be up-to-date on the latest developments in medical treatment and psychological assistance relevant to HIV. (The reader is referred to Chapter Two of this book, David Ostrow's excellent review of current medical understanding.)

It is also crucial that the clinician meet the individual where he is in terms of needs, capacities, and responsive style. An individual recently diagnosed will likely be in shock initially, but if he is also symptomatic, he may need to make immediate decisions about treatment and sharing information about his illness. Similarly, he may need to make important employment and financial decisions. This individual's adaptive time line is compressed, and the opportunity to gradually develop an understanding of the disease and its meaning will take a back seat to the need for immediate interventions.

Likewise, an individual who has been aware of, but in denial about, his diagnosis will inevitably experience greater trauma at the point at which symptoms emerge. He may present much like the individual just described, despite the time he has had to adjust to his illness. Some individuals take comfort in establishing a scientific and theoretical knowledge base about the disease, and there is some evidence to suggest that this will improve the doctor-patient relationship as well as the course of treatment. Others may be more in need of emotional support, and establishing social contacts will be most important. Still others will need to focus first on identifying providers, financial concerns, immediate loss issues, or issues about disclosure. Naturally, as with all psychotherapy candidates, the individual's personality and personal style will largely circumscribe their treatment options as well as the clinician's optimal approach. A fine and empathic attunement to the client is necessary in all cases.

Preexisting Conditions

Individuals with psychiatric problems prior to infection are more likely to have them after infection. The most severe problems will usually occur among this group. It is estimated, for example, that 78 percent of HIV-infected individuals diagnosed as depressed had a history of depression prior to HIV infection diagnosis. Gay men have been shown to have lifetime prevalence rates for major depression in the 25 to 35 percent range and for alcohol and substance abuse in the range of 25 to 40 percent, both significantly above that found in the general population. These estimates are about comparable for both HIV-positive and HIV-negative individuals. Current rates of alcohol abuse are now actually comparable to the general population, however. This fact may reflect the recent seriousness with which the gay community has taken messages about the danger of alcohol abuse, both as a risk factor in unsafe sexual practices and as a problem in its own right.

Anxiety disorders have been shown to be likewise elevated among gay men, with the exception of Panic Disorder and Obsessive-Compulsive Disorder, again at levels comparable for seropositive and seronegative individuals. It is beyond the purpose of this chapter to discuss the possible reasons for these findings, although the experience of marginalization and oppression described previously may offer some meaningful suggestions.

PHASE I: THE WORRIED WELL

Although uninfected, the normative gay man is likely to be worried about infection to a greater or lesser degree. He is also likely to have experienced multiple losses as a result of AIDS. One recent study found that approximately 90 percent of gay men in the sample had been tested for the HIV antibody, and that the average gay man had lost two lovers or close friends *and* three casual friends or acquaintances to AIDS. In 1992 in San Francisco, as many as 43 percent of the gay male population was infected with the virus. For the newly emerging closeted gay man, for the sexually active gay man, for the gay man unresolved about his sexuality, and for anyone who has gay friends or acquaintances, anxiety about HIV is virtually inevitable, given these astounding rates of loss and infection.

Adjustment disorders are in fact the most common diagnosis in all phases of infection, affecting two-thirds of one outpatient sample, for example. Among the uninfected, anxiety is the most common symptom of an adjustment reaction or disorder. Similarly, uncertainty about exposure to the virus is more related to a depressive response than is certainty, of either a positive or negative antibody finding. This may seem surprising at first glance. How could an individual with a seropositive diagnosis be less depressed than one not yet diagnosed? The finding seems to reflect the centering power of predictability; we will discuss this later on.

A common scenario involves a man who develops a fear that he has been infected. This may begin with a dream, a conversation about HIV, knowledge that an acquaintance or friend has been infected, an article in the newspaper, or even some positive event in his life—in short, as with other anxiety reactions, the precipitant may vary widely. Research has shown that the individual who is most likely to have an anxiety reaction in this phase is the one who has least well integrated his sexual identity into his personality and lifestyle. Although he is likely to have a low-risk sexual history, he has engaged in covert and guilt-producing sexual behavior since adolescence, typically, and is socially iso-lated. This man is likely to have greater levels of conflict about being gay, might not self-identify as gay despite the fact that he is sexual with other men, and is not open about his sexual orien-tation.

ALLEN

Allen was thirty-five and a successful middle-level manager when he sought my help related to extreme distress he'd been experiencing about AIDS. Allen had been in psychotherapy with me previously, and had made significant gains in his interpersonal capacities and in adapting to a gay identity. He had also begun to allow emotional expression without feeling shame, a new experience for him. He had left treatment at the point at which he began to explore his anger with his father. He had related a history of physical and emotional abuse, but could not tolerate further work in this area at that time.

For nine months before his second intake, he'd had nightmares about being infected, had found himself sweating excessively, and had had chronic bouts of diarrhea. He was so distraught that he had put off being tested again for the HIV antibody, fearing that he could not handle the inevitable news that he was infected. In addition, he had told no one about his fears, not even his lover of one year.

He finally scheduled a therapy appointment while awaiting the antibody test results. He was quite fearful at intake, had continued to have sweats, diarrhea, and sleep disturbance, and was distracted most of the time. In the current round of treatment, it became clear that his anxiety about AIDS coincided with at least two events: first, the deepening of his commitment to a lover and consequently to the "gay" lifestyle, and second, a visit with his lover to his family home in an ultra-conservative and highly Christian Missouri town. Though Allen had not yet come out to his parents, his lover behaved with them in a way that made it clear that the two were partners.

Allen's mother at one point fled dinner in tears, and thereafter refused to be in the same room with the two of them. His mother had remained distant since the visit. Allen felt guilty that he had neither tried to comfort his mother nor confronted her to discuss the circumstances. He berated himself heavily for these failings, and also began to have significant suicidal ideation. In addition to his work in session, he was encouraged to talk to his lover, who was apparently quite supportive, about these feelings. As a result of a heated argument between the two of them, he finally did so.

During the course of treatment, in addition to learning he was HIV seronegative, he also discovered how conflicted he was about the meaning of his sexuality and its place in his life. Although he'd found a behavioral adaptation to his homosexuality, he had not come to emotional terms with that reality—he had avoided it. By bringing his lover home to his parents, he was doing unconsciously what he could not consciously choose to do. And his parents got the message. But, as was typical in this family, nothing was discussed.

The result was tremendous anxiety about his parents' love and approval, linked as well to unresolved issues concerning his parents' response to him as a child. This anxiety was unconsciously converted to anxiety about AIDS, emblematic of the intense ambivalence and guilt Allen felt about his homosexuality.

The dynamics in this case are consistent with descriptions in the literature of anxiety and its etiology, corresponding to this phase. It is important to note that symptoms of anxiety are often similar to some of those that may indicate HIV infection, such as sweating and diarrhea. Consequently, the clinician must be careful not to collude with an individual's fears before medical confirmation of infection is established.

Poor resolution of adjustment disorders in this phase has been linked to a history of psychological disturbance, increased social isolation, and decreased perceived acceptance from peers or family, as well as to guilt related to sexual behavior or lifestyle. Consequently, individuals in this phase should be encouraged to look at the nature of their adjustment to sexual orientation and identity, including guilty or self-denigrating feelings; to become less isolated; and to get treatment for long-standing psychological problems.

Considering that rates of substance use and abuse may be elevated in this community, careful assessment of these behaviors is important. Alternative measures for dealing with stress, as well as identifying stressor sources and options, may be useful.

Testing

The question of testing is an important one and should be discussed at length both before referral for testing is initiated and while awaiting results. Research has shown that a sudden diagnosis without consent or pre-counseling is likely to be particularly traumatic for the individual, and may more readily lead to suicidal responses. The process of deciding and proceeding to get tested usually engenders anxiety for the gay man. This has been shown to be influenced in part by the extent to which the individual has, or believes he has, engaged in unsafe sexual practices.

Uncertainty about exposure to the virus, again, has been linked to higher levels of depression. As the guidelines for "safer sex" are not definitive, regarding the risk of oral sex for example, most sexually active gay men will have some concern. Those who have engaged in receptive anal intercourse without the protection of a condom are most at risk both for infection and for anxiety about it, all other factors being equal.

Bereavement

AIDS-related bereavement has been found to be another significant problem for gay men seeking psychotherapy in this and other phases of HIV infection. As noted previously, the average gay man experiences a high rate of personal loss due to HIV-related deaths of friends and acquaintances. Symptoms may include those commonly associated with Posttraumatic Stress

Disorder (PTSD), including emotional numbing, sleep disturbance and nightmares, hopelessness, loss of meaning in life, and suicidal ideation. Additionally, there may be significant survivor guilt and, perhaps more troubling, a sense of inevitability concerning personal infection with the virus.

This latter symptom is very important, as it may lead to high-risk sexual behaviors and substance use and abuse, which has been linked to greater risk of infection. Likewise, self-blaming and self-punishment have been shown to increase the likelihood of high-risk sexual behavior. Consequently, the therapist should emphasize that infection is not inevitable and encourage the exploration of underlying feelings in such a response, especially those related to self-blame. It is also reasonable to encourage discussion of the impact on the individual of the infection of others around him. Survivor guilt and trauma response may have a significant impact on perceptions of the inevitability of infection.

VINCENT

Vincent came to therapy confused and disorganized. He'd lost several friends and a former lover to AIDS within the last year, and his most recent lover had died of the disease. He'd expressed no emotion since the loss three months earlier and reported feeling like he was "numb" all the time. He also had few hopes for the future, and wondered how and why he'd escaped infection himself. He was particularly troubled by the way he'd handled his lover's recent death. His partner, apparently understanding how difficult the final phase of his illness was for Vincent, or perhaps needing to emotionally distance himself from Vincent before dying, had insisted that another friend, not Vincent, be with him in his final weeks of life.

Vincent moved out of their apartment, with both enormous misgivings and profound relief. He had had trouble comforting his lover without breaking into tears. He therefore believed he had failed him in his hour of need and berated himself severely for his cowardice and emotionality. He was naturally also quite angry with his lover, for leaving him as well as for depriving him of their final moments of closeness. He could not possibly experience his anger while feeling so guilty, however.

The losses he'd sustained were emotionally overwhelming. He could neither cry nor rage, and instead felt confused, anxious, hopeless, and without direction. In the course of treatment, his emotional reaction was validated. He was able to slowly unleash the "explosive" emotions he'd suppressed. In the process, he uncovered childhood messages received from his father about emotion as weakness and about the need to know how to do things without experience and without anyone's help. The combination of effects had proven too much for him.

Once he discovered the sources of his emotions and allowed them to flow more freely, and once he understood his own innocence, he could proceed with a difficult but feasible period of grieving.

Again, there is evidence in this instance of early traumatic events and childhood lessons serving as sources for later conflicts. This is almost inevitably the case for the gay man seeking psychotherapeutic treatment. It is also common for survivors to feel guilt as well as anger. These feelings can be profoundly confusing and may contribute to the emotional numbing noted here. The therapist in this case must encourage discussion of events and responses in a way that normalizes and validates the individual's experience, while connecting responses to pertinent events both current and historical.

In summary, the clinician in this phase should focus on the following:

- What are the current complaints, symptoms?
- What is the individual's psychological symptom history and history of treatment?
- At what stage is he in adopting a gay identity?
- How does he feel about his sexuality and identity?

- What is his history of experience as a child and gay man?
- Are there links from that experience to current symptoms?
- What has been his experience with HIV?
- Has he sustained losses as a result of the illness?
- How does he construe the meaning of HIV?
- Are physical symptoms possibly psychogenic?
- Is a referral for medical evaluation appropriate?
- Is he socially isolated?
- Has he been tested or is he fearful of or anticipating a test result?
- How does he perceive his likelihood for risk? Is that realistic?
- Does he understand the safer sex guidelines and follow them?
- If not, why not?
- Is he using or abusing substances?
- Does he need alternative coping and stress-reducing strategies?
- To what extent is he in immediate crisis? Suicidal?

PHASE II: SEROCONVERSION AND DIAGNOSIS

This phase is typically marked by shock, denial, and intense anxiety. The man who has recently learned that he is HIV-positive is likely in crisis. Enormous consequences and decisions may face him, not the least of which is whom to approach for support and treatment. He may have multiple fears, including worry about job and financial security, fear of rejection by friends and family, fears of discovery, anxiety about the illness itself as well as the likelihood of eventual death, and concerns about isolation versus intimacy. Symptoms may include distractibility, poor short-term memory, and disorientation.

As with any crisis, the clinician's responsibility is to delineate and reflect the client's circumstances and concerns while establishing a trustworthy therapeutic alliance; to help identify problems and potential resources; and to develop action plans related to immediate needs. Does the individual have sound treatment options? Are there necessary resources yet to be identified? Which decisions must be made now, and which can be deferred in order to allow a period of careful consideration? Of particular importance is the question of isolation versus support. The individual should be guided to determine whom he might approach for assistance. Such support has been shown to be related to a more positive prognosis and to decreased hopelessness, depression, and distress.

EVAN

Evan was twenty-five, a recent college graduate, and two years into a course of personal therapy with me when he was diagnosed as HIV-positive. The diagnosis was unexpected and devastating. Evan had worked through many difficult issues related to self-esteem, his relationship with his family, assertiveness, and compulsive sexuality in the course of treatment. He had been poised on the brink of a significant career, long debated and prepared for, and was supremely optimistic about the future.

Upon diagnosis, however, he became intensely anxious, regressing to earlier emotional coping mechanisms. He began to obsess about possible symptoms but would tell no one of his distress. He felt powerless and hopeless in the face of yet another life challenge. The recent respite from distress, which had resulted from the hard personal work he'd accomplished over a two-year period, seemed a giant lie to him now. Having worked so hard to individuate from his parents both emotionally and financially, the specter of a renewed dependence on them was a severe narcissistic blow, as well. He was determined not to pass the disease on to anyone else, but his former compulsive sexual behaviors were once again compelling.

In session, he was often angry and emotionally saturated. He felt the need to address all issues at once, and responded with confusion, panic, and suicidal ideation. By initially distinguishing his immediate needs from those questions that could be put off, he was able to gain some perspective. Though difficult for him, choosing one issue at a time helped him to focus and problem-solve, as well as to grieve, at a more manageable pace. He spent many sessions focused on very pragmatic concerns, whereas much of the previous work had tended to be emotionally focused. An emotional focus proved to be overwhelming for him initially, but over time he was able to approach his emotional responses within the context of particular issues he needed to address. Although he felt compelled to throw up his hands in despair, his previous successes were used as evidence of his ability to cope and make good decisions, as well as to tolerate intense emotion.

Differentiating the disease from his self-worth proved very important; it helped to significantly decrease suicidal feelings and his compulsion to be sexual in order to validate himself as valuable and desirable. He decided to put off notifying his family, but was able to avail himself of local resources for information and support. These actions strengthened him emotionally and provided necessary elements for his treatment and adjustment. He eventually became active in an organization designed to inform others about available resources for the HIV infected. With the exception of continuing to need to manage this serious illness, he was ultimately functional at virtually the same level as he'd been before diagnosis.

Among the most troubling concerns for the individual in this phase are the questions of who should know and how they will react. Identifying even one likely support can make a world of difference. In many localities, county health departments and other AIDS service organizations (ASOs) are available to provide free support groups as well as legal and medical information and referral. These groups, as well as broader social support, have been shown to be effective in easing adaptation to HIV and in decreasing hopelessness and depression, and participation should be encouraged. The clinician should therefore become apprised of such resources, as locally available.

Appraisal and Coping

The individual's coping style will likely become more evident in this phase, as he is pressed to respond to overwhelming circumstances. It has been shown that some coping strategies are more advantageous than others. To the extent that the individual appraises the situation as relatively controllable—that problems can be identified and effectively addressed, for example—he is more likely to develop an "involved" response. Such a response, wherein the client is actively involved in responding to problems, has been linked to lower levels of depression. Those who respond more passively or with detachment show higher rates of depression.

Men in this phase are likely to experience a compelling challenge to core beliefs about safety, self-esteem, and life meaning and purpose. The world no longer makes sense in the way it once did. Having an answer to "why" at this stage, whatever the answer, has been related to improved coping. "Active behavioral" coping, as opposed to "active cognitive" coping, is advantageous as well. Hence, the individual who attempts only to evaluate, and not to act, is more at risk for Obsessive-Compulsive Disorder and rumination. Likewise, purely emotionally focused coping has been linked to a sense of loss of control, whereas problem-focused coping increases the sense of control and therefore positive adaptation. Nonetheless, a focus on emotional coping is essential and, with selective attention, is negatively related to symptoms. This can be seen in the case example noted above.

A person's beliefs and style of approach make an enormous difference in positive adaptation to the disease. Although emotional working through in therapy can be quite helpful, a wholly emotional perspective may be overwhelming to the client, just as thinking alone will not resolve problems satisfactorily. The client must therefore be encouraged to identify those aspects of the circumstances over which he may exert control, to develop action plans relative to these circumstances, and to selectively explore emotional issues related to the circumstances as they come up. An avoidant response, which has been linked to a greater degree of psychological symptoms and poorer adaptive response in the long run, should be discouraged. It is also true, however, that personal style will determine the extent of comfort with any particular focus. The individual must always be approached individually and at his own pace, to avoid both a disruption in the therapeutic bond and an overwhelmed response to the circumstances.

There is an inevitable conflict in the treatment of serious illness, related to optimism as opposed to realism. Shouldn't we encourage an optimistic orientation to the illness? Research has shown that such an outlook is likely to have positive effects. But when does blind optimism become counterproductive? At what point is a particular level of denial no longer healthy? At what point is a focus on the illness to the exclusion of other activities and orientations likely to adversely affect adaptation to the disease? The clinician must proceed cautiously in uncovering denial in these circumstances. Clients will typically approach pertinent issues only as they are ready to do so.

Some denial is essential to continued functioning, and is common for all of us. As we board a jet, for example, we do not review in our minds the last story we heard about a plane crash, unless we want to create stress for ourselves and encourage rumination for the course of the trip. Likewise, it is essential for HIV-infected individuals to compartmentalize concerns and pending decisions to some extent, in order to cope effectively. Selective attention to emotional concerns, as well as to perceived consequences of illness, is often appropriate, especially considering that an individual may survive with HIV for many years.

An individual who wishes to avoid any discussion of the disease or the problems related to it, however, should be gently reminded that there are positive options of which he may not be able to avail himself without such a focus. It should be noted that delaying indefinitely the need to do the emotional, cognitive, and behavioral work in response to the disease will likely make matters worse.

Potential for Suicide

Individuals with a serious illness have been found to be at greater risk for suicide, especially if the illness involves a malignancy or the central nervous system. Among individuals infected with HIV, suicide risk is estimated to be as much as sixty-six times that of the general population. Such behavior is more likely during the phase of initial shock from diagnosis, for those who are socially isolated and fearful, and for those who do not receive follow-up counseling and support. The following predictive risk factors have been identified:

- Multiple psychosocial stressors
- Perceived social isolation
- Perceiving oneself as a victim
- Reliance on denial as the central and only defense
- Substance abuse
- Perceived unavailable social support
- History of psychiatric illness
- History of suicide attempts
- Acute crises in the course of infection
- CNS dysfunction
- Catastrophic loss

Therapists must be prepared to assess and discuss suicidal ideation early in treatment. They must be clear on the procedures they will utilize, including assessment, "no-harm" contracting, and hospitalization, for example.

As with any suicidal ideation, the therapist's leverage is based in part on the client's ambivalence. The therapist should help to identify the immediate precipitant—a drop in T-cell count, a recent loss, chronic isolation, and so on. Discussion should focus on the likely transience of such feelings, the impact for survivors, and the importance of focusing on manageable rather than global concerns, and should encourage the expression of feelings. An evaluation for antidepressant medication may be in order.

It is very important that therapists not collude with a hopeless or despairing outlook. We should also be prepared to act decisively, and quickly, should suicide appear to be an imminent threat.

In this phase, the clinician should focus on the following:

- To what extent is there an immediate crisis?
- How do I help the client prioritize immediate versus longer-term decisions?
- What are the immediate resource needs, and where can they be met?
- What can the individual do to gain a sense of control?
- What are the options for personal support? Groups? Friends?
- Who can and should be notified now? Who can be informed later, if at all?
- Are there pertinent cognitive symptoms? Should these be normalized or further evaluated?
- What does the infection mean to and about the individual?
- Is the diagnosis cuing up old issues or history for the individual?
- How do I help the client compartmentalize emotion to avoid feeling overwhelmed?
- Is the client avoiding the reality of the diagnosis?
- What is his understanding of the disease and disease course, treatments, and so on?
- Does he need a medical evaluation or evaluation for anxiolytic or antidepressant medications?
- Does he need assistance with suicidal ideation or intent?
- What is(are) the action plan(s)?

PHASE III:
THE WORRIED INFECTED

Because the asymptomatic phase is indefinite in both duration and outcome, it appears to be the most stressful phase, according to several sources. Affective disorders are most likely among those infected but asymptomatic. It has also been shown that the perceived number of symptoms on self-report and having no one to talk to about one's circumstances are related to greater levels of depression. These findings may seem both contradictory and surprising in some ways. We might expect those who are symptomatic or who have developed full-blown AIDS to be the most emotionally affected by stress. Likewise, if symptoms are linked to depressive responses, why would asymptomatic individuals show more distress?

It appears to be uncertainty that influences stress most profoundly. And it is *perceived* symptoms rather than actual symptoms that are correlated with the depressive response.

The lack of predictability of future events may be the most troubling aspect of this period. Given the time remaining, does one strive to accomplish professional goals, plan to retire early, take that long-planned dream trip, buy a house, settle down with one's lover, leave a relationship for one more rewarding? What will be the financial ramifications of these decisions? Who should be informed of the illness and at what point? These decisions are quite difficult to make when one's time line could be six months, five years, or even fifteen or more years. The potential of the newest treatments may make these decisions even more complex. The question often comes down to choosing between preparing to die and living life to the fullest. It is enormously difficult to do both. And while one waits for the onset of symptoms, it is easy to imagine that every rash, cold, flu, or bout of acne or diarrhea is the beginning of the symptomatic phase.

PAUL

Paul was forty-seven years old at the time of intake. He complained of malaise, sleep disturbance, and some anxiety. He had known of his HIV-positive diagnosis for about one year. He felt he'd adjusted well, having proceeded with medical evaluations and prophylactic treatments, and having tolerated prescribed medications without significant side effects. His lover, who was also HIV-positive, was generally supportive, and the two seemed to be carrying on as if nothing was really wrong.

Still, Paul had lately had nightmares in which he was in great danger or had developed appalling symptoms of the disease. In one frankly symbolic dream, Paul was about to take a long-desired cruise, but as he approached the gangplank it disappeared, leaving him to stare into the dark and chilly water below, with the feeling that his falling in was inevitable.

Initially, the only anxiety Paul could substantially describe involved his fear about what would happen to his son by a former marriage. The two were very close, and the boy was only nine at the time. Paul was obsessed with how and when to tell his son about the illness. As he explored this dilemma, he also realized that he was fearful of telling the boy's mother, who might then refuse visitation.

He hoped that he could just continue as always, without disclosure, but then began to wonder about early retirement; the possibility of being disabled; who would die first, he or his lover; and of course, what would happen to his son. These worries were just beneath the surface of the calm he projected to friends and was convinced of himself. By beginning with the anxiety around his son, he was eventually able to uncover other anxieties and, with careful pacing, to address them more realistically.

Though painful, this process was necessary, and it eventually allowed his anxiety to be ameliorated. It also allowed him to take further steps in preparing realistically for his future and that of his family.

Individuals in this phase are less likely to turn to their families for support than are those either HIV-negative or those with full-blown AIDS. It has also been noted that gays and lesbians in general are more likely to turn to friends than to family for support. Those with supportive family involvement typically have better adjustment, however. Again, the intense stress of this period greatly increases the likelihood that unresolved issues related to childhood and family will emerge. The individual in this phase may be able to delay the point of notifying family members about his illness, but he is likely to be struggling with what to do about that question and when to do it. The client may not raise this issue in therapy; he may require the guidance of the therapist to remind him of the work to be done in this area.

The clinician working in this phase of the illness should attend to the following questions:

- To what extent is the individual perceiving the onset of symptoms?

- Is he accurate in his evaluation? Do physical symptoms need to be evaluated medically?

- Are there depressive or anxiety symptoms that require treatment?

- What are his greatest fears?

- To what extent is the individual isolated? How can this be addressed?

- What decisions does the client struggle with? Are they realistic?

- Is there business from the past that he must work through in this phase?

- What losses has the individual sustained? Does he need to grieve these?

- How does he perceive the future? Is that realistic?

- What are the job and financial concerns?
- Who needs to know about his condition? How can he prepare to discuss it?
- Is he getting appropriate and reasonable medical treatment?
- Has he considered contact with his family of origin?
- Does he need additional social support?
- Is he suicidal?

PHASE IV:
SYMPTOMATIC HIV AND AIDS

Although infected individuals may show early symptoms, such as shingles and those similar to influenza, for example, the "symptomatic phase" referred to here is that period in which the immune system becomes more fully compromised and therefore increasingly unable to protect the individual from opportunistic infection.

This stage of advanced immunosuppression has been commonly defined by a CD4 cell count of under 200, although other considerations have recently emerged as potentially more significant. The onset of symptoms is, in any case, variable.

It is in the symptomatic phase that the clinician must be particularly alert to differential diagnostic concerns. In one study, evidence of cognitive impairment was found in 87 percent of AIDS patients. Central nervous system impairment is very likely for the individual with AIDS. Although depression is associated less with this phase than with the asymptomatic phase, symptoms of cognitive impairment resulting from HIV-1 Associated Dementia Complex, formerly known as AIDS Dementia Complex, may become more apparent. These symptoms tend to coincide with other immunosuppressive constitutional conditions and opportunistic infections. Although cognitive impairments have been identified prior to this phase, they are typically milder and less disruptive during earlier phases. Some of the

Distress in this phase is often related to the effects of medical treatments and to the progression of symptoms and their meaning in relation to the future. A first bout with an immune-related disorder, as the immune system becomes increasingly dysfunctional, can be quite troubling. At this point, the individual may begin to take up issues of spirituality in earnest. He may also become more involved with his family of origin; perceived support from family will likely decrease anxiety about dying. Those who are able to gain the support of family during this period have shown better adjustment. The individual may begin to withdraw from more active involvement in the world. Energy levels begin to wane, and simple tasks such as mounting stairs may become quite difficult. Consequently, the individual must face repeated losses of capacity and must adjust to increasing dependence on others. Although he is also likely to receive medications for his physical condition, the pharmacological treatments for HIV have not shown evidence of significant effects on mood.

It has been noted that it is significantly more difficult psychologically to let go of something not yet achieved and to adjust to asynchronous life events than to let go of attained status or adjust to developmentally appropriate life events. The individual in this phase, or even somewhat prior to this phase, may need to grieve the loss of a prominent career, retirement, intimate relationship, and so on, whether achieved or forever beyond reach. He must establish a new "narrative" for his life that can leave him with a positive sense of meaning and accomplishment. The therapist can assist in reviewing individual successes great or small, the qualities of personality that the client and others have shown appreciation for, and inevitably, the strength the individual has shown in the face of adversity. The therapist can also elucidate the ways in which the illness has fostered personal growth. While helping the client to view his accomplishments positively, the therapist must also be willing to acknowledge losses and to allow the grieving process to proceed in a manageable way.

The individual at this stage may begin to bargain with the notion of suicide, determining in advance the point at which his life will not be worth living to him. Such a response is not unusual, and should be seen as an attempt to gain mastery in response to the loss of control and the increase of painful circumstances. Such "deal making" may actually be useful in restoring a sense of instrumentality. However, it is important that the clinician not collude with the client's desire to die before other options have been fully explored. All reasonable steps should be taken to provide treatment for anxiety and depressive responses, and to explore their etiology. Such feelings may be temporary, and related to a particularly stressful period.

The partner's or caregiver's role is likely to become more stressful and demanding during this phase. Changes in relationship habits and in sexual relations with the patient are common, for example, and almost half will experience a change in their role in relation to the infected individual. The therapist may be called on to help caregivers identify adjunctive assistance, to have conjoint sessions to discuss changes in the relationship and difficult decisions faced by the patient and his family, or to cope with the many losses faced by all. The reader is referred to Chapter Seven for a more detailed discussion of family and couples interventions.

The therapist working in this phase should attend to the following questions:

- Is there evidence of central nervous system involvement that warrants further assessment?
- Is the client competent to understand his condition and make treatment decisions?
- Is the client struggling with losses or repeated losses of capacity or others?
- How does he perceive his future?
- What are his greatest concerns?

- Has the individual been able to come to terms with the meaning of his illness?

- Do caretakers and significant others need to be more involved in treatment?

- Does the individual need help in preparing to say good-bye, to die, and to mourn these losses?

- Can the individual's family be supportively involved?

- Is the client struggling with increased dependency? How does he construe this fact?

- Is he considering suicide or assisted death?

- Has he considered a wish to end treatment with you?

- What is your countertransference reaction? Do you need consultation or assistance?

Termination of Treatment

It is in this phase that the therapist will inevitably face the termination of therapy, if it has not ended previously. Although it would be ideal to have a planned termination, this may not always be possible. Often, the individual's medical symptoms will suddenly preclude office visits or even hospital consults. Naturally, the patient may also die suddenly. The therapist will face, in addition to feelings of loss related to the patient, the need to make decisions about the appropriateness of atypical interventions, such as phone sessions, hospital visitation, and so on.

It is important for us to be acutely aware of our response in this phase, as denial may be as likely as a mournful response. We must approach termination squarely, in the open, in order for the patient to fully benefit from our assistance. This is the point at which the "real" relationship may become more prominent. Therapists should distinguish the ethical and legal boundaries from those boundaries designed to insulate us from pain. We must let the patient go without making him gone, in a manner of speaking. This may create for the heartiest therapist a real challenge—to allow a more human side to emerge.

Occasions to cry with a patient or to hug him, for example, may become more reasonable options. The therapist should continue to focus on the needs and best interests of the patient, of course. The point is to avoid a preemptive closing off of the relationship.

It is also true that the therapist may not know the fate of clients who terminate before the symptomatic or end stage of illness. This absence of information may be worrisome, yet it is important to allow the client to determine what contact with the therapist is desired, where possible. An open invitation to let the therapist know how the patient is doing, or to drop a line if desired in the future, may be a good suggestion at termination.

We have reviewed the social, psychological, and medical aspects of treatment for the gay man's HIV-related mental health concerns. Much of the work of psychotherapeutic intervention for the gay man will have its foundation in the individual's history of marginalization and discrimination. This will be a potentially significant source of conflict and suffering for the individual as well. Additional stressors are generated by the culture's response to HIV and the stigma associated with infection.

As we have seen, each stage of illness is often related to specific concerns, risk factors, and treatment needs. The therapist should remain apprised of developments in the medical and psychiatric treatment of the disease, as available research findings and treatments change rapidly. The therapist should also be aware of special considerations around termination.

The role of the therapist in the treatment of HIV can be quite stressful. It is important that we as therapists be aware of our own strengths and limitations. We should expect to need occasional or ongoing consultation to review our response to case load, losses, and other concerns that might arise. Burnout is a real risk that should be monitored. The reader is referred to

Chapter One on transference and countertransference for a more thorough review of these issues.

NOTES

P. 118, *Research has even shown that lesbian women:* Steffensmeier, D., & Steffensmeier, R. (1974). Sex differences in reactions to homosexuals: Research continuities and further developments. *Journal of Sex Research, 10*(1), 52–67.

P. 118, *The reasons for this fact are at once fascinating and elusive:* Morin, S., & Garfinkle, E. (1978). Male homophobia. *Journal of Social Issues, 34*(1), 29–47.

P. 119, *Gay men, on the other hand, may learn from an early age:* Sanders, D. (1980). A psychotherapeutic approach to gay men. In J. Marmor (Ed.), *Homosexual behavior: A modern reappraisal* (pp. 342–356). New York: Basic Books; Coleman, E. (1982). Developmental stages of the coming-out process. In W. Paul, J. Weinrich, J. Gonsiorek, & M. Hotvedt (Eds.), *Homosexuality: Social, psychological and biological issues* (pp. 149–158). Thousand Oaks, CA: Sage.

P. 119, *A recent study showed that 58 percent of gay men:* Herek, G., & Greene, B. (Eds.). (1995). *Medical perspectives on lesbian and gay issues: Vol. 2. AIDS, identity and community: The HIV epidemic and lesbians and gay men.* Thousand Oaks, CA: Sage.

P. 120, *The disease has also been called the "gay cancer":* Shilts, R. (1987). *And the band played on: Politics, people and the AIDS epidemic.* New York: St. Martin's Press.

P. 120, *Reflecting a predictable response of the public to a new and devastating scourge:* Herek, G. (1990). Illness, stigma and AIDS. In P. Costa & G. VandenBos (Eds.), *Psychological aspects of serious illness: Chronic conditions, fatal diseases, and clinical care* (pp. 103–150). Washington, DC: American Psychological Association.

P. 121, *Gregory Herek, a social psychologist, has studied the sources of both homophobia:* Herek, G. (1990). Illness, stigma and AIDS. In P. Costa & G. VandenBos (Eds.), *Psychological aspects of serious illness: Chronic conditions, fatal diseases, and clinical care* (pp. 103–150). Washington, DC: American Psychological Association.

P. 122, *Ronald Reagan did not mention AIDS publicly:* Herek, G. (1990). Illness, stigma and AIDS. In P. Costa & G. VandenBos (Eds.), *Psychological aspects of serious illness: Chronic conditions, fatal diseases, and clinical care* (pp. 103–150). Washington, DC: American Psychological Association.

P. 123, *Such action is consistent with the moralistic view:* Goffman, E. (1963). *Stigma.* Englewood Cliffs, NJ: Prentice Hall.

P. 125, *Gays have frequently been seen as mysterious:* Paul, W. (1982). Social issues and homosexual behavior: A taxonomy of categories and themes in the anti-gay argument. In W. Paul, J. Weinrich, J. Gonsiorek, & M. Hotvedt (Eds.), *Homosexuality: Social, psychological and biological issues* (pp. 29–56). Thousand Oaks, CA: Sage.

P. 125, *These ascriptions have been associated with other stigmatized groups:* Goffman, E. (1963). *Stigma.* Englewood Cliffs, NJ: Prentice Hall.

P. 125, *A history of psychiatric musings . . . is well known to most gay:* See for example Socarides, C. W. (1978). *Homosexuality.* New York: Aronson.

P. 125, *Modern research with unbiased samples proved these conclusions erroneous:* Marmor, J. (Ed.). (1980). *Homosexual behavior: A modern reappraisal.* New York: Basic Books; Gonsiorek, J. C. (1982). Results of psychological testing on homosexual populations. In W. Paul, J. D. Weinrich, J. C. Gonsiorek, & M. E. Hotvedt (Eds.), *Homosexuality: Social, psychological and biological issues* (pp. 71–80). Thousand Oaks: Sage.

P. 126, *In addition, the issue of "concealability":* Goffman, E. (1963). *Stigma.* Englewood Cliffs, NJ: Prentice Hall.

P. 127, *People with AIDS have been shown to be more negatively evaluated:* Herek, G. (1990). Illness, stigma and AIDS. In P. Costa & G. VandenBos (Eds.), *Psychological aspects of serious illness: Chronic conditions, fatal diseases, and clinical care* (pp. 103–150). Washington, DC: American Psychological Association.

P. 128, *It is not unusual for a gay man:* Malyon, A. (1982). Psychotherapeutic implications of internalized homophobia in gay men. *Journal of Homosexuality,* 7(2/3), 59–70.

P. 128, *That history is likely to include experiences:* O'Connor, M. (1992). Psychotherapy with the gay or lesbian adolescent. In S. Dworkin and F. Gutierrez (Eds.), *Journey to the end of the rainbow: Counseling gays and lesbians* (pp. 3–22). Alexandria, VA: American Counseling Association Press.

P. 130, *We know, for example, that most gay men:* Cass, V. (1979). Homosexual identity formation: A theoretical model. *Journal of Homosexuality, 4,* 219–236.

P. 132, *Some individuals take comfort in establishing a scientific:* Rabkin, J. G., Remien, R. H., & Wilson, C. (1994). *Good doctor, good patient.* New York: NCM.

P. 133, *Individuals with psychiatric problems prior to infection:* Atkinson, J., & Grant, I. (1994). Natural history of neuropsychiatric manifestations of HIV disease. In L. S. Zegans & T. J. Coates (Eds.), *Psychiatric manifestations of HIV disease. The Psychiatric Clinics of North America, 17*(1), 17–34.

P. 133, *It is estimated, for example, that 78 percent:* Markowitz, J., Rabkin, J. G., & Perry, S. (1994). Treating depression in HIV-positive patients. *AIDS, 8,* 403–412.

P. 133, *It is beyond the purpose of this chapter:* Atkinson, J., & Grant, I. (1994). Natural history of neuropsychiatric manifestations of HIV disease. In L. S. Zegans & T. J. Coates (Eds.), *Psychiatric manifestations of HIV disease. The Psychiatric Clinics of North America, 17*(1), 17–34.

P. 134, *One recent study found that approximately 90 percent of gay men:* Herek, G., & Glunt, E. (1995). Identity and community among gay and bisexual men in the AIDS era: Preliminary findings from the Sacramento men's health study. In G. Herek & B. Greene (Eds.), *Medical perspectives on lesbian and gay issues: Vol. 2. AIDS, identity and community: The HIV epidemic and lesbians and gay men* (pp. 55–84). Thousand Oaks, CA: Sage.

P. 134, *Adjustment disorders are in fact the most common diagnosis:* O'Dowd, M., Biderman, D., & McKegney, F. (1993). Incidence of suicidality in AIDS and HIV-positive patients attending a psychiatry outpatient program. *Psychosomatics, 34*(1), 33–40.

P. 134, *Similarly, uncertainty about exposure to the virus:* Ostrow, D. G., Monjan, A., Joseph, J., VanRaden, M., Fox, R., Kingsley, L., Dudley, J., & Phair, J. (1989). HIV-related symptoms and psychological functioning in a cohort of homosexual men. *American Journal of Psychiatry, 146*(6), 737–742.

P. 134, *Research has shown that the individual who is most likely to have an anxiety reaction:* Miller, D., & Riccio, M. (1990). Non-organic psychiatric and psychosocial syndromes associated with HIV-1 infection and disease. *AIDS, 4*(5), 381–388.

P. 136, *Poor resolution of adjustment disorders in this phase:* Miller, D., & Riccio, M. (1990). Non-organic psychiatric and psychosocial syndromes associated with HIV-1 infection and disease. *AIDS, 4*(5), 381–388.

P. 137, *Research has shown that a sudden diagnosis:* Miller, D., & Riccio, M. (1990). Non-organic psychiatric and psychosocial syndromes associated with HIV-1 infection and disease. *AIDS, 4*(5), 381–388.

P. 137, *This has been shown to be influenced in part by the extent:* Ostrow, D. G., Monjan, A., Joseph, J., VanRaden, M., Fox, R., Kingsley, L., Dudley, J., & Phair, J. (1989). HIV-related symptoms and psychological functioning in a cohort of homosexual men. *American Journal of Psychiatry, 146*(6), 737–742.

P. 137, *AIDS-related bereavement has been found to be another significant problem:* McKusick, L. (1988). The impact of AIDS on practitioner and client:

Notes from the therapeutic relationship. *American Psychologist, 43*(11), 935–940.

P. 137, *Symptoms may include those commonly associated with Posttraumatic Stress Disorder:* Schwartzberg, S. (1992). AIDS-related bereavement among gay men: The inadequacy of current theories of grief. *Psychotherapy, 29*(3), 422–429.

P. 138, *This latter symptom is very important:* Cabaj, R. (1994). HIV and substance abuse in the gay community. In S. Cadwell, R. Burnham, & M. Forstein (Eds.), *Therapists on the front line: Psychotherapy with gay men in the age of AIDS* (pp. 405–426). Washington, DC: American Psychiatric Press.

P. 138, *Likewise, self-blaming and self-punishment:* Miller, D., & Riccio, M. (1990). Non-organic psychiatric and psychosocial syndromes associated with HIV-1 infection and disease. *AIDS, 4*(5), 381–388.

P. 140, *This phase is typically marked:* Ross, M. (1990). Psychovenerology: Psychological aspects of AIDS and other sexually transmissible diseases. In D. G. Ostrow (Ed.), *Behavioral aspects of AIDS* (pp. 19–39). New York: Plenum.

P. 140, *He may have multiple fears:* Zegans, L. S., Gerhard, A., & Coates, T. J. (1994). Psychotherapies for the person with HIV. In L. S. Zegans & T. J. Coates (Eds.), *Psychiatric manifestations of HIV disease. The Psychiatric Clinics of North America, 17*(1), 149–162.

P. 140, *Symptoms may include distractibility:* Miller, D. (1990). Diagnosis and treatment of acute psychological problems related to HIV infection and disease. In D. G. Ostrow (Ed.), *Behavioral aspects of AIDS* (pp. 187–204). New York: Plenum.

P. 141, *Such support has been shown to be related to a more positive prognosis:* Ostrow, D. G., Monjan, A., Joseph, J., VanRaden, M., Fox, R., Kingsley, L., Dudley, J., & Phair, J. (1989). HIV-related symptoms and psychological functioning in a cohort of homosexual men. *American Journal of Psychiatry, 146*(6), 737–742; Miller, D. (1990). Diagnosis and treatment of acute psychological problems related to HIV infections and disease. In D. G. Ostrow (Ed.), *Behavioral aspects of AIDS* (pp. 187–204). New York: Plenum.

P. 142, *These groups, as well as broader social support:* Tunnel, G. (1994). Special issues in group psychotherapy for gay men with AIDS. In S. Cadwell, R. Burnham, & M. Forstein (Eds.), *Therapists on the front line: Psychotherapy with gay men in the age of AIDS* (pp. 237–254). Washington, DC: American Psychiatric Press; Miller, D. (1990). Diagnosis and treatment of acute psychological problems related to HIV infections and disease. In D. G. Ostrow (Ed.), *Behavioral aspects of AIDS* (pp. 187–204). New York: Plenum.

P. 143, *Such a response, wherein the client is actively involved:* Folkman, S., Chesney, M., Pollack, L., & Coates, T. (1993). Stress, control, coping and depressive mood in human immunodeficiency virus-positive and -negative gay men in San Francisco. *Journal of Nervous and Mental Disorders, 181,* 409–416.

P. 143, *The world no longer makes sense:* Schwartzberg, S. (1992). AIDS-related bereavement among gay men: The inadequacy of current theories of grief. *Psychotherapy, 29*(3), 422–429.

P. 143, *"Active behavioral" coping:* Miller, D. (1990). Diagnosis and treatment of acute psychological problems related to HIV infection and disease. In D. G. Ostrow (Ed.), *Behavioral aspects of AIDS* (pp. 187–204). New York: Plenum.

P. 143, *Hence, the individual who attempts only to evaluate:* Miller, D. (1990). Diagnosis and treatment of acute psychological problems related to HIV infections and disease. In D. G. Ostrow (Ed.), *Behavioral aspects of AIDS* (pp. 187–204). New York: Plenum.

P. 143, *Likewise, purely emotionally focused coping:* Folkman, S., Chesney, M., Pollack, L., & Coates, T. (1993). Stress, control, coping and depressive mood in human immunodeficiency virus-positive and -negative gay men in San Francisco. *Journal of Nervous and Mental Disorders, 181,* 409–416.

P. 145, *Individuals with a serious illness:* O'Dowd, M., Biderman, D., & McKegney, F. (1993). Incidence of suicidality in AIDS and HIV-positive patients attending a psychiatry outpatient program. *Psychosomatics, 34*(1), 33–40.

P. 145, *suicide risk is estimated to be as much as sixty-six times:* Miller, D., & Riccio, M. (1990). Non-organic psychiatric and psychosocial syndromes associated with HIV-1 infection and disease. *AIDS, 4*(5), 381–388.

P. 145, *The following predictive risk factors have been identified:* Miller, D. (1990). Diagnosis and treatment of acute psychological problems related to HIV infection and disease. In D. G. Ostrow (Ed.), *Behavioral aspects of AIDS* (pp. 187–204). New York: Plenum; Forstein, M. (1994). Suicidality and HIV in gay men. In S. Cadwell, R. Burnham, & M. Forstein (Eds.), *Therapists on the front line: Psychotherapy with gay men in the age of AIDS* (pp. 111–146). Washington, DC: American Psychiatric Press.

P. 146, *It is very important that therapists not collude:* Markowitz, J., Rabkin, J. G., & Perry, S. (1994). Treating depression in HIV-positive patients. *AIDS, 8,* 403–412.

P. 146, *We should also be prepared to act decisively:* Forstein, M. (1994). Suicidality and HIV in gay men. In S. Cadwell, R. Burnham, & M. Forstein (Eds.), *Therapists on the front line: Psychotherapy with gay men in the age of AIDS* (pp. 111–146). Washington, DC: American Psychiatric Press.

P. 147, *Because the asymptomatic phase is indefinite:* O'Dowd, M., Biderman, D., & McKegney, F. (1993). Incidence of suicidality in AIDS and HIV-positive patients attending a psychiatry outpatient program. *Psychosomatics, 34*(1), 33–40; Catalan, J. (1988). Psychosocial and neuropsychiatric aspects of HIV infection: Review of their extent and implications for psychiatry. *Journal of Psychosomatic Research, 32*(3), 237–248.

P. 147, *Affective disorders are most likely:* O'Dowd, M., Biderman, D., & McKegney, F. (1993). Incidence of suicidality in AIDS and HIV-positive patients attending a psychiatry outpatient program. *Psychosomatics, 34*(1), 33–40.

P. 147, *It has also been shown that the perceived number of symptoms:* Ostrow, D. G., Monjan, A., Joseph, J., VanRaden, M., Fox, R., Kingsley, L., Dudley, J., & Phair, J. (1989). HIV-related symptoms and psychological functioning in a cohort of homosexual men. *American Journal of Psychiatry, 146*(6), 737–742.

P. 147, *It appears to be uncertainty that influences stress:* Ostrow, D. G., Monjan, A., Joseph, J., VanRaden, M., Fox, R., Kingsley, L., Dudley, J., & Phair, J. (1989). HIV-related symptoms and psychological functioning in a cohort of homosexual men. *American Journal of Psychiatry, 146*(6), 737–742.

P. 149, *Those with supportive family involvement:* Catania, J., Turner, H., Kyung-Hee, C., & Coates, T. (1992). Coping with death anxiety: Help-seeking and social support among gay men with various HIV diagnoses. *AIDS, 6*(9), 999–1005.

P. 150, *In one study, evidence of cognitive impairment:* Catalan, J. (1988). Psychosocial and neuropsychiatric aspects of HIV infection: Review of their extent and implications for psychiatry. *Journal of Psychosomatic Research, 32*(3), 237–248.

P. 150, *These symptoms tend to coincide with other immunosuppressive constitutional conditions:* Becket, A., & Kassel, P. (1994). Neuropsychiatric dysfunction: Impact on psychotherapy with HIV-infected gay men. In S. Cadwell, R. Burnham, & M. Forstein (Eds.), *Therapists on the front line: Psychotherapy with gay men in the age of AIDS* (pp. 147–163). Washington, DC: American Psychiatric Press.

P. 151, *Evidence of apathy, irritability, and a rigid, inflexible style:* Becket, A., & Kassel, P. (1994). Neuropsychiatric dysfunction: Impact on psychotherapy with HIV-infected gay men. In S. Cadwell, R. Burnham, & M. Forstein (Eds.), *Therapists on the front line: Psychotherapy with gay men in the age of AIDS* (pp. 147–163). Washington, DC: American Psychiatric Press.

P. 151, *Motor impairments, including weakness in the lower extremities:* Becket, A., & Kassel, P. (1994). Neuropsychiatric dysfunction: Impact on psychotherapy with HIV-infected gay men. In S. Cadwell, R. Burnham, & M. Forstein (Eds.), *Therapists on the front line: Psychotherapy with gay men in the age of AIDS* (pp. 147–163). Washington, DC: American Psychiatric Press;

Ostrow, D. G. (1990). Psychiatric aspects of AIDS: An overview. In D. G. Ostrow (Ed.), *Behavioral aspects of AIDS* (pp. 9–17). New York: Plenum.

P. 152, *Rapid onset of symptoms should also suggest:* Ostrow, D. G. (1990). Psychiatric aspects of AIDS: An overview. In D. G. Ostrow (Ed.), *Behavioral aspects of AIDS* (pp. 9–17). New York: Plenum.

P. 152, *It has been noted that individuals at this stage of the disease:* Becket, A., & Kassel, P. (1994). Neuropsychiatric dysfunction: Impact on psychotherapy with HIV-infected gay men. In S. Cadwell, R. Burnham, & M. Forstein (Eds.), *Therapists on the front line: Psychotherapy with gay men in the age of AIDS* (pp. 147–163). Washington, DC: American Psychiatric Press.

P. 152, *He must understand the nature of his illness:* Becket, A., & Kassel, P. (1994). Neuropsychiatric dysfunction: Impact on psychotherapy with HIV-infected gay men. In S. Cadwell, R. Burnham, & M. Forstein (Eds.), *Therapists on the front line: Psychotherapy with gay men in the age of AIDS* (pp. 147–163). Washington, DC: American Psychiatric Press.

P. 152, *Although assisted death is not uncommon:* Forstein, M. (1994). Suicidality and HIV in gay men. In S. Cadwell, R. Burnham, & M. Forstein (Eds.), *Therapists on the front line: Psychotherapy with gay men in the age of AIDS* (pp. 111–146). Washington, DC: American Psychiatric Press.

P. 153, *Although he is also likely to receive medications:* Markowitz, J., Rabkin, J. G., & Perry, S. (1994). Treating depression in HIV-positive patients. *AIDS, 8,* 403–412.

P. 153, *It has been noted that it is significantly more difficult psychologically to let go:* Linde, R. (1994). Impact of AIDS on adult gay male development: Implications for psychotherapy. In S. Cadwell, R. Burnham, & M. Forstein (Eds.), *Therapists on the front line: Psychotherapy with gay men in the age of AIDS* (pp. 25–52). Washington, DC: American Psychiatric Press.

P. 153, *He must establish a new "narrative":* Shelby, R. (1994). Mourning within a culture of mourning. In S. Cadwell, R. Burnham, & M. Forstein (Eds.), *Therapists on the front line: Psychotherapy with gay men in the age of AIDS* (pp. 53–80). Washington, DC: American Psychiatric Press.

P. 154, *Such a response is not unusual:* Forstein, M. (1994). Suicidality and HIV in gay men. In S. Cadwell, R. Burnham, & M. Forstein (Eds.), *Therapists on the front line: Psychotherapy with gay men in the age of AIDS* (pp. 111–146). Washington, DC: American Psychiatric Press.

P. 154, *Changes in relationship habits:* Miller, D. (1990). Diagnosis and treatment of acute psychological problems related to HIV infection and disease. In D. G. Ostrow (Ed.), *Behavioral aspects of AIDS* (pp. 187–204). New York: Plenum.

5

TREATING ETHNIC MINORITY INDIVIDUALS

Fernando J. Gutierrez

It is not my intent here to pull any punches or sugar-coat my perspective. What I do promise is to give you a realistic and honest view from one gay ethnic minority perspective. As is often the case, the sole ethnic minority must speak for all minorities, so I apologize if my perspective is one you don't share. You may wish to take what you want and leave the rest.

In a community in which I once worked, ethnic minorities made up the majority of HIV-related cases, yet most of the resources went to white Anglo–oriented services staffed by white Anglo staff who, for the most part, had little or no training in working with ethnic minority groups. In that service area, 758 of the 1,443 cases of HIV and AIDS, or more than half, were ethnic minorities: Latinos (470), African American (195), Asian/Pacific Islander (72) and Native American (11). Yet the four minority programs shared $70,000 of county funding, of which 50 percent went to administrative costs. This left less than $9,000 per program for direct services to ethnic minority clients out of a fiscal year budget of $681,000. If you looked at the county budget and where most of the money was going, you would think that AIDS was only a white gay male disease. Clearly there is a political problem in the way that such programs are funded.

As a gay, Caucasian ethnic minority, originally from Cuba, I have found it quite frustrating to work in the AIDS field. To focus on the culturally sensitive treatment of clients with HIV or AIDS seems rather naive to me when in fact the biggest problem is really the infrastructure within which the ethnic minority clinician must operate. That is why my journey has taken me from establishing the first emotional support group for HIV for this county's Latinos to law school. My recent focus has been to expend my energy not on primary care but as a member of my county's Commission on AIDS. The commission's task is to oversee all planning of HIV/AIDS services, to ensure coordination of access and quality of care; to review, assess, and identify deficiencies in current and proposed HIV and AIDS care and education programs in the county; and to identify gaps in services.

It is very difficult for a clinician to work within the political environment just described and to contain the anger and frustration toward the system in order to provide a serene and safe environment for the client. It is not surprising then that the first chapter of this book focuses on transference and countertransference, and very accurately suggests that there may come a time when a clinician will need to change roles completely, moving from working directly with clients or even leaving the area of HIV work because of burnout. In my case, I decided to move to the policymaking arena.

OBSTACLES IN DEALING WITH THE INFRASTRUCTURE

Most ethnic minority clinicians are the only ethnic minority clinicians on the staff. We have been hired to provide culturally sensitive services, yet our treatment designs and protocols may be challenged because they don't fit the traditional medical model, or we are provided little or no resources with which to do our jobs. We are often placed in the middle between the service delivery systems and the client. The clients' unmet needs make continuing demands of us while the inadequate resources and support force us to become creative in meeting all the demands placed on us as clinicians. We share the same stresses that middle-level managers often face in corporate organizations, with the same risks of burnout.

During my first year of providing services to Latinos/as, I worked as a volunteer, as there was no funding for emotional support groups for this group. The local AIDS project was privately funded by donations. There were no ethnic minority staff members, except for the receptionist, and I was the only ethnic minority member on the board of directors of the project. It quickly became evident to me that the project's services to ethnic minorities were nonexistent. As the funding for the project grew, I began to make demands on the board to pressure the executive director to hire an ethnic minority staff person. There was much support from other board members, but not enough to succeed. The next staff person that was hired was considered a "minority," a white woman. This is typical of many AIDS projects across the country, as I have learned at national conventions where these programs are described.

When these organizations are challenged about their hesitancy to provide services to ethnic minorities, their answer boils down to: "We acknowledge that we don't have the cultural sensitivity in our programs to deal with the specific needs of these populations, and we are burned out with all the work that we already have to do" (meaning the work with white gay males). This becomes what I describe as the "Pontius Pilate" approach to service delivery, because in a sense what the policymakers and administrators are saying is, "We wash our hands of the problem." The excuse is that the services are open to all clients. Yet if these services are not culturally sensitive and relevant to all clients, only the clients that the program matches in composition of staff and style of service delivery will feel welcome and use the services.

I ultimately approached the director of a Latino/a health education program at a local hospital, and we began an association. Proposed support meetings could not take place at the hospital because there was no space, despite the fact that the hospital had a psychiatric unit. I held the meetings at a substance abuse agency for which I consulted, which predominantly served African Americans. This arrangement worked out during the first year; however, in the following year, a new executive director came on board, and he asked me to find another meeting space.

The next year, the health education program found funding for my services; however, there was still the issue of inadequate space. Our group roamed from room to room at the hospital, often meeting in a room that was separated from the next meeting room by only a folding curtain. Alcoholics Anonymous meetings were held in the next room, often with much applause and laughter. Imagine trying to conduct relaxation techniques training or asking a client to self-disclose his pain about his HIV status under these conditions. I finally gave the hospital an ultimatum: find me adequate space, or I will be forced to resign. No adequate space was forthcoming, so I resigned.

This support group had taken the pressure off the local AIDS project to deal with providing emotional support services to Latinos/as. When I resigned, the pressure was back on the project to do something about the lack of services to ethnic minorities. The director of the AIDS project contacted someone at one of the local mental health agencies and convinced her to ask the county for a grant to start an emotional support group. The grant was funded, not for Latino gay men but for a part-time provider for perinatal AIDS prevention education for women, who would also conduct the emotional support group for the Latino men.

The county statistics showed that of the 476 cases of HIV and AIDS within the Latino/a community, only 6 cases (cumulative reporting from 1983 to 1995) of HIV and AIDS came from a parent at risk of contracting HIV. Did these statistics warrant that a heterosexual Latina woman should be hired to focus predominantly on parent-at-risk issues? Would it not have made more sense to hire a gay Latino male (I was not looking for the job, by the way) who might be able to reach the 327 homosexual and bisexual clients, 41 homosexual and bisexual IV drug users, 39 heterosexual IV drug users, and 39 clients infected through heterosexual contact?

What happened at this agency can occur only in communities where ethnic minorities are disempowered. Few minority group members belong to boards, commissions, and policymaking infrastructures. Many of the ones that do belong have been so transculturated into the white Anglo culture that they often go along with the program rather than stand up for the rights of the ethnic group that they represent.

The best intervention to address the issue of a poor infrastructure is for the community to take a look at its own attitudes and prejudices toward different ethnic minority groups. One way to do this is to have a diversity training consultant do a program with the Health Services Department administration using awareness training exercises such as those developed by Judy Katz, in order to explore how the administration institutionalizes racism in its decision making and program development.

There are other obstacles that prevent people with AIDS from seeking professional help, such as cultural differences.

CULTURAL DIFFERENCES

Culture is defined as "acquired knowledge which people use to interpret experience and generate social behavior." It includes a social group's observable pattern of behavior, customs, way of life, ideas, values or beliefs, definition of reality, attitudes, and habits. Culture is what a group develops in order to solve its problems of survival in the external environment as well as its problems of internal integration. The learning of culture is simultaneously a behavioral, cognitive, and emotional process.

The deepest level of culture is the cognitive level, in that the perceptions, language, and thoughts that a group comes to share become the causal determinants of feelings, attitudes, values, and overt behavior.

Perceptual Differences

Anthropologists have shown that cultures differ in terms of value orientation. For example, the Anglo culture is grounded on one's ability to conquer nature. We can go to the moon or even send a telescope to Jupiter. The Hispanic culture is more fatalistic. One can often hear a mother lamenting, "This is the cross I have to bear." Native Americans, on the other hand, approach life in an attempt to live in harmony with nature.

Asian cultures often relate hierarchically within families or formal organizational structures. There is much respect for elders as well as for persons in authority, such as the counselor. In contrast, within the white Anglo culture, relationships are linear, and peer associations are valued over hierarchical ones.

These differences in values affect the way a client pursues clinical services. For example, white Anglos who are used to conquering nature will likely be very assertive in the pursuit of not only the services but also the funding for those services. They will likely also view the clinician as a peer who is there to help clients attain their goals. Ethnic minorities approaching the relationship from a more hierarchical perspective may hesitate to make a request of the clinician for fear of being disrespectful or to avoid burdening the clinician with their problem. They may not assert their rights because the group's needs may be impinged upon by an individual need. In a culture where group identity has a higher value than individual identity, asserting one's needs may be seen as self-centered and disrespectful of the group.

Because of these differences, clinicians must understand how the target group of their services operates in the world so that they can convey acceptance and respect for that culture. They need to learn how to invite members of that particular ethnic group, directly or indirectly, to use the services and engage in intimate relationships such as counseling or psychotherapy. They need to understand that in some cultures, it could be considered a taboo to bring personal information or problems to a stranger. "Los trapos sucios se quedan en la casa" (the dirty laundry remains at home).

Clinical service delivery programs often assume that as long as the clinician can speak the language, the program will be able to reach the client. The following example provides a humorous yet vivid illustration of how textbook information alone cannot fill the gap in communication.

At a recent statewide conference on Latino/a health and leadership, an AIDS hotline counselor shared an incident that occurred at his agency. A Latino man called the AIDS hotline quite upset and told the Anglo hotline counselor who knew some Spanish: "Se me callo la mano." Literally translated this means "My hand fell off." Thinking that this man had been in an industrial accident, the hotline counselor recommended to the caller that he hang up and call 911. The caller was confused because he didn't see his situation as so drastic; he just wanted someone to talk to. What the caller said had actually meant was, "My wrist went limp." This is a vernacular expression. The caller had just realized that he was gay and wanted to talk to someone about this shocking self-discovery.

The various ethnic groups in this country have different issues related to their specific culture. In this chapter, I am going to focus on African Americans, Latinos/as, and Asians, the largest groups affected by AIDS/HIV and the groups with whom I have had the most experience.

Working with African Americans

Over 10 percent of AIDS cases in the United States due to male-to-male contact have occurred among African-American men. Among African Americans, 36 percent of the cases are attributed to homosexual or bisexual activity, 38 percent to intravenous injection contamination, and 12 percent to hetero-sexual contact.

The stigma of homosexuality in the African-American culture and the absence of a large openly gay subculture that would buffer such intolerance create a community environment where bisexuality is commonly preferred to homosexuality as a label for sexual identity. Some African-American men may engage in recreational homosexual behavior to obtain physical pleasure; others engage in homosexual behavior for economic reasons or to satisfy the sexual drive during imprisonment; and still others engage in homosexual behavior because they are gay.

In counseling African-American men, the clinician must be careful not to assume that the fact that a person engages in same-sex behavior means that the person is gay. The clinician will do better to ask clients to identify where in the sexual spectrum they belong, so as not to antagonize the client or jeopardize the coun-selor-client relationship.

For example, during a group session, I commented on how the group represented all the different at-risk groups. Lamont, an African-American man, became angry at me because he felt that I had assumed that he was gay simply because he had become infected through same-sex contact. Actually, I had counted Lamont as a heterosexual male who engaged in same-sex behavior; Lamont had misunderstood this, and I had to explain to him what I'd intended.

African-American gay and bisexual men who are uncomfort-able about publicly disclosing their homosexual behavior are more likely to engage in unprotected anal intercourse. High-risk sexual behavior strongly correlates with marginal status. Mar-ginal status includes low income, getting paid for sex, and IV drug use.

Positive intervention objectives for clinicians treating African-Americans include the following:

1. Reduction of discomfort regarding homosexuality or bisexual-ity as viewed within the African-American community

2. Increase of racial pride, given that many of these individuals feel ostracized from the African-American community and adopt identities that conform more to the white Anglo gay/lesbian culture in order to fit into that cultural group

3. Strengthening of the clients' beliefs that condom use should become normative within the African-American subculture.

CHARLES

Charles was an African-American man who felt alienated from the gay world and the heterosexual African-American world as well as from the heterosexual white Anglo world. His presenting complaints were depression, feelings of isolation, and problems with intimacy. Charles had gone to an African-American counselor but had felt uncomfortable with him because of Charles's own internalized oppression as an African American and a gay person. Charles had gone to two white therapists but discredited them because of their race. I discussed with Charles how he might discredit me because I am Caucasian, as a way to have him explore how he uses people's characteristics to discredit them in the same way that he feels discredited from the African-American community and the gay community due to his own unique characteristics.

The goal of the clinician in working with someone like Charles is to have him own all the characteristics of himself and to embrace each of those characteristics in order to solidify his fragmented identity. This action helped Charles with his intimacy problems and helped him to stop projecting his feelings of difference, which caused him to feel distant from others.

Thomas Parham once stated that as long as Black people are subjected to racist and oppressive conditions in this society, and are forced to compromise their Blackness in order to assimilate successfully, they will need therapeutic assistance to deal with these issues. To this scenario one can add the African American's sexual orientation. With a same-sex orientation, African Americans must compromise not only their racial identity but their sexual orientation in order to fit into the respective ethnic and sexual communities.

One way that a clinician can help ethnic minority clients is to become familiar with the ethnic resources that are relevant for that particular client. For example, if a client is bisexual, the clinician should explore the resources available not only within the white bisexual community but within the bisexual African-American community. Clients may be too anxious to do this exploration on their own. Giving clients leads as to where the resources are can break the ice. A clinician thereby will also be role modeling assertiveness in the pursuit of these resources.

Maintaining a Level of Comfort

It is important for clinicians to focus at the level of cultural awareness at which the client feels comfortable. Clients may be embarrassed to admit to a person of their own ethnic group or sexual orientation that they are having difficulty accepting that part of their identity. Although a group format with all participants from the same sexual orientation and ethnic background as the client may eventually be beneficial to the ethnic minority client, a group may initially be too threatening for that client. Individual counseling may be more appropriate at this phase.

People with HIV/AIDS have to deal not only with issues of ethnic identity and sexual orientation but also with the fact that they have been infected. Being a "person with AIDS" or a seropositive person may be a difficult new identity for that client, who is already going through the grieving process about the loss of normal health. The clinician must be patient and supportive in helping the client to move through stages of acceptance for each aspect of identity with which the client is feeling discomfort.

W I N O N A

Winona was infected by her husband, who was an IV drug user. She was angry that her husband did not take better care of himself in order to protect her. Her husband died of AIDS. As a mother of three children, Winona had to deal with the fact that her children could potentially be orphaned. Her oldest son was chemically dependent, and Winona, as usual, kept putting others' needs ahead of her own.

Winona was overwhelmed with the loss of her husband, the loss of her health, her new identity as a person with HIV, her son's addiction, and the need to find a guardian for her children in the eventuality of her death. It is hard enough to lose a loved one, but to have to grieve that loved one while at the same time knowing that the person infected the bereaved with a deadly virus can be quite traumatic.

The impact of this news on Winona's life and that of her family required much support and assistance from the clinician in sorting through Winona's feelings and finding solutions to her concerns about her children. In Winona's case, the local AIDS Legal Services office was helpful in putting her in contact with an attorney who could draft a will or living trust whereby Winona could assign a guardian to her children in the event of her death. This intervention facilitated the removal of a burden for Winona so that she could continue her grieving process without as much of the concern for her children's future welfare.

Working with Latinos

As when working with African Americans, the clinician needs to be sensitive with Latino men, in particular, as to labels of sexual orientation. Latino/a culture has a strong Catholic religious base. Sex-role differences may cause a lack of availability of female partners, because the Latino/a cultures expect women to refrain from sexual activity except for procreation, whereas men are expected to express their machismo in the form of sexual conquests. This can actually be a cultural benefit to gay and bisexual Latino men because it increases the pool of partners for these subcultures within the overall culture. Despite the fact that homosexual behavior occurs, however, it is not condoned or approved of within the culture.

For many ethnic minority groups, bisexuality may be an alternative to being gay. It provides a cover for people while allowing them to express their same-sex needs. This was certainly true in my case. I was in the Air Force ROTC program at Michigan State University in 1972. My draft number was fourteen, and it was during the Vietnam War, so I felt I had no choice but to join the military. I often received comments from my commanding officers that I was the only cadet who was neither married nor engaged. I felt so much pressure that I came out to the Air Force and was given an honorable discharge despite the fact that I had won two Outstanding Commander Awards and was runner-up for Outstanding Cadet.

Two years later my sister was married, and again I was the only one in my sister's wedding party who was neither married nor engaged. Latino/a parents expect grandchildren; they want their children to marry as soon as possible to propagate the family, so I found a woman who had dated only gay men and married her after disclosing to her that I was gay. We thought the relationship could work. The more I accepted my gayness, however, the more permission and desire I had to have a male relationship.

Counseling can help to move the client from a bisexual perspective to a gay perspective if that is the true desire of an individual, as it was for me.

JUAN

Juan was a married man with no children who attended an emotional support group for Latino men with HIV/AIDS. During our sessions, his wife would sometimes come into the room and interrupt the session because Juan had forgotten to take his medication. This behavior was being triggered by the fact that his wife sensed that many of the men in the room were gay and that her husband was dealing with his sexual orientation. Juan and his wife had come from El Salvador and had experienced many losses as a result of the civil war. Juan's wife had to separate from her family and friends. Juan's mother lived with them, and Juan's wife did not get along with her. She felt very isolated. We had to arrange for counseling for Juan's wife to take place at the same time that Juan was in his group session so that Juan's wife could have some support about her own needs and wants and Juan could participate in the group without interruption.

During the group time, we talked about gay sexual orientation and what that meant for the group. As Juan owned his gay identity more and more, one of the members of the group commented that Juan was "soltando las trenzas" (undoing his braids). This became a group saying, and when I introduce the topic of exploring a gay sexual orientation I now introduce it as *soltando las trenzas.*

Within Latino cultures, sex-role differences are acted out in the gay and bisexual subcultures, in relation to what type of sexual activity a person will engage in. The macho person will be active as the anal inserter but will refuse to be a receptor. He will also allow his penis to be sucked by another man but will not suck another man's penis. This macho inserter role has also created a myth within the Latino culture that "as long as I remain the inserter, I do not need to use condoms and will not be infected with the AIDS virus."

Gay people within the Latino/a culture may also believe that if you are not heterosexual, you cannot behave in the manner customary for your own gender, so gay people within the Latino/a culture often adopt gender roles of the opposite sex by cross-dressing or engaging in opposite gender-typical behavior—effeminacy for men and butch behavior for women. These types of behaviors are also prevalent among gays and lesbians within the white Anglo culture, but as the gay movement in the United States has become stronger, there has been less emphasis on cross-dressing and on cross-gender behavior. Economic opportunities for gays and lesbians in the heterosexual white Anglo culture may also put pressure on gays and lesbians to conform to gender-typical behavior, so gays and lesbians in the white Anglo culture generally have more freedom than Latinos/as to separate gender roles from sexual orientation.

Camp talk has been described as gays referring to one another by women's names and pronouns. The significance of camp in the gay community in general and in the Latino/a community in particular has been attributed to the fact that camp talk changes the real, hostile world into one that is controllable and safe. If you reject me for my dress and effeminate behavior, I know why you are rejecting me. I am flaunting my feminine side at you. I am also protecting the core of my sexual orientation and self by giving you something external for which to reject me. Another role of camp is to bring a lighter side to the hostility that gays and lesbians receive for being who we are.

Sometimes, clinicians will be placed in roles that challenge notions learned in their training. When I was asked to be a participant in a drag show at a retreat for Latino gays, I had to make several psychological decisions. First, I had to consider my own discomfort in dressing as a woman. Next, I had to evaluate how dressing as a woman was going to affect my role and effectiveness as a clinician facilitating the retreat. For example, I had fantasies of losing my authority as a group leader. Third, and most important, I aspire to be a judge someday, and I didn't want this potentially harmful image of me in drag to become more generally known.

Being a Caucasian Latino with an advanced level of education sets me apart from many other members of the Latino/a community, including the gay and lesbian community. I made the decision to align with the group by participating in the drag show. I attempted to not do anything that I would later regret or feel had cost my dignity. Still, *respeto* (respect) is an important aspect of Latino/a culture. I weighed whether my participation would enhance or diminish this respeto in the eyes of the participants. It turned out that it was a positive decision because it brought me closer to their cultural experience.

Therapists need to have enough distance from their clients to be effective. In working with ethnic minorities, however, the role of therapist can be distancing in itself because ethnic minorities may not be familiar with the process of therapy or with going to a stranger to talk about their problems. By participating in the drag show I modeled vulnerability to the group and gained the participants' trust. This decision was also congruent with the Latino/a cultural norm of *personalismo*, which refers to the cultural preference for having more informal personal relationships with others as opposed to hierarchical, distant professional relationships.

Another area in which personalismo is important is in the expectations the Latino/a client has of the counselor. In the Anglo culture of psychodynamic psychotherapy, one is taught to maintain distance from the client, not to accept gifts from the client, and not to get too personally involved with the client. In the Latino/a culture, if you do not get somewhat personally involved with clients, they will consider it a rejection of them and a disrespect for the gift of friendship that they are offering you.

DANIEL

Daniel was a member of my first emotional support group for Latino men with HIV/AIDS. He had to be hospitalized at one point because of a bout with *Pneumocystis carinii* pneumonia. When he came back to the group, he expressed anger and disappointment that I had not gone to the hospital to visit him. After all, that is what family would have done. I had not understood that this was an expectation of this particular client. In fact, I also had some countertransference. I had visited other clients in the hospital in the past, so why not him? This particular client tended to be critical and negative, so I did not feel particularly warmly toward him. What I needed was to step back and look at why he was that way. Many people with AIDS develop dementia and lose the filtering inhibitory capabilities that stop most of us from saying everything we think and feel, some of which may not be socially acceptable or appropriate.

This experience has made me more sensitive to such issues as I continue to work with people with HIV/AIDS.

Other concerns regarding how personal to get with a client have to do with accepting small gifts or invitations to eat or have refreshments at their home.

One day, I made a home visit, and the client offered me coffee. Cognizant of the fact that declining such an invitation was culturally disrespectful, I accepted her offer. I heard her whispering to her daughter because she did not know how to make coffee. I asked her how she had coffee when she had it, and she said that she made instant. I told her that instant was fine and was able to divert a crisis.

This was a situation where we were both bound by the culture even if neither of us felt culturally tied to the ritual. I am usually in a hurry, and sometimes the social ritual of sharing a cup of coffee may take more time than I really have. However, if one is going to work within ethnic minority groups, one needs to make the time to incorporate some of these rituals. Agency administrators must allow counselors who work with ethnic minorities the flexibility to make the time for these clients, which may even entail reducing that counselor's client load.

Working with Asian Americans

Asians and Pacific Islanders (APIs) make up 3 percent of the U.S. population, yet the incidence of AIDS was only .7 percent as of 1993. In comparison, African Americans represent 12 percent of the population and 32 percent of AIDS cases; Latinos/as represent 9 percent of the U.S. population and 17 percent of AIDS cases. At the same time, the incidence of AIDS for APIs is increasing at a higher rate than among whites. It is suspected that underreporting may be a significant factor among APIs because of the stigma of AIDS and the cultural value of family honor that is so strong among these cultural groups.

A common theme, identified among gay APIs in treatment programs during the 1980s, is the cultural ambivalence reflected in their identity. Many of these individuals were found to feel pressure to choose between their Asian and gay identities.

In working with API gay and lesbian clients, as well as with other ethnic minorities, Connie Chan suggests that a clinician look at the following variables:

1. Is the client an immigrant or American born?
2. To what ethnic group does the client belong?
3. What are the specific cultural values of the client, this group, the client's family?
4. Does the client follow traditional or nontraditional customs?
5. What is the client's socioeconomic status?
6. What is the client's level of bilingualism?

Sally Jue and Craig Kain have also suggested that a clinician take into consideration the client's level of education.

Work with Asian Americans should include the exploration of the stigma of being gay or lesbian and of being exposed to HIV/AIDS within the API culture. API clients will need support in exploring their sense of isolation from family and community as well as racism and homophobia from the white Anglo heterosexual and gay and lesbian communities.

MANUEL

Manuel is a twenty-six-year-old Filipino man who is living by himself. He moved out of his parents' house when he was twenty-two in order to allow himself more privacy for his social life. Manuel is gay.

His moving out was a cause of concern to his family, as they expected him to live at home until he married, which is typical of the culture. Manuel initially came to counseling to work through his dual gay and Filipino identity; however, during the course of the treatment, he went to get a blood test and found out that he was HIV-positive. Even though he was twenty-six years old, Manuel had a shy, child-like quality about him. There was a side of him that wanted to be an adult, and there was another side that was afraid to express itself.

Manuel worked as a shift manager for a fast-food restaurant. He dated a physician. When the physician had his friends over, Manuel felt very out of place because of the differences in education and income between him and the physician and the physician's friends. Manuel complained that the physician did not want to make a commitment.

I pointed out to Manuel that it was not only the physician but Manuel himself who was ambivalent about his commitment to him. Manuel seemed intent on pleasing others at his own expense. One of the things that Manuel had to begin to establish was an individuated self. He seemed stuck in his image of himself as an adolescent without the right to make decisions for himself about his life.

The news of being HIV-positive exacerbated his fears of coming out to his family. His sister knew that he was gay, but the rest of the family did not know. He was close to his sister, who was a college student majoring in medical technology. They shared a bond because both of them were more transculturated than their parents, so there was a cultural generational division. Manuel wanted to tell his sister about his HIV status, but he didn't want to upset her while she was in school, and he was not sure if she would honor his request for confidentiality, even though she had not disclosed his gayness.

For Manuel, as for many clients who are HIV-positive, disclosure of his HIV status was an important issue. These clients need to explore the rationale for disclosure of their HIV status, and they need support as they attempt to make these disclosures to the significant others in their lives.

Notice that Manuel had to deal with several issues: his dual identity as a Filipino and a gay man, the normal developmental process of transitioning from adolescence to young adulthood, his psychological separation from his family within the cultural context, and his HIV status.

It was evident that Manuel was very isolated. After individual work with Manuel regarding some of these issues, I encouraged him to seek out an API support group that he could join. Manuel went to a group meeting and came back reporting that he didn't feel comfortable going there because nobody there was like himself. This can be a typical reaction for someone who is coming out. "I will reject you before you reject me. I'm also afraid that if I join the group, I will be forced to commit to the group's values and norms." After exploring these feelings with Manuel, I encouraged him to continue going to the group without making any commitments. Eventually, Manuel began to feel more comfortable in the group.

I also suggested to Manuel that he go to an API store that sold dolls; I wanted him to get a doll that he could use as a representation of his inner child. The closest doll that Manuel could find to represent his ethnic identity was a Kung Fu doll. The doll's arms moved and were supposed to be in a Kung Fu pose; however, as Manuel displayed the doll for me, the doll's arm was twisted with the palm of the hand upward and bent down, in an effeminate fashion. I kidded Manuel about how appropriate the doll was and how it depicted his gay side. Manuel became defensive because this depiction of overt gayness was threatening to him. This incident opened up an opportunity to explore his fear directly.

Manuel also wanted me to give him permission to destroy this doll. I told Manuel that if he wanted to destroy the doll, he could make that decision, and that I could not make it for him. Manuel struggled for several sessions about whether or not he would destroy the doll. He finally made the decision not to destroy the doll; he even began to like it. Part of the homework assignment with the doll was for him to become acquainted with his inner child. Here was a new "object" in his life that he needed to become acquainted with, just like the scared inner child that he had been ignoring all these years.

As the therapy progressed, I suggested to Manuel that he might want to use the doll to work through the feelings of having been infected with the AIDS virus. I suggested that he symbolically infect the doll with the virus so that he could experience the moment of infection to draw out the feelings. Manuel reported that this part of the counseling had been difficult but that it had been an important and moving experience. As Manuel learned to accept his HIV-positive status, I began to encourage him to seek out a support group for HIV-positive API gay men. This would likely help him to integrate all the different aspects of his identity.

Heterosexual Asian Americans must face the AIDS epidemic as well, as this case example illustrates.

K I M

Kim worked at an AIDS hospice as a housekeeper. When she started working there, she was supposed to have gone through a safety training in handling materials, but because she was monolingual in Korean only, she did not attend the training. Kim pricked herself with a used needle that had blood on it from an AIDS client who lived in the hospice. Kim panicked at the thought she might be infected. She was a single mother who had a daughter in junior high school. Like Winona, she was concerned about what would happen to her daughter if she developed AIDS.

In counseling, I helped Kim to learn not to catastrophize. At this point, Kim was one of the "worried well." My role consisted of providing Kim with the best available information regarding transmission and the hope that she may not have been infected. There was nothing Kim could do immediately because of the incubation period of HIV. She needed to wait until enough time had elapsed for her to be tested.

During the waiting period, I assisted Kim by teaching her relaxation exercises and helping her vent her anxiety. I also did some rational-emotive counseling with her to help her contain the anxiety and not catastrophize, as there was no clear evidence that she had been infected. I also referred Kim to an attorney so that she could protect her rights as an employee of the company, because it appeared that the company was negligent in not providing safety instructions to Kim in her language.

Fortunately, Kim's test turned out negative. We were able to celebrate the news, and left it open for Kim to be tested in another six months and come back if the test turned out positive.

Because of cultural differences, clients may not be privy to their legal rights in this country. It may be helpful for the counselor to make the client aware of these issues and to provide appropriate referrals. This can be empowering to a client, but it can also add to the anxiety if the client's culture discourages a confrontive approach to problem solving. The therapist needs to present clients with their options in a way that does not communicate an expectation of confrontation, as clients may then feel torn between their culture and trying to please the therapist.

SPECIAL ISSUES

Research has revealed that many ethnic minority clients tend to prefer a concrete, directive, problem-solving approach. Sally Jue and Craig Kain suggest that the focus should thus be on information and referral, advocacy, and assistance with social services, rather than on discussions of feelings and life histories. This approach conforms to Maslow's hierarchy of needs. For many ethnic minorities, issues revolve around the basic needs of food and shelter, whereas counseling is a higher-level need. Many Anglos have their basic needs already taken care of, so they can focus on the higher-level needs of identity and self-actualization, which psychotherapy can help address. If a clinician assists ethnic minority clients with their basic needs, they will be accepting the clients at the level at which they are presenting themselves. At the same time, we are not only helping clients to move on to the higher-level tasks of identity and self-actualization, but we are doing so in a way that creates trust and respect between the clinician and the clients.

Using Structured Activities

Structured activities may be useful in certain circumstances. For example, one of the activities that I conducted with my emotional support groups included a presentation on the wellness model. For many people who have been exposed to HIV/AIDS, the reason for exposure may have been an unhealthy lifestyle. For many ethnic minorities who feel disenfranchised from society, and even for gay men who are professionals but have lost that sense of commitment to self and others in their lives, the future is not that important to them. They develop a present-life value orientation that calls for immediate gratification without concern for the consequences. "If I die tomorrow, so what? I don't see a bright future ahead of me anyway, so why not enjoy today?"

The wellness model provides a good base from which such clients can take a look at the different aspects of their life. It includes a focus on the spiritual, emotional, psychological, financial and occupational, physical, and social values in living. These topics, as well as the relevant issues of identification in sexual orientation, can all be discussed within the relevant cultural context of the ethnic minority group to which the person belongs. The clients in the cases previously discussed in this chapter provide examples.

In Manuel's case, he took a look at where he was going occupationally. He had always wanted to pursue a college education, so he decided to enroll in college classes.

Lamont, on the other hand, expressed a void in his spiritual life. There was a local African-American Baptist church that began to do ministry with brothers and sisters who were HIV-positive or had AIDS. I provided support for Lamont to pursue an association with that church and encouraged him to contact the coordinator of the ministry so that he could connect individually at first. Then when he felt comfortable, he could join the other parishioners participating in the ministry.

Juan and the other members of the Latino emotional support group began a custom of going out to a coffee shop after the meeting. This provided Juan with a social outlet.

During one session of the support group, I introduced a blown-up picture of the AIDS virus to the group and placed the picture on a chair. Then I asked each group member to sit across from the picture and confront the AIDS virus and tell it what he was feeling about its being in his body.

The physical component of wellness is very easy to address: it includes looking at healthy ways of eating and changing one's habits to include proper amounts of rest and relaxation. The members of the emotional support group were taught relaxation exercises. Members also had the opportunity to share with each other different symptoms and treatments so that they could anticipate them and identify what was happening to them physically.

Psychologically, many of the group members who were dealing with chemical dependency issues or with issues of dementia could discuss what was happening to them mentally. Referrals to appropriate resources for assessment and treatment of these issues were helpful to these clients.

Dealing with Internalized Shame

People with HIV/AIDS and gays, lesbians, and bisexuals often carry internalized shame about who they are. At a retreat, I introduced an exercise to have the participants look at their sexual orientation and embrace it. Music is very important in the lives of ethnic minorities, so I chose a song to lead the exercise. Because the group was bilingual, I chose a song titled "Love Is All It Takes" by Romanovsky and Phillips, two gay composers. The song is about a man singing a lullaby to his children the day before he is supposed to go to court to attempt to get custody.

In the song, the father is expressing a wish that the court would see him the way his children see him and the way he sees himself, as opposed to the way society stereotypes him to be. The song was a powerful tool because it validated the goodness in the gay father. The group could identify with the father; they could own the goodness inside themselves and feel the sadness that others could not see that goodness as well.

During the exercise, participants hugged their pillows, which represented their inner child. Not long after the song started, one could hear the sobbing (and the healing) that this song was creating for the participants. This exercise was too much for one of the participants, and he took care of himself by leaving the room. I asked one of the retreat facilitators to go after him to make sure he was OK. After the exercise was over, the group processed what they had felt. The young man who left the room talked about his sense of isolation because he felt so distant from his family. He wanted to feel close to them. However, the fear of rejection from his family for being gay kept him emotionally separated.

Familismo, or sense of family, is an important value within the Latino/a culture. Having a characteristic such as a gay, lesbian, or bisexual orientation can be especially traumatic for Latinos/as because this characteristic sets them apart from their families as well as their society.

Dealing with Death

Relationship to death can differ from culture to culture. In the Anglo culture, for example, there is much discomfort with the concept of death. After all, when one dies is not something that is under one's control. Latinos/as, on the other hand, take a more fatalistic approach to death. Some of the cultural rituals actually imply looking forward to it, such as the *Dia de los Muertos* (Day of the Dead) and the Mexican folk art figures of skeletons playing dominoes around a card table while smoking cigars. There is an assumption of life after death.

Sometimes, Latinos/as in particular express discomfort about joining the emotional support groups at the local AIDS projects because of the somber manner in which those groups treat death. Minority clients should be supported in dealing with the full range of emotions they may feel about death, from the humorous to the sad. The task of death is acceptance. Too much emphasis on the somber aspects of death may communicate negative messages to a client who is experiencing the inevitable. Too much levity may also indicate denial of the pain of disengaging from loved ones. Clinicians need to work through their own issues with regard to death in order to assist their clients in dealing with it.

Counseling ethnic minorities with HIV/AIDS can be a multilayered proposition. Clinicians must be eclectic in their approach in order to address the different needs of these clients within both a culturally and sexually relevant context. These treatments must include interventions that confront issues of stigma related to being from an ethnic minority group; being gay, lesbian, or bisexual; and having an HIV-positive or AIDS status. We need to help our clients deal with their family and community as well as to develop a positive identity so that they can integrate all aspects of their lives. Lastly, these clients and their significant others must be introduced to techniques of community empowerment that will allow them to confront the insensitivities of the mainstream culture and to obtain the necessary resources that these groups deserve.

NOTES

P. 165, *In that service area . . . ethnic minorities:* Santa Clara County Health Department. (1995, June 30). *Santa Clara Valley Health and Hospital System surveillance report: Cumulative AIDS cases ending June 30, 1995.* Santa Clara, CA: Author.

P. 165, *Yet the four minority programs share $70,000:* Motoyor, M. (1995). *Santa Clara County Commission on HIV and AIDS annual report, 1994–1995.* Santa Clara, CA: Author. Statement quoted from M. Madsen, Director of AIDS and HIV Health Services.

P. 166, *The commission's task is to oversee all planning of HIV/AIDS services:* Motoyor, M. (1995). *Santa Clara County Commission on HIV and AIDS annual report, 1994–1995.* Santa Clara, CA: Author.

P. 168, *The county statistics show . . . a parent at risk of contracting HIV:* Santa Clara County Health Department. (1995, June 30). *Santa Clara Valley Health and Hospital System surveillance report: Cumulative AIDS cases ending June 30, 1995.* Santa Clara, CA: Author.

P. 169, *awareness training exercises such as those developed by Judy Katz:* Katz, J., & Ivey, A. (1977). White awareness: The frontier of racism awareness training. *Personnel and Guidance Journal, 55,* 485–489.

P. 169, Culture *is defined as "acquired knowledge":* Spradley, J. (1979). *The ethnographic interview.* Austin, TX: Holt, Rinehart and Winston.

P. 169, *Culture is what a group develops . . . its problems of internal integration:* Fetterman, D. (1989). *Ethnography step by step.* Thousand Oaks, CA: Sage.

P. 169, *The learning of culture is simultaneously . . . overt behavior:* Schein, E. (1990). Organizational culture. *American Psychologist, 45,* 109–119.

P. 170, *Anthropologists have shown . . . conquer nature:* Kluckhohn, F., & Strodtbeck, F. (1961). *Variations in value orientation.* New York: HarperCollins.

P. 170, *within the white Anglo culture, . . . peer associations are valued over hierarchical ones:* Kluckhohn, F., & Strodtbeck, F. (1961). *Variations in value orientation.* New York: HarperCollins.

P. 172, *Over 10 percent . . . 12 percent to heterosexual contact:* Peterson, J. L. (1995). AIDS-related risks and same-sex behaviors among African-American men. In G. Herek & B. Greene (Eds.), *Medical perspectives on lesbian and gay issues: Vol. 2. AIDS, identity, and community: The HIV epidemic and lesbians and gay men* (pp. 85–104). Thousand Oaks, CA: Sage.

P. 172, *The stigma of homosexuality in the African-American culture . . . sexual identity:* Doll, L., Peterson, J. L., & Carrier, J. (1991). Male homosexuality and AIDS in the United States. In R. Tielman, M. Carballo, & A. Hendriks (Eds.), *Bisexuality and HIV/AIDS* (pp. 27–39). Amherst, NY: Prometheus.

P. 172, *Some African-American men . . . because they are gay:* Delamater, J. (1981). The social control of sexuality. *Annual Review of Sociology, 7,* 263–290.

P. 172, *African-American gay and bisexual men . . . unprotected anal intercouse:* Peterson, J. L. (1995). AIDS-related risks and same-sex behaviors among African-American men. In G. Herek & B. Greene (Eds.), *Medical perspec-*

tives on lesbian and gay issues: Vol. 2. AIDS, identity, and community: The HIV epidemic and lesbians and gay men (pp. 85–104). Thousand Oaks, CA: Sage.

P. 172, *Positive intervention objectives . . . African-Americans include the following:* Peterson, J. L. (1995). AIDS-related risks and same-sex behaviors among African-American men. In G. Herek & B. Greene (Eds.), *Medical perspectives on lesbian and gay issues: Vol. 2. AIDS, identity, and community: The HIV epidemic and lesbians and gay men* (pp. 85–104). Thousand Oaks, CA: Sage.

P. 173, *Charles:* Case study reprinted from Gutierrez, F., & Dworkin, S. (1992). Gay, lesbian and African American: Managing the integration of identities. In S. Dworkin & F. Gutierrez (Eds.), *Counseling gay men and lesbians: Journey to the end of the rainbow* (pp. 141–156). Alexandria, VA: American Counseling Association Press.

P. 173, *Thomas Parham once stated:* Parham, T. (1989). Cycles of psychological nigrescence. *Counseling Psychologist, 17,* 187–226.

P. 177, *The macho person . . . another man's penis:* Carballo-Dieguez, A. (1995). The sexual identity and behavior of Puerto Rican men who have sex with men. In G. Herek & B. Greene (Eds.), *Medical perspectives on lesbian and gay issues: Vol. 2. AIDS, identity, and community: The HIV epidemic and lesbians and gay men* (pp. 105–114). Thousand Oaks, CA: Sage.

P. 177, *This macho inserter role . . . "the AIDS virus":* Carballo-Dieguez, A. (1995). The sexual identity and behavior of Puerto Rican men who have sex with men. In G. Herek & B. Greene (Eds.), *Medical perspectives on lesbian and gay issues: Vol. 2. AIDS, identity, and community: The HIV epidemic and lesbians and gay men* (pp. 105–114). Thousand Oaks, CA: Sage.

P. 178, *Economic opportunities . . . from sexual orientation:* Gutierrez, F. (1994). Gay and lesbian: An ethnic identity deserving equal protection. *Law and Sexuality: A Review of Lesbian and Gay Legal Issues, 4,* 195–247.

P. 178, Camp talk *has been described:* Bronski, M. (1984). *Culture clash: The making of a gay sensibility.* Boston: South End Press.

P. 178, *Another role of camp . . . who we are:* Grahn, J. (1984). *Another mother tongue.* Boston: Beacon Press.

P. 179, *the Latino/a cultural norm of* personalismo: Morales, E. (1992). Counseling Latino gays and Latina lesbians. In S. Dworkin & F. Gutierrez (Eds.), *Counseling gay men and lesbians: Journey to the end of the rainbow* (pp. 141–156). Alexandria, VA: American Counseling Association Press.

P. 181, *A common theme, identified among gay APIs in treatment programs during the 1980s, . . . choose between their Asian and gay identities:* Choi, K., Salazar, H., & Lew, S. (1995). AIDS risk, dual identity, and community response among gay Asian and Pacific Islander men in San Francisco. In G. Herek & B. Greene (Eds.), *Medical perspectives on lesbian and gay issues: Vol. 2. AIDS, identity, and community: The HIV epidemic and lesbians and gay men* (pp. 115–134). Thousand Oaks, CA: Sage.

P. 181, *Connie Chan suggests . . . look at the following variables:* List reprinted from Chan, C. (1992). Cultural considerations in counseling Asian American lesbians and gay men. In S. Dworkin & F. Gutierrez (Eds.), *Counseling gay men and lesbians: Journey to the end of the rainbow* (pp. 115–134). Alexandria, VA: American Counseling Association Press. Copyright © ACA. Reprinted by permission. No further reproduction authorized without written permission of the American Counseling Association,

P. 181, *Sally Jue and Craig Kain have also suggested:* Jue. S., & Kain, C. (1989). Culturally sensitive AIDS counseling. In C. Kain (Ed.), *No longer immune: A counselor's guide to AIDS* (pp. 131–148). Alexandria, VA: American Counseling Association Press.

P. 185, *Research has revealed that many ethnic minority clients . . . problem-solving approach:* Jue. S., & Kain, C. (1989). Culturally sensitive AIDS counseling. In C. Kain (Ed.), *No longer immune: A counselor's guide to AIDS* (pp. 131–148). Alexandria, VA: American Counseling Association Press.

P. 185, *Maslow's hierarchy of needs:* Kagan, J., & Havemann, E. (1968). *Psychology: An introduction.* Orlando: Harcourt Brace.

P. 187, *"Love Is All It Takes":* Romanovsky, R., & Phillips, R. (1991). Love is all it takes. On *Be political not polite* [Record]. Santa Fe, NM: Fresh Fruit Records.

P. 188, Familismo, *or sense of family:* Morales, E. (1992). Counseling Latino gays and Latina lesbians. In S. Dworkin & F. Gutierrez (Eds.), *Counseling gay men and lesbians: Journey to the end of the rainbow* (pp. 125–139). Alexandria, VA: American Counseling Association Press.

FOR FURTHER READING

Carballo-Dieguez, A. (1989). Hispanic culture, gay male culture and AIDS counseling implications. *Journal of Counseling and Development, 68*(1), 26–30.

Chan, C. (1195). Issues of sexual identity in an ethnic minority: The case of Chinese American lesbians, gay men, and bisexual people. In A. R. D'Augelli & C. J. Patterson (Eds.), *Lesbian, gay, and bisexual identities over the lifespan: Psychological perspectives* (pp. 87–101). New York: Oxford.

Chan, C. (1989). Issues of identity development among Asian-American lesbians and gay men. *Journal of Counseling and Development, 68*(1), 16–20.

Golden, C. (1987). Diversity and variability in women's sexual identities. In Boston Lesbian Psychologies Collective (Eds.), *Lesbian psychologies: Explorations and challenges* (pp. 18–34). Urbana: University of Illinois Press.

Gutierrez, F., & Perlstein, M. (1992). Helping someone to die. In S. Dworkin & F. Gutierrez (Eds.), *Counseling gay men and lesbians: Journey to the end of the rainbow* (pp. 259–275). Alexandria, VA: American Counseling Association Press.

Loiacano, D. Gay identity issues among Black Americans: Racism, homophobia, and the need for validation. *Journal of Counseling and Development*, *68*(1), 21–25.

Rust, P. C. (1996). Managing multiple identities: Diversity among bisexual women and men. In B. A. Firestein (Ed.), *Bisexuality: The psychology and politics of an invisible minority*. Thousand Oaks, CA: Sage.

Tafoya, T. (1989). Pulling the coyote's tale: Native American sexuality and AIDS. In V. Mays, G. W. Albee, & S. F. E. Schneider (Eds.), *Primary prevention of AIDS: Psychological approaches* (pp. 280–289). Thousand Oaks, CA: Sage.

6

TREATING HIV-POSITIVE WOMEN

Kathleen J. Goggin and Judith G. Rabkin

Although the need to confront progressive disease and premature mortality in the context of personal, family, and community devastation are common to all who live with HIV illness, the situation of HIV-positive women requires special consideration. With exceptions, the life course, current living circumstances, social bonds, and perceived options of HIV-positive women differ dramatically from those of HIV-positive men, often to the point where the common bond of their illness is overshadowed. Although many sources of assistance are equally useful for HIV-positive men and women, such as generic community-based organizations offering support groups, meals, recreation, and access to medical information, women need supplementary services and considerations to address their particular needs. Even though most issues we include here are not *unique* to women (for example, disclosing one's HIV status to a child, or "permanency planning" regarding custodial care of a child), they are largely the province of women, if only by default.

In our roles as psychologists conducting clinical research over the past several years, we have worked with several hundred patients with HIV illness, including Hispanic, Caucasian, and African-American HIV-positive women. From this work, we have identified common underlying issues of concern to HIV-positive women. In this chapter, we will present these issues and offer therapeutic techniques to deal with each.

PROBLEMS IN RESEARCH ON WOMEN

Women were not included in the major epidemiologic studies and clinical trials conducted in the 1980s for several reasons, some more justifiable than others. On a practical level, affected women were hard to find and thus to recruit for studies. Although the increases in rate of infection among women has in recent years been higher than for men, the actual numbers are substantially lower. In 1984, when the Multicenter AIDS Cohort Study (MACS) enrolled five thousand men in five sites across the country, only 293 women with AIDS nationwide (6 percent of all cases) had been identified by the Centers for Disease Control and Prevention (CDC). In 1985 and 1986, when the first clinical trials of antiretroviral drugs were undertaken, only 530 and then 923 women were identified as having AIDS, (7 to 8 percent of the total). It wasn't until 1992 that the first natural history study of HIV disease in women commenced. According to the *HIV/AIDS Surveillance Report*, by 1995, women constituted about 18 percent of newly diagnosed cases (13,800 out of 75,800 cases in all).

In the 1980s, women of childbearing age (which includes almost all HIV-positive women) were excluded from all clinical trials of investigational drugs unless they were sterilized or otherwise unable to have children, according to FDA rules, until the compound in question was shown to have presumptive evidence of efficacy. This extreme concern about unknown risks to fetuses from investigational drugs, paternalistic as it was, was no doubt heightened by the thalidomide disaster in the 1970s. This rule also applied to investigational drugs for HIV. Consequently, women were not included in the 1980s clinical trials of AZT, aerosolized pentamidine, and other medications being studied for HIV illness. With increasing recognition on a national level of the consequent neglect of women's health needs, federal policy changed for all trials, including HIV trials.

In the 1990s, there has been a new awareness of the need to enroll women in trials of HIV-related treatments. However, success has been elusive, and the number of women currently participating in trials remains disappointing. This is partly due to the suspicions of many HIV-positive women, especially ethnic minority women, of research in general. It is also related to the likelihood that HIV-positive women as a group are less informed as medical consumers, are less likely to "take charge" of the medical management of their illness, and have less access to trials because of such practical barriers as costs of transportation and lack of baby-sitters. HIV-infected women who are aggressive about getting the best available health care may be more resistant than men to studies with placebo arms, at least in our own experience.

In order for more women to be successfully enrolled in trials of new HIV medications, they may need special outreach to understand their rights and obligations as research subjects, to learn how to find out about ongoing trials and how to persist in the often onerous task of actually getting accepted in such trials.

Therapists can help women become informed research participants by helping them to explore their thoughts, feelings, and past experiences with research. We have found that validating negative experiences while encouraging problem solving and assertive approaches is an effective strategy. Role-playing can further enhance assertiveness skills while improving self-esteem and mastery. Therapists can also play an important role in educating women about research and specific research opportunities.

PSYCHOSOCIAL CHALLENGES

There are few absolutes when working with HIV-positive women. In general, HIV-positive women present with a variety of psychosocial problems, some HIV related, some not. Many problems will be amplified by HIV, others will have little to do with the woman's medical status. Some situations, such as abusive relationships, will require immediate attention. Although getting out of the relationship may be a desirable goal, it is not always possible. At the very least, a plan for staying safe should be developed and implemented before a crisis presents itself.

As is true of work with HIV-positive men, working with HIV-positive women will require therapists to be more flexible than they might otherwise be in a "traditional" therapeutic relationship. They will often be called on to address many issues that typically are within the domain of the social worker, the family therapist, or the interpreter of medical information. Therefore, therapists must become knowledgeable about the transmission, prevention, medical, psychological, and sociopolitical issues faced by HIV-positive women. Due to the unpredictable nature of the disease and women's often heavy caregiving responsibilities, therapists will need to be flexible about the scheduling and site of appointments, as women may need to change appointments or require home or hospital visits. In short, the successful therapist must be willing to respond with great flexibility to the client's changing circumstances and needs, especially with progressive HIV illness.

Safer Sex: Staying Healthy

In most cultures, it is not easy for women to initiate conversations with their partners about sexual behavior and health practices. In the U.S., it is particularly hard among ethnic groups where HIV is overrepresented and where feminism has had little impact. In both Latino and African-American communities, women seldom have equal power in relationships, and even raising the subject of condom use may provoke abuse, rejection, or both. These power disparities have led major research programs to develop techniques such as viricides and the "female condom," which women can use for protection without having to count on the cooperation (and in the former instance, knowledge) of their partners. However, viricide research is still in the experimental stage, and women today have little recourse if their partners resist requests or refuse to practice safer sex. Heterosexual transmission is also more likely (for biological reasons) from men to women than the reverse, so women are in greater jeopardy for infection than their partner if only one is HIV-positive.

For the therapist working with "at-risk" women, it is important to adopt a partnership stance that includes sufficient psychoeducation (for example, in safer sex techniques) without making judgments. Women may need help in developing negotiation skills to enable them to practice safer sex. In some cases, bringing the partner into the therapeutic setting to facilitate open discussions can be helpful.

The literature has identified a multitude of financial, emotional, and cultural factors that interfere with a woman's ability and motivation to adhere to safer sex techniques. A crucial first step toward changing this situation is to provide a safe and supportive environment that facilitates uncovering the specific factors that influence a woman's ability to practice safer sex. Once these factors have been identified, individual strategies can be developed to deal with each barrier. Women's communication and assertiveness skills can be greatly improved by role playing appropriate safer sex interactions. This technique can be especially helpful, as it allows the woman to gain mastery while enhancing her self-esteem.

Testing for HIV

Women at risk for HIV report a number of reasons for and against getting tested. In the second decade of AIDS, it is increasingly recognized that early diagnosis, prophylaxis, and treatment can delay illness progression. However, many women still choose not to know. They may be struggling with more immediate demons such as drug addiction, or they may have other more immediate crises to address, such as poor housing, the threat of losing custody of their children, or problems with welfare benefits. Many get tested when they are in prison on drug-related charges or in drug rehabilitation programs. Some use the information to help themselves get and stay clean. One of our research participants, a forty-one-year-old HIV-positive woman with a long history of drug abuse, explained how getting a diagnosis helped her turn her life around:

> It saved my life. The kind of life that I was living before I got arrested, before I found out I had the virus, I was dead but I didn't lay down. And today I'm not living that way. You know, I've been thrown from cars, I've been cut up, I've been raped, I mean, the whole nine. So I look at it like it saved my life because I don't have to go out and do the same things that I was doing. It gave me my heart back. It gave me my feelings back, which I didn't have before.

Other women we have worked with have used their diagnosis as an excuse to get high. One forty-five-year-old woman shared her story with us: "It [the diagnosis] was devastating, really devastating and I felt like getting more high. . . . I knew it was high risk, I was doing high-risk behavior, but I didn't believe that I had the virus. And then I was ignorant to really what it was, so I thought it was a death sentence or a quick death."

For an addicted woman, an HIV diagnosis brings with it many painful realities. If she decides to get clean, she must deal with the consequences of her past drug-using behavior. This may include revisiting old family conflicts, attempting to be reunited with children who have been removed by family members or the courts, and facing her own personal insecurities and fears. If she is serious about getting clean, she will have to deal with a drug rehabilitation system that is overtaxed in general and not geared toward women, especially women with children. If she has children with her, she will have to find someone to care for them while she is in treatment. If there are no readily available family or friends who will provide care, she is left with few options beyond foster placement. At this point, many women delay or refuse treatment because they fear the loss of their parental rights.

The lucky woman who somehow navigates her way into treatment will have to deal with the feelings of guilt, anger, hopelessness, and uncertainty that often accompany early sobriety and an HIV-positive diagnosis. Attaining sobriety is difficult in its own right; in the face of HIV it is even more complicated.

For some nonsubstance-addicted women, testing is simply confirmation of a long-held belief that they are HIV-positive. Many know that they are or were at risk and fully expect to test positive. Others have no idea that they were exposed and find out their status only after they or a sexual partner become ill or when they give birth to an HIV-positive child. In some cases, the discovery is by chance, as it was for one of the women in our study, who found out her HIV status after donating blood for her daughter's surgery.

Coming to Terms with an HIV-Positive Diagnosis

Once women know their HIV-positive status, the issue of how they became infected arises. For some women it is an easily answered question of past risky behavior, usually unprotected sex or shared needles. For others, this becomes a painful acknowledgment that their husband or sexual partner lied to them and put them at risk without their knowledge or consent. Feelings of anger, betrayal, and helplessness are common. As one woman who was infected by her bisexual husband told us: "My husband just used me. He used me. I was speaking to a bisexual, an older man, and he tells me, 'I'm sorry to say, but your husband just used you, that's all he did, used you for show and tell.' And I believe that. I honestly believe that. For his family, you know. Don't do that, because *I loved you!* I mean, intensely loved. How can you use a person like that? But, he did."

Others had some idea that they were at risk, but were powerless to protect themselves. "There had been lots of abuse in our relationship, lots of abuse, mental and physical. And my partner, he has had many sexual partners, and I was pregnant and they offered the test and I just volunteered to take it. And wow, I was positive. I told him about it, but he denied the whole thing, even though I knew what he was all about. He still hasn't gotten tested."

And some are the victims of violent crime. "I was raped in '89. . . . He pulled a gun out on me and he raped me. So I was like, I couldn't believe it. . . . He's been arrested cause he's done it quite a few times. Matter of fact, he just got out of jail this year for doing it to another girl. I know that's how I got it, cause nine months later came him [my son] and three months later came the shingles. I've never done IV drugs, no transfusions, and all the other sex was safe. It was him."

Some women are angry because they feel they were betrayed by HIV/AIDS education campaigns that left them out and therefore sent the message that they were not at risk. "I wasn't involved with men, just women, so I really didn't think, ya know, that I could get it. I'm pissed, really pissed that nobody told me I could get it from another woman. If I'd known, I'd have been more careful."

Regardless of how they came in contact with the virus, HIV-positive women who seek treatment will require a safe environment in which to explore their often conflicting feelings. An effective therapist will provide a supportive environment that includes sufficient HIV/AIDS education to reduce unrealistic fears while promoting self-exploration. As described previously, many HIV-positive women are angry at partners who have infected them. When possible and appropriate, the therapist can play an important role in preparing the woman to share her feelings with her partner. Care should be taken to ensure that the woman will not face any violence as a result. If violence is possible, the focus of treatment should become the procurement of a safe environment. If, as is often the case, the partner has already passed away, Gestalt techniques can be very helpful in reducing unresolved grief. We have experienced good success with having patients write a letter to their partner explaining their feelings. Group therapy or support groups can be extremely helpful for women. Such settings allow them to identify with others in their situation, to hear how others have sought solutions to similar problems, and to learn about new strategies and options.

Women will need to mourn the loss of their long-term future. This issue will come up over and over again throughout treatment as the woman struggles with accepting her foreshortened life. Therapy is one of the only places where this conversation can take place without repercussions. Simply allowing the woman to talk is very powerful. Let us stress that this can be a very slow process. However, when appropriate, guiding the woman to set short-term obtainable goals can help to restore her perspective and reduce feelings of helplessness.

Mental Health Considerations

Although the available research is sparse, it appears that HIV-positive women without histories of substance abuse are not significantly more likely than matched HIV-negative women to have a psychiatric disorder. One study of HIV-positive women in the military found that "sexual functioning was disrupted in a majority." New-onset Hypoactive Sexual Desire Disorder was, in fact, the most common psychiatric disorder identified in this sample of twenty women.

HIV-positive women (and men) with current or recent substance abuse are much more likely than members of the general population or matched groups to have other (non–drug-related) psychiatric problems. In a study conducted in New York, Lipsitz and colleagues evaluated the psychiatric status of thirty HIV-positive and thirty-seven HIV-negative drug-using women. Rates of major depression or dysthymia or both were high in both groups (26 percent and 30 percent, respectively). At least in this study, substance abuse rather than HIV status seemed to be the major reason for high rates of depressive disorder.

Regardless of whether or not they have an "official" psychiatric diagnosis, HIV-positive women are likely to experience distress at various points in the disease process and may need and want mental health services. Those with children may need help with parenting skills in general, with such HIV-related problems as disruptive behavior by uninfected children who are frightened and angry by what is happening to their family, and with management issues regarding an HIV-positive child.

In our experience, HIV-positive minority women are often reluctant to take any psychotropic drugs, including antidepressants such as Prozac. If in recovery, they are worried about re-addiction, even when assured that antidepressant medications are not addictive. Even women who have a clear-cut significant depressive disorder may resist the recommendation for medication as the standard of care, and request counseling instead. Although women can and have benefited greatly from participation in support groups run by and for gay men (and in the 1980s they had no other option), women's support and therapy groups seem more valuable. Particularly for minority women (and non–English-speaking women), such groups appear to be appreciated and successful in helping HIV-positive women to develop self-esteem, parenting and assertiveness skills, hope, and a sense of community.

Seeking Treatment

Although there are still reports surfacing which state that HIV-positive women die sooner than men, it is becoming increasingly clear that this is largely due to the fact that women typically seek diagnosis and treatment later in the disease process, rather than to some unknown biological difference that hastens death in women. In fact, a recent *New England Journal of Medicine* article demonstrated that there was no difference in disease progression or survival associated with sex, race, IV drug use, or socioeconomic status among 1,372 HIV-positive patients seen at an inner-city clinic.

So why do women seek diagnosis and treatment later in their illness than men? Often, it is due to ignorance, denial, or their partners' failure to disclose their HIV status so that women are unaware that they are at risk and do not get tested until mysterious symptoms arise. Frequently the true cause of these symptoms is not immediately identified by physicians because many women (especially middle-class women) were not, and to some extent are still not, seen as at risk for HIV. Complicating the diagnostic picture is the fact that many of the early symptoms of HIV infection in women are problems of the reproductive tract that can have many causes other than HIV. Although medical professionals are becoming more informed about HIV-related conditions in women, some still fail to see HIV as a possible cause in women who do not come from one of the typical "high-risk" groups (in other words, IV drug users, sex workers, and partners of IV drug users).

MARY

Mary, a thirty-seven-year-old Hispanic woman who worked with us, told this story. Mary had struggled with symptoms of fatigue, dizziness, sore throat, and dry mouth for several months before she finally decided to seek testing:

> I was going through a lot of stress, hair loss and I was going because of the thrush, but I didn't know it was thrush. It's just that I had this dry mouth and this ugly tongue which no one was able to explain to me what it was. I had the skin biopsy and lots of other tests and Dr. D said it could be a possibility of lupus, but she wanted to start me on medication. I went for a second opinion with a specialist which didn't do any tests, but that's another story. I went to six or seven specialists and no one could pinpoint anything. I don't understand the medical— sometimes they screw-up royal. . . . Finally by the sixth doctor, I said, give me an HIV test, just for the hell of it. Nobody suggested it, I just decided, take the test for the hell of it. I never thought I'd be positive.

Another major reason for women's postponing of diagnosis and treatment, one that is difficult for many health care providers to understand or appreciate, is the issue of priorities. Many of these women have been hard hit—by their families, communities, and life experiences. To them, HIV/AIDS is just another problem in a problematic life. They were physically and sexually abused as children, started using drugs when they were very young, and have been homeless, in prison, and the victims of physical attacks. Some have had children who are now being raised by family members or the courts. Many have tried to take back control of their lives by quitting drugs and getting psychological help. Others still struggle to see the benefit in quitting drugs only to face what they see as a death sentence. Many of these women simply don't have the skills to quit drugs for good. Because of their life experiences, a lot of these women already had limited hope for their future. Now they have to face HIV as well.

Women sometimes delay seeking treatment because of fear. They may worry that staff or other patients at the clinic will recognize them and find out that they are infected. Many, especially African-American women, distrust the health care system in general and especially when it comes to HIV. Women with children may be fearful that seeking treatment will lead to disclosure of their diagnosis and subsequently cause their children to become targets of discrimination. This is especially true if one or more of the children is also infected. Women often fear that their HIV-positive status, especially when accompanied with a history of drug abuse, will be used by the child welfare system to revoke their parental rights.

Women, especially women of color, are usually the primary caretakers of their families. These duties, which may include caring for an infected mate, relative, or child, can interfere with a woman's ability and motivation to seek treatment for herself. Women in abusive relationships, who typically struggle with low self-esteem, are also unlikely to seek diagnosis and treatment.

Therapists working with HIV-positive women who are struggling to establish appropriate medical care must provide a supportive, nonjudgmental environment that promotes self-exploration and enhances self-esteem. Therapists need to work with women to explore the women's feelings about, and past experiences with, health care professionals, and to validate negative experiences. Women will need to be empowered to take an active role in their health care and to establish a partnership with their medical professionals. In many cases, this will include educating women about their disease and treatment options, as well as identifying unrealistic fears. Some clients will benefit from role-playing to practice assertive approaches to dealing with health care professionals. We have found that the most successful therapists have established relationships with several HIV/AIDS health care providers and can offer referrals to competent and compassionate providers when appropriate.

Many women put the care of their child(ren), especially an HIV-positive child, before their own. Others simply feel too overwhelmed by caretaking responsibilities to follow through with their own treatment. In either situation, women need to get the message that they are better mothers, wives, and partners if they take care of themselves first. Even a woman who sees everyone's needs as more important than her own will be motivated to care for herself if she believes that she will no longer be able to care for others if she doesn't. Encouraging women to identify members of their social network who can aid in child care, or referring them to a community-based organization that provides child care or respite care, can also be very helpful.

Caregiving

HIV illness itself is a constant up-and-down struggle. Women are likely to feel great one day and horrible the next. Dealing with one's own illness is hard enough, but most women have somebody else to care for—a partner, child, family member, or friend. If it is a partner that they are caring for, it is typically the person who infected them. If they were unknowingly put at risk by this person, they are likely to have conflicting feelings of anger, resentment, love, and pity. Caring for an infected child is not only difficult and trying in terms of the amount of effort demanded. It can also rekindle feelings of guilt, shame, anger, and loss. One young mother of three we worked with described her struggles with caring for her two-year-old HIV-positive daughter: "My little one is sick. She's got the virus and right now she's got the herpes in her mouth. She can't even eat. It's not fair, she's just a baby. . . . I kinda blame myself for my daughter being sick. And it's because of me that she's suffering. [crying] I'm scared I'm gonna lose her. And I try not to cry in front of the kids, but sometimes I feel like I'm going to explode."

Caring for an ill person is an exhausting job; caring for more than one ill person can be overwhelming. HIV-positive women are often single mothers with more than one child. They live with other chronic stressors related to poverty, fragmentation of family, or child behavior problems (common in both their HIV-infected and uninfected children). If she has a male partner, he is typically not the father of all of her children and is most likely HIV-positive as well. He may or may not be helpful with the children and may be in failing health himself.

Caregiving demands often interfere with a woman's ability to seek and receive adequate care for herself. The needs of the caregivers were examined by Claude Mellins and Anke Ehrhardt in a study of twenty-five African-American and Hispanic families in New York City with at least one HIV-positive child. (The caregivers were either the biological mothers who were HIV-positive themselves, or foster parents who were not.) Compared to foster parents, the HIV-infected mothers reported more social isolation, more financial problems, and, perhaps most urgent, too little respite from child care.

HIV-positive mothers don't often get enough practical support (including baby-sitting) or encouragement from friends and relatives. Consequently, they are often unable to leave their children long enough to attend to their own needs for relaxation, social activities, recreation, or even health care.

Clearly, women with significant caregiving demands need support. Although they would likely benefit from individual or group therapy, the very nature of their problem usually precludes them from seeking and attending sessions. One successful solution to this problem is to offer child care during individual sessions or a separate children's group during group sessions. Quite often this is the only way to ensure some sort of regular attendance. Another good option is to refer the woman to a community-based organization that offers respite care, and then schedule sessions around its services. Two less-desirable but workable options are to allow the woman to bring her children to the sessions or to make home visits. However, both of these options reduce privacy in therapy and do not capitalize on the naturally reinforcing effect of the built-in break from child care provided by the first three options.

Once the initial hurdle of scheduling is overcome, therapy will need to focus on allowing the woman to vent. While this sounds simplistic, we have found that a substantive amount of time in the early sessions is best spent simply empathizing with the woman's experience. Often therapists are pulled to try to quickly fix problems, knowing that their time with the client may be limited. HIV-positive women may experience this as simply another person who is demanding something of them. The bottom line is to go slowly and listen.

When it is clearly time to start problem solving, it is essential to focus on *small* obtainable goals. Many aspects of an HIV-positive woman's life may be out of control. As previously discussed, identifying people in her social network who can help out and locating community-based organizations with useful services can go a long way in improving the situation. In most situations, aiding the woman in identifying ways she can take breaks while still caring for her loved ones is helpful. Examples include taking a hot bath *alone*, video movies for the kids, and quiet time once everyone is in bed or at school. We have had some success with relaxation training for motivated women.

Bereavement

The prenatal use of AZT has been shown to reduce rates of transmission from 25 to 8 percent. Regardless of the rate, the threat or reality of multiple deaths within the family raises the level of distress for all its members, infected or not. Most HIV-positive women have already lost someone in their family to AIDS. If it isn't their husband or boyfriend, it is their brother, sister, cousin, parent, or child. Many families suffer multiple losses to AIDS. Often, there is little time to mourn one loss before another occurs. One of the women in our study told us her story: "I lost my husband back in '91. . . . Then my cousin passed and I waited a year after to tell anyone [about me]. Then I told my sister who I think is HIV, but she won't test. . . . Then my sister-in-law was full-blown AIDS and she passed. And my mother, my mother knows, but tries to pretend she don't."

Bereavement typically brings feelings of loss, anger, and isolation. Some women feel abandoned and helpless after the loss of their partner. Many have never been on their own or had to care for themselves before, and are uncertain about their ability to survive without their partner. One of the women we worked with shared her feelings with us: "He was the light of my life! I miss him, we did everything together. I know I should be over him by now, but I miss him, every day I miss him. He did everything for me and I don't know what to do now that he is gone."

Others struggle to understand their conflicting feelings of loss and anger toward a deceased partner who infected them with or without his knowledge.

When a child dies, it is especially difficult. Regardless of the illness or the circumstances, parents typically blame themselves for their child's death. When a child dies of AIDS, self-blame is a particularly difficult and painful hurdle to overcome. Women who were infected without their knowledge or consent usually experience a resurgence of anger and contempt for the person who infected them. They often blame themselves as well. Women who had engaged in risky behavior feel guilty, ashamed, and worthless. Most are alone to deal with this loss as their husbands or boyfriends have either moved on or already died. Depending on to whom the woman has chosen to disclose her

HIV-positive status, she may have limited support from others as well. Women are often distracted from their own grieving process as they attempt to help their other children deal with the loss of their sibling. Without support, women with substance abuse histories also risk relapse.

Therapists working with bereaved HIV-positive women will need to provide a supportive environment where feelings of loss, anger, guilt, and shame can be explored. Adopting a family systems perspective, in which the family is viewed as an interwoven system that changes every time a piece of it changes, can be helpful in understanding the impact a loss has had on the family. Further, because the woman is likely to be the head of the household and primary caregiver, it is important to discuss how other members are coping with the loss. Support groups that have children's groups attached can also be extremely useful to bereaved families.

We have found Gestalt techniques, such as creating some meaningful ceremony in which a private good-bye is delivered, especially helpful in dealing with unresolved grief. Creating a new family ritual that honors the loved one can also be very helpful. One of us worked with a family of five in which the mother and youngest child were infected. The three older children were aware that their little brother was ill and going to die, but they still struggled with the reality of his death. Even after repeated explanations, they had trouble understanding where he had gone and that he would not be coming back. The mother, drawing on her cultural and religious background, helped the children build a shrine for their little brother. Every day, they had to replace the small offerings of food and drink and ensure that the candle continued to burn. Occasionally she would overhear one of her children talking to their little brother, explaining that it was really quiet without him around or telling him about something that had happened at school that day. Over time, the children came to an understanding that their brother had gone to heaven and was watching over them.

TOUGH CHOICES

HIV-positive women face many tough choices. HIV-positive men are faced with some of the same decisions (such as disclosure in intimate relationships), but others, by default or design, ultimately fall within a woman's domain (such as disclosure to children, permanency planning, and pregnancy).

Sexuality

Although there are almost no systematic data available, results from relatively small samples of HIV-positive women suggest that a significant number are not interested in sexual relationships with men. In one study of IV drug-using women recruited from a New York City infectious disease clinic, 31 percent identified themselves as lesbian or bisexual. In a study we are currently conducting, we have so far interviewed fifty women, the large majority of whom are African American or Hispanic. When asked about their sexual orientation, 31 percent described themselves as lesbian or bisexual. One possible explanation for this surprisingly high percentage is the fact that many of these women have been in prison, where "gay for the stay" is a recognized phenomenon; perhaps this orientation has carried over into post-prison community life.

These and other women may feel that men (and sex) are to blame for their current circumstances. Their anger, together with the exigencies of holding together their health and their family, have made sexual activity low on their list of priorities. Other women may avoid sexual behavior out of fear of disclosing their HIV status to potential partners.

Although celibacy works for some women, others find it a very lonely solution, and they long for a relationship or simply miss sex. Many find it helpful to remove the problem of disclosure altogether by going to HIV-positive social events or dances.

Therapists working with HIV-positive women who are experiencing troubles in this area will need to aid in the full explo-

ration of the women's thoughts and feelings about sexual relationships. Basic education about sexuality and women's bodies is
sometimes helpful. Underlying fears of rejection or abandonment often interfere with women's desire for sexual relationships.
Changes in body composition due to wasting, medication side
effects, and opportunistic infections can also interfere with
women's sexual desire and feelings of attractiveness. If the primary barrier to sexual desire is fear of rejection, identifying and
role-playing appropriate strategies may be helpful.

Pregnancy

One of the most controversial issues surrounding HIV-positive
women is that of pregnancy. Some HIV-positive women decide
to become pregnant or to continue a pregnancy out of a need
to experience a life-affirming act, to please a mate, or in hopes
that the baby will live on as a legacy. For many, their identity
and self-worth are linked to their reproductive capacity. Other
HIV-positive women will firmly state that they have no intention of having a child now that they have learned of their HIV-
positive status. All struggle with feelings of sadness and loss,
often feeling cheated when they confront the issues of having a
child. In the past, many health care professionals have
approached this personal struggle as a public health issue with
a single solution: "Don't get pregnant." However well inten-
tioned, such messages continue to frame women as vectors of
disease who produce "innocent victims." If nothing else, such
messages often don't work.

Therapists working with HIV-positive women who are considering pregnancy will need to establish a trusting, nonjudgmental relationship in which the women can openly explore their
thoughts and feelings. For the therapist, the emphasis must be
on the right of the woman to make her own decision. A full
exploration of cultural, religious, and personal beliefs about
abortion, children, illness, and family may be very helpful in
identifying hidden motivations and barriers. Information about

medical options to reduce the likelihood of maternal transmission and the odds of giving birth to an infected child should be provided. Often others (husband or partners) are pushing for the woman to have a child. If this is the case, complicated relationship issues will probably need to be dealt with before a reasoned decision can be reached. Once all the factors have been uncovered, we have found the behavioral technique of listing pros and cons of the different options to be very helpful in reaching a decision.

Disclosure

Deciding how, when, and to whom to disclose is a difficult process that takes both time and energy. Fear of disclosing often prevents HIV-positive women from seeking much-needed emotional and instrumental social support from family and friends who are unaware of their situation. This is true, of course, for men as well, but women with children often have greater needs for assistance from family and friends in terms of everyday living. Women who decide not to disclose report that it is safer not to tell anyone, but they also state that keeping the secret prevents them from developing and maintaining close relationships and leaves them with deep feelings of loneliness and isolation. Further, not telling often prevents HIV-positive women from doing the work necessary to adjust to the reality of their own foreshortened lives. It also robs the family members of time to adjust to the situation and prevents them from rendering much-needed support.

Instead of actively dealing with the situation, HIV-positive women who struggle with disclosure often anxiously wait for an accident to happen. They hope that someone close to them will find their medication or take a medically related phone call that ends the secret keeping. In the worst cases, HIV-positive women wait until too late, and family members find out when the women are hospitalized with a critical or even terminal diagnosis. These situations are extremely difficult for adult family members to handle, but they can be overwhelming and sometimes devastating to children.

Disclosing to Children

When children are told about a family member's HIV-positive status early and repeatedly, they have the best chance of adjusting to and effectively dealing with the situation. Most children, when given the chance, adapt to the worst of situations. Conversely, children struggle to understand deathbed explanations and postmortem stories of a missing parent. Clearly, parents know their children best and are the most accurate judges of what their children need to know. However, it is often the case that their struggles with how to tell their children prevent them from telling a child who needs to know. Women often have misconceptions about what information their children can handle or understand, and they question what good the information will do their child. They are also concerned that their children will not keep the information private, and fear the ramifications of others knowing, in terms of stigma directed at the mother or the child. Women also fear having to disclose how they became infected with the virus, because of the social stigma associated with most modes of transmission. Lastly, women (and men) in our society fear discussions about death in general, and especially discussions about their own death.

If it is difficult for mothers to tell their children of their own illness, it is even more painful to have to tell children that they are infected. This can be a major point of contention between the parent (typically the mother) and the child's health care providers, who characteristically feel it is in the child's best interest to be informed. Sometimes the child will spend years going regularly to the hospital for routine checkups, for inpatient stays during acute illness episodes, and for regular intravenous treatments, without the mother ever offering a medical explanation. Mothers experience many of the same sources of reluctance that apply to disclosing their own status: fear that the child will tell others, fear of stigma, fear that the child will be rejected by his or her classmates and neighbors. In addition, some feel that it is unfair to burden the child with the information and that the child gains no advantages from knowing.

Therapists working with HIV-positive women who are struggling with disclosure to their child(ren) will need to "support the secret" and the woman's right to decide when to tell. Letting women know that they are the best judge of when the right time is will go a long way in helping them to make a move. Exploring the woman's fears about disclosure will often reveal fears of being rejected and of having to explain how they became infected. It is often quite helpful to explain and practice age-appropriate responses to likely questions. Role-playing the disclosure can be key to reducing fears and increasing mastery. Identifying members of the woman's social network who can be present during the disclosure can reduce her anxiety and feelings of being alone to handle the situation. This network includes the therapist, when appropriate.

Several families we have worked with instituted family meetings prior to the disclosure so that the family already had an established mechanism for dealing with family problems. Some families find it easier to start educating their children about HIV/AIDS before the disclosure so that the words themselves are not so powerful. Others found the courage to disclose in the knowledge that they would then be able to educate their children about HIV and protect their children from becoming infected even after the mothers' death. Many of the mothers we work with have found disclosing easier after they became regular members of HIV/AIDS support groups or community-based organizations, which helped them gain a sense of community and hope.

Disclosure to children is a complicated task that involves a multitude of interrelated issues. Although we have reviewed some of the key points here, a thorough discussion is beyond the scope of this chapter. Interested readers are referred to Mary

Tasker's excellent book *How Can I Tell You?* and the thoughtful work of Michael Lipson.

Disclosing in Intimate Relationships

Deciding if, how, and when to disclose HIV status in intimate or potentially intimate relationships is a difficult task for all HIV-positive individuals. Women's struggles with this issue are complicated by many factors. Some women, especially African-American women, have a limited pool of acceptable mates (in other words, non–drug-abusing, non-incarcerated) to choose from. Some also depend on much-needed financial support from their boyfriends. For both emotional and financial reasons, many are weary of taking a chance and possibly "scaring a good one away." Others believe that disclosure of HIV will lead to further disclosure of a drug use or prostitution history that they fear will make them unattractive to a prospective partner. Others are in early recovery from drug addiction or abuse; they fear that the stress of possible rejection will send them into relapse. Some fear physical and emotional abuse if they disclose.

By far the most common reason for not telling is fear of rejection. Most of these women already have multiple challenges to their self-esteem (poverty, poor education, unemployment, discrimination, and so on) and are unsure of their worth as a mate. Many simply believe that the presence of a progressive, life-threatening, often disfiguring, communicable disease makes them unlovable and unacceptable.

Regardless of the circumstances, if an HIV-positive woman is currently engaged in risky sex with a partner of unknown or HIV-negative status, the therapist cannot ignore the situation. The preferred option is to help the patient to engage in safer sex and to tell the partner. Ultimately, if the patient continues to place others at risk and refuses to change her behavior, the therapist may have to insist on notification as a condition for continued work together.

Permanency Planning

Each year, more children lose their mothers to AIDS than to auto accidents. One of the most difficult decisions HIV-positive women with children face is what will happen to their children after their death. Facing this issue requires women to admit to themselves that they are going to die and that their children will need care from someone else. After struggling to have and care for their children, women often have great difficulty facing the reality that somebody else will be raising them. They feel cheated and angry that someone else will be there to see their child's first day of school, first date, or first job.

Many women assume that a family member (sister or mother) will automatically take care of their children after their death, and therefore don't feel any need to plan how this will happen. This approach to permanency planning often leads to unnecessary confusion, fear, grief, and stress for all of those involved.

For many women, it is difficult to think about the idea of somebody else raising their child, no matter how close and trusted the person. However painful, this is where the process begins. Therapists can help greatly by encouraging the woman to contemplate what she wants to have happen to her child(ren) after she has died. She will need to be aided in dealing with many questions:

- Who will be the best caretaker for her child(ren)? Is that person likely to accept the responsibility of raising her child(ren)?

- Will this person be able to cope with the added burden of one or more children? Of an HIV-positive child?

- Will the child(ren) be safe and well taken care of?

- If the mother has more than one child, will the children be able to stay together?

- How does she go about making plans? Will she need to involve a lawyer?

- How will she ask the prospective guardian if he or she will assume responsibilities for the mother's child(ren)?

- How does she tell her child(ren)? Does she have to tell her child(ren)?

- What sort of contact should the future caregiver and child(ren) have now?

Women will need to talk to someone about what will happen. They are likely to choose a trusted family member, friend, therapist, case worker, or cleric for this purpose. These conversations provide much-needed support and allow women a chance to think through their prospective plans. Once a prospective guardian is identified, that person will need to be approached with the idea. Some women find it easier to have all the information about formal guardianship plans and what benefits are available for the care of the children assembled before they speak to the potential guardian. Others decide that working together to locate this information is a helpful first step in a successful transition to new and changing roles.

Once plans have been made, the decision of how, when, and whether or not to tell children must be made. Some women, especially those who have already disclosed their HIV-positive status to their children, decide to share their guardianship plans. As a part of the process, many decide to allow contact, (such as sleepovers or weekend trips) with the future guardian. Others, usually those who have chosen not to disclose their HIV-positive status, decide not to share their plans with their children.

Like the decision to disclose, these are extremely personal decisions that only the parent can make. The important message for parents is that they can make guardianship plans that will ensure the care of their children after their death without having to disclose. The exact order of these steps is less important than getting through them. Women who complete guardianship plans report a great sense of relief and peace, knowing that their children will be well cared for after their death.

Interaction with Medical Professionals

Poor people, especially inner-city minority women, often have difficult experiences with the health care system. Many lack ongoing relationships with specific physicians or clinics, and instead tend to get most of their family's medical needs addressed in emergency-room situations. Such visits are often characterized by long waits, rotating staff, and impersonal care, especially if the presenting complaint is not "emergent" and the medical staff considers the family's use of the emergency room a misuse of the medical system. In turn, patients find the experience difficult, stressful, and frustrating, and often develop deep-seated reservations about the benevolence of the medical community in general.

Many HIV-positive women have no academic background to prepare them to learn about their complicated disease. Some never completed high school, and many never held down a job. These women, though street savvy, struggle with understanding their medical conditions and medications. They may also have personality styles that interfere with interpersonal relationships and their ability to work with medical teams. Drug-abusing women, like drug-abusing men, can be frustrating and difficult to deal with. They may be insatiably needy and demanding during one period, and then disappear from the health care system only to turn up with drug-aggravated medical conditions that dismay and infuriate their health providers. Speaking as a physician who treated hundreds of currently addicted HIV-infected patients, P. A. Selwyn cautioned: "We need to understand that our patients cannot begin the long and difficult process of recovery from addiction until they are ready to do so themselves. Our role as care providers is to be there, to bear witness, to be willing to accompany patients through their illness, and to refrain from passing judgement. We can neither save them nor do we have the right to condemn them."

Feelings of aversion among care providers toward substance-abusing patients may be intensified if the patient in question is an HIV-infected mother whose care of her children does not meet their standards. Their injunctions to the mother to stop shooting up because it is bad for her and her children—as if this idea hadn't occurred to her—is at best ineffective and often undermining to the mother's attempts, however flawed, to get health care for herself and her children.

Due to the overcrowded setting in which care is delivered, practitioners may make hasty interventions before appropriate trust has been established, which leaves women feeling judged rather than understood. In addition to the issue of continued drug use, these situations are likely to arise around issues of pregnancy and refusal to take prescribed medications. After one or more such encounters, women may choose to stay away, rather than risk the shame and embarrassment of another such episode.

Medical practitioners and HIV-positive women will need to take the necessary time to establish trusting partnerships. HIV-positive women, working with their health care providers, will need to educate themselves about their conditions and treatment options to ensure that they can become effective consumers of their medical care. For their part, physicians need to recognize the medical conditions common to women. Disorders in HIV-positive women often involve problems of the reproductive tract, so women also require good gynecological care. Accordingly, a close working relationship between gynecologist and primary care provider is important.

Clearly, HIV-positive women face a multitude of challenges. Even so, these women are often remarkably resilient. As some will tell you, they have been to hell and back, and life, even with HIV, is better now. Working with them is never boring, and often inspirational. Many have a thirst for life that reminds you to put your priorities in order and value every day that you're alive.

NOTES

P. 196, *some more justifiable than others:* Cooper, E. B. (1995). Historical and analytical overview of policy issues affecting women living with AIDS: A blueprint for learning from our past. *Bulletin of the New York Academy of Medicine, 72* (summer suppl.), 283–299; Wiener, L. S. (1991). Women and HIV: A historical and personal psychosocial perspective. *Social Work, 36,* 375–378; Corea, G. (1992). *The invisible epidemic: The story of women and AIDS.* New York: HarperCollins.

P. 196, *(13,800 out of 75,800 cases in all):* Centers for Disease Control and Prevention (CDC). (1995, June). *HIV/AIDS surveillance report, 7*(1), 8–13.

P. 198, *working with HIV-positive women will require:* Winiarski, M. G. (1991). *AIDS-related psychotherapy.* New York: Pergamon Press.

P. 199, *The literature has identified a multitude:* Kalichman, S. C. (1995). *Understanding AIDS: A guide for mental health professionals.* Washington, DC: American Psychological Association.

P. 202, *An effective therapist will provide a supportive environment:* Kloser, P., & Craig, J. M. (1994). *The women's HIV sourcebook: A guide to better health and well-being.* Dallas: Taylor.

P. 203, *New-onset Hypoactive Sexual Desire Disorder:* Brown, G., & Rundell, J. (1990). Prospective study of psychiatric morbidity in HIV-seropositive women without AIDS. *General Hospital Psychiatry, 12,* 1–6.

P. 203, *In a study conducted in New York, Lipsitz and colleagues evaluated:* Lipsitz, J. D., Williams, J. B., Rabkin, J. G., Remien, R. H., Bradbury, M., el Sadr, W., Goetz, R., Sorrell, S., & Gorman, J. M. (1994). Psychopathology in male and female intravenous drug users with and without HIV infection. *American Journal of Psychiatry, 151,* 1662–1668.

P. 204, *a recent* New England Journal of Medicine *article demonstrated:* Chaisson, R. E., Keruly, J. C., & Moore, R. D. (1995). Race, sex, drug use, and progression of HIV disease. *New England Journal of Medicine, 333,* 751–756.

P. 207, *educating women about their disease . . . identifying unrealistic fears:* Denenberg, R. (1994). Special concerns of women with HIV and AIDS. In W. Odets & M. Shernoff (Eds.), *The second decade of AIDS.* New York: Hatherleigh Press.

P. 208, *needs of the caregivers were examined:* Mellins, C., & Ehrhardt, A. (1994). Families affected by pediatric AIDS: Sources of stress and coping. *Journal of Developmental and Behavioral Pediatrics, 15,* S54–S60.

P. 209, *Regardless of the rate, . . . all its members, infected or not:* Connor, E. M., Sperling, R. S., Gelber, R., Kiselev, P., Scott, G., O'Sullivan, M. J.,

VanDyke, R., Bey, M., Shearer, W., Jacobson, R. L., Jimenez, E., O'Neill, E., Bazin, B., Delfraissy, J. F., Culnane, M., Coombs, R., Elkins, M., Moye, J., Stratton, P., & Balsley, J. (1994). Reduction of maternal-infant transmission of human immunodeficiency virus type 1 with zidovudine treatment. *The New England Journal of Medicine, 331,* 1173–1180.

P. 212, *results from relatively small samples of HIV-positive women:* Lipsitz, J. D., Williams, J. B. W., Rabkin, J. G., Remien, R. H., Bradbury, M., el Sadr, W., Goetz, R., Sorrell, S., & Gorman, J. M. (1994). Psychopathology in male and female intravenous drug users with and without HIV infection. *American Journal of Psychiatry, 151,* 1662–1668.

P. 212, *In one study of IV drug-using women:* Lipsitz, J. D., Williams, J. B., Rabkin, J. G., Remien, R. H., Bradbury, M., el Sadr, W., Goetz, R., Sorrell, S., & Gorman, J. M. (1994). Psychopathology in male and female intravenous drug users with and without HIV infection. *American Journal of Psychiatry, 151,* 1662–1668.

P. 212, *In a study we are currently conducting:* Goggin, K. J., Engelson, E., Rabkin, J. G., & Kotler, D. P. (1996). *Relationship of mood, endocrine and sexual disorders in HIV-positive women: An exploratory study.* Manuscript submitted for publication.

P. 213, *"Don't get pregnant":* Bayer, R. (1995). Women's rights, babies' interests: Ethics, politics, and science in the debate of newborn HIV screening. In H. L. Minkoff, A. DeHovitz, & A. Duerr (Eds.), *HIV infection in women.* New York: Raven Press.

P. 216, *Mary Tasker's excellent book . . . work of Michael Lipson:* Tasker, M. (1992). *How can I tell you?* Bethesda, MD: Association for the Care of Children's Health; Lipson, M. (1993). What do you say to a child with AIDS? *Hastings Center Report, 23,* 6–12.

P. 218, *Each year, more children lose their mothers:* Boyd-Franklin, N., Steiner, G. L., & Boland, M. (Eds.). (1995). *Children, family, and HIV/AIDS: Psychosocial and therapeutic issues.* New York: Guilford Press.

P. 220, *P. A. Selwyn cautioned:* Selwyn, P. A. (1995). Caring for HIV-infected drug users: A provider's perspective. *Bulletin of the New York Academy of Medicine* (summer suppl.), 211–216.

7

TREATING COUPLES AND FAMILIES WITH HIV
A Systemic Approach

Douglas S. Rait, Joan M. Ross, and Stephen M. Rao

There is little question that HIV-related disorders constitute the major public health threat in our lifetimes. However, despite evidence that serious illness can adversely affect family functioning, the role of the family as a context for the psychological and psychiatric management of HIV disease has not been well articulated. Not only do family members typically provide direct patient care and emotional support, share in decision making, and assume financial costs, but they frequently are also the primary source of health beliefs and behaviors. Whereas traditional psychiatric approaches have paid only nominal attention to the importance of the family's role in serious medical illness, there is a growing interest in applying family systems concepts and practice to working with the medically ill. At the same time, changing trends in health care toward briefer hospital stays, greater reliance on outpatient care, and the strengthening of community health care services also prompt a renewed examination of the family's potential to contribute to the overall care of the person with HIV disease.

This chapter is intended to complement other established clinical approaches by providing an overview of premises for a family systems approach to the person with HIV disease, a developmental view of the family's responses to the illness at various points in its course, a model for assessing couples and families, and a practical guide to consultation and clinical interventions based on family systems principles. In our combined experience, we have worked with patients and families facing HIV disease for a combined twenty-five years in academic medical centers and community agencies. With the Centers for Disease Control and Prevention (CDC) reporting that 1 in every 250 persons in the United States is infected with HIV and 1 in every 9 AIDS cases worldwide is a U.S. citizen, we believe that it is necessary for all therapists to become proficient in treating the psychosocial and systemic problems associated with HIV disease.

Just as the AIDS epidemic has exacted a monumental toll of human anguish, the secondary epidemic of psychosocial distress among the partners, relatives, and close friends of patients with HIV disease deserves special concern. For the sick person and his or her family, HIV-related disorders present a challenge that invariably creates profound discontinuity in their lives. Familiar family patterns and functional roles are disrupted, producing complex problems at every level of daily functioning from the completion of mundane household chores to questions of fundamental existential importance. At the same time, a rapidly expanding population of children and adults with HIV disease and their families are being forced to confront difficult practical and interpersonal demands resulting from this illness. Finally, because of the stigma presently attached to AIDS, families often struggle in isolation and secrecy with explosive and painful issues relating to shame, guilt, discrimination, acute medical crises, chronic disease processes, and death and bereavement.

Although there has been a dramatic growth in the literature pertaining to the medical, psychiatric, and social aspects of AIDS, research on the family context of HIV disease is still scarce. Studies have shown that the most frequent sources of stress in relatives of homosexual AIDS patients were fears of contracting AIDS, simultaneous revelations of sexual orientation and sexual activity, the notoriety of the disease, helplessness, loss, and grief. A study looking at the sequelae of AIDS-related death in the gay community in New York City showed a strong association between significant symptoms of psychological distress and AIDS-related bereavement in partners and friends of the victims.

Several reports on the partners of HIV-infected gay men and the relatives of HIV-infected children have documented a range of psychosocial problems related to the illness, and case studies have described the acute psychological reactions of gay partners to the diagnosis of AIDS including panic, rage, and fear. Clinical experience suggests that many of these features are also common among relatives of heterosexual people with HIV. A survey of major pediatric AIDS centers demonstrated that anxiety, depression, and grief ranked as the primary preoccupations among parents and caretakers (for example, extended family, adoptive parents, foster parents). Locating a home and placement for an HIV-infected child can also create a major family problem.

In order to broaden the agenda for health care providers working with the HIV-infected population and to promote more family-oriented research in this area, the National Coalition on AIDS and Families issued general principles relating to the treatment of persons with HIV and AIDS. These principles (presented in Table 7.1) reflect a commitment to extend the focus of health care policy and patient care.

In emphasizing the family systems context of HIV, these principles serve as the basis for a more comprehensive, biopsychosocial approach to the person with HIV disease.

A FAMILY SYSTEMS APPROACH TO THE PERSON WITH HIV DISEASE

Whereas persons who are HIV-infected are frequently classified according to major risk groups, there is no typical family of the person with HIV disease. Because the two primary risk groups

Table 7.1
1989 General Principles of the
National Coalition on AIDS and Families

- AIDS affects families and not just the individual who contracts the disease.

- The family plays a key role in education, prevention, and attitude change regarding AIDS.

- The family must be seen as the unit of care in the treatment of AIDS. Families need to be educated regarding this role and be provided the support required to be effective.

- The impact on the family continues beyond the illness and death of the infected member.

- Special attention must be given to the needs of low-income families and minority families because these families, with multiple burdens, suffer severely from the AIDS epidemic.

- The impact of the AIDS epidemic on families, and the reaction of families, will vary with ethnicity, religion, race, and social class.

- Efforts must be made to reduce the stigma, discrimination, and isolation of families with an HIV-infected member.

- Preventative and educational efforts must be rational, pragmatic, and supportive of healthy sexuality.

- Decisions regarding the psychosocial aspects of prevention and treatment must be based on solid theory and research.

- Social policy regarding AIDS must recognize and respond to the strengths and needs of families.

Source: E. D. Macklin (Ed.). (1989). *AIDS and families: Report of the AIDS Task Force Groves Conference on marriage and the family* (pp. 269–270). New York: Harrington Park Press. Copyright © 1989 by Harrington Park Press. Reprinted by permission.

for HIV infection have been homosexual men and IV drug users, traditional descriptions of who constitutes "family" are inadequate. In defining the family context of the person with HIV disease, we must consider a more inclusive definition that comprises the biological family as well as those individuals who functionally form the system of support for the person with HIV infection. The range of family systems can therefore include gay couples; a gay man and his family of origin; a bisexual or heterosexual man or woman and his or her heterosexual partner or spouse; bisexual couples; serocongruent and serodiscordant couples; the immediate and extended family members (parents, grandparents, siblings, children) of IV drug users; networks of friends, parents, and relatives of HIV-infected children; hemophiliacs and their families; the families of persons who received HIV-contaminated blood transfusions; and relatives of prisoners and prostitutes.

Family therapists have described this emergent family as the "problem-defined system." From this perspective, family may consist of the relevant group of people who, were it not for the person's illness, would otherwise have little reason for being together. Our clinical experience indicates that the available family tends to correlate with particular risk factors as well as with the phase of illness. For example, at the time of HIV-positive diagnosis, only a partner may be present, whereas in advanced stages, the available and relevant family may expand to include parents, siblings, extended family, and friends.

In addition to adopting a broader definition of family, we can look at three fundamental premises that underlie a family systems perspective on HIV disease:

1. *HIV disease is an illness that affects other family members.* Second only to the patient, the family generally takes on the burden of the day-to-day management of the illness, shares in decision making, and incurs the significant financial and social costs related to HIV/AIDS. No matter how physically involved family members are, they inevitably become *hidden patients* who may

experience a range of transient psychological difficulties in trying to cope with the present stresses and later sequelae associated with HIV disease. In addition, the family facing HIV disease
must contend with the isolation fueled by social stigma and discrimination.

2.   *The family with a member with HIV disease is in transition.*
The clinical course of the HIV-related conditions is episodic,
consisting of a variety of acute and chronic challenges that must
be addressed. Throughout the course of the illness, the family
must continually adapt to the specific stresses associated with the
illness. Family members report little respite from the relentless
awareness that a life hangs in the balance. At the same time, roles
among family members frequently shift, requiring members to
learn new skills and assume additional responsibilities. As a
result, periodic instances of confusion and distress are to be
expected as family members explore new alternatives in accom-
modating themselves to HIV disease.

3.   *The family's capacity to cope with stresses associated with HIV
disease can contribute to the patient's psychosocial adaptation.* Because
families function as the primary context of health and illness,
family members can serve as resources in the overall care of the
sick person. Their solutions to the problems produced by HIV-
related disorders may therefore promote the healthy adaptation
of its members or induce greater distress. As a result, one goal
of treating a person with HIV disease is to identify ways that
family members can purposefully participate in patient care.

These basic premises highlight the interdependence of patient
and context and the extent to which HIV disease compels the
family to accommodate while maintaining its own stable, coher-
ent functioning. The biopsychosocial paradigm orients health
care professionals to better recognize the reciprocal relationships
between biological, psychological, and social levels of functioning. Therefore, we propose a family systems approach to the

person with HIV disease because it addresses the interactions among the illness, the infected person, family context, and treatment providers.

FAMILIES AND THE COURSE OF HIV DISEASE

If HIV-related disorders constituted a single, isolated stressful experience, they might be handled more easily. However, HIV disease represents a "disorder of change" in that the sick person and family must struggle to solve a series of both generic and idiosyncratic problems posed over the duration of illness. Like all diseases, HIV follows a life course of its own, and the stages of illness and treatment, in part, define the issues facing the family and help anticipate points of expected psychological distress.

Each stage is generally associated with practical and psychosocial tasks that family members must face and master. These transition points include medical workup and diagnosis, sudden changes in medical status, changes in treatment, reentry to daily life, recurrence of opportunistic infections, progression to clinical AIDS diagnosis, and death and bereavement. The clinical course of HIV disease can also be condensed into three broader stages—acute, chronic (with or without symptoms), and resolution—yet within each stage, it rarely follows in an invariant sequence.

A four-step paradigm for understanding family transitions related to sickness and disability has been proposed, describing (1) a period of stability in which the family operates in a patterned, balanced fashion, (2) a challenge to this pattern by the illness, (3) a period of exploration in which the family gropes for and experiments with different ways to respond to the change, and (4) an eventual reorganization at a new level of balance. We therefore view the family's ensuing behaviors in reaction to HIV disease in a family member as efforts to master the crisis and to restore order in the face of continual life threat rather than as signs of incipient psychopathology.

Acute Stage

The initial workup for and subsequent confirmation of seropositivity, symptomatic phase, or AIDS are shattering events, leaving the sick person fearful and anxious. The diagnosis also represents a tremendous crisis for the person's "significant others"—lovers, family members, and friends. Although generalizations can be drawn from what occurs following the diagnosis of other life-threatening conditions, the initial practical and emotional problems associated with HIV disease are likely to be more complicated.

For example, at the point where a member of a risk group elects to test for HIV, the implications of doing so will invariably affect family relationships. If the choice is made privately, the ensuing secrecy inevitably creates barriers in significant relationships until the results are confirmed. If the decision to be tested is openly shared, this choice will also affect the couple's or family's decisions regarding activities in a range of domains (social, sexual, financial). At the same time, when testing for HIV disease, individuals inevitably confront concerns related to the infection of partners and spread of contagion to other family members.

If seroconversion has occurred, the patient and partner are faced with critical challenges. Difficult choices about disclosure must be made, all of which can influence current relationships with partners, family members, friends, and colleagues. Couples may postpone informing others in order to consolidate their own strategies regarding the illness. Decisions regarding safe sex and other precautions need to be negotiated, often including substantial changes in lifestyle. The initiation of these discussions can be daunting, and family members may collude with each other in avoiding expressing their fear of contagion or feelings of sadness, panic, shame, and anger.

Relatives of the recently diagnosed person with serious illness frequently describe extreme levels of distress, including feelings of shock, disbelief, powerlessness, and despair. We have often heard family members confronting the diagnosis of HIV disease report that they feel out of control, scared, and furious. They also describe themselves as sad, overwhelmed, unprepared, and uncertain about what actions to take. They may also find themselves feeling lonely and isolated.

While personally struggling with the disastrous implications of HIV disease, families initially face two related tasks that are important for the welfare of the sick person: (1) constructing an emotional system of support, and (2) managing the transition into the medical culture. In some families with AIDS, already fragile relationships may not be able to bear the burden and fear associated with the confirmation of illness. The couple's relationship may be further distressed by questions regarding fidelity, sexual orientation, substance abuse, threat of infection, trust, and responsibility. However, just as the crisis poses an attack on the patient and the family system that can result in fragmentation and disintegration, the acute crisis can also draw strengths and resources from within the family. In these instances, it is not uncommon to see friends and relatives close their ranks and organize themselves protectively around the sick person.

Whether family members have been involved at an early or later stage, they may confront the uncomfortable fact that they were unaware of or were denied access to information about the patient's lifestyle, sexual orientation, and HIV risk status. Issues of secrecy, ambivalence over homosexuality, and troubles with empathy in the parents of infected gay men are not uncommon. In heterosexual and bisexual couples, there is great potential for feelings of betrayal, shame, and confusion regarding the hidden promiscuity of the partner. With HIV-infected drug users, the issues may be quite different, as their family members frequently know about the risk involved in their relative's personal choices. Nevertheless, their families often report feelings of helplessness and demoralization regarding the possibility of behavior change. Irrespective of their ties to the HIV-infected person, friends and family invariably face multiple implications of the confirmation of HIV disease status in a family member.

Chronic Stage

Once the initial shock of diagnosis subsides, family members may find that they have an opportunity to regain their footing and prepare for the frequently protracted period of the illness. The chronic stage can be quite lengthy and punctuated by unpredictable acute medical and emotional crises. As a result, this stage confronts patients and their family members with new challenges.

During this time, the illness literally enters the home, and the practical routines of both family life and ongoing medical care must be managed. As with most chronic illnesses, significant strains on finances, time, and other resources are common, and tend to be experienced as more burdensome as the realities of long-term care become more explicit. The primary task for the family at this juncture is to shift gears and change from what might have been an adaptive, crisis-oriented response to a coping strategy that supports the ongoing social, emotional, and economic functioning of all family members.

During this chronic stage, the sick person's illness remains a powerful organizer and regulator of family life. The family's social life frequently contracts and becomes primarily illness- and family-centered. Although the potential for family disruption is strongly associated with both the severity and length of the illness, chronic dysfunction is often related to the sick person's former position in the family and his capacity to rejoin the family in that role.

For example, in a case of a mother with AIDS and an HIV-infected father, their fifteen-year-old daughter gradually assumed more parenting responsibilities for the younger two children, thereby interfering with her own age-appropriate activities (schoolwork, dating, and so on). In such a situation, family responsibilities may require temporary or permanent reshuffling to compensate for the patient's incapacitated status. In general, changes in the sick person's capabilities can lead to increased role conflicts among family members.

Most family members report that they never fully relax during the chronic period and that they are perpetually in a state of readiness for the emergence of any acute crisis. Patients and family members are frequently on alert for those telltale symptoms, such as lymphadenopathy, fever, night sweats, diarrhea, weight loss, chills, and shortness of breath, that can catapult the family system back into a period of crisis over the diagnosis of AIDS. Comments such as "I worry at every little sign of congestion" or "When he doesn't feel like eating, I start to get nervous" are not uncommon. Yet these concerns are not at all unfounded. For example, we have treated families who coped only briefly with chronic-stage stressors because their HIV-infected relative succumbed quickly to a sudden, acute infection. Many patients and family members report that their vigilance regarding physical changes can become a primary preoccupation that inhibits healthy functioning in other important areas such as work and socializing.

The presence of more visible, difficult-to-disguise symptoms (such as wasting, Kaposi's Sarcoma, and AIDS-Related Dementia) compels the sick person and his or her immediate family to address the issue of broader disclosure and explanation. Whereas asymptomatic patients and their families were initially more able to manage the flow of information regarding the patients' health status, their secret may no longer be easy to hide. Disclosure is invariably associated with a loss of control and privacy, and it has been well documented that there are substantial social and economic implications that often follow open discussions of HIV status. In one case, an HIV-infected child was excluded from school and sports activities after a hospitalization for *Pneumocystis carinii* pneumonia. As children, gay men, members of ethnic minorities, and drug addicts are already disenfranchised within the larger society, the stigma of HIV status can fuel even greater discrimination and ostracism. Many family systems, whatever their configuration, also risk fracture as they attempt to manage the burgeoning impact of AIDS on their lives.

Finally, time takes on a different quality during the chronic stage. No matter how capably the family accommodates to these changes prompted by the illness, stability and familiarity may be favored over the dread associated with change. Family members are often reluctant to make radical changes in the fabric of family life, fearing that the introduction of novelty might upset the delicate balance they have established. Whereas some aspects of the HIV disease experience can be described as a roller coaster, this extended period is frequently characterized as a state of limbo. The chronic period has been described as "neutral time," a period during which neither patient nor family allow themselves to truthfully anticipate the future.

Resolution Stage

Just as the diagnosis of AIDS confirms the progressive and deteriorating course of the illness, the appearance of serious opportunistic infections or significant decrements in cognitive functioning signal the sick person's fatal decline. When the illness enters the end stage and the patient's condition is viewed as terminal, the family squarely faces its own imminent dissolution. Patients with AIDS dementia complex or other central nervous system conditions may experience difficulty in communication, resulting in frustration and despair on the part of caretakers. As the demands increase due to the sick person's disabling condition, the capacity of caretakers to feel effective in their patient-care roles frequently diminishes. For example, the mother of a young gay man with HIV disease expressed feelings of guilt, regret, and failure when she decided that she could no longer care for him due to his rapid deterioration in physical and cognitive functioning.

Regardless of what hardships have been endured, the practical and emotional impact of physical decline and impending death is unparalleled. In some families we have treated, this final stage elicits heroic last efforts to save the patient by any means, including one case where the sister insisted that her brother with end-stage AIDS be given transfusions to extend his life despite his wishes to the contrary. In other families, the news of imminent death prompts the beginning of a process of distancing and denial sometimes described as a "conspiracy of silence." Well-intentioned strategies aimed at protecting other family members from the extraordinary pain and discomfort of the moment can also backfire, leaving patient and family feeling disconnected from each other as the resolution phase progresses. This subtle process of disengagement by both patient and family can, in turn, foster either a natural process of letting go or a premature grieving on the part of family members, reduced involvement in decision making related to medical care, increased family conflict, and the exclusion of the patient in discussing his or her own death.

There is no greater problem for the family than death; it sends an emotional shock wave throughout the family. Members are affected by the loss no matter how old they are or how close they are to their families. In the case of AIDS-related death, each carries with it its own special meaning, be it the death of a lover, child, friend, parent, sibling, or grandchild. Family tasks for adapting to each of these different kinds of losses include the shared acknowledgment of the reality of death, the experience of grief, the reorganization of the family system, and a reinvestment in other relationships and life pursuits.

Given the stigma attached to AIDS-related deaths, secrecy unfortunately leaves many gay men isolated at the point of death. A family's disapproving distance may not only exclude a bereaved gay lover but also complicate the family's own grieving process. Clinicians working with the families of AIDS victims have identified psychological problems secondary to loss that can include an over-idealization of the dead family member, continued secrecy regarding details of the death, and enduring feelings of guilt, shame, and blame. Researchers have also found greater rates of traumatic stress response, demoralization, sleep problems, and increased use of recreational and sedative drugs to be associated with bereavement in the partners and friends of gay men who had died. In almost every instance, the enduring impact of AIDS-related death extends well beyond the burial and the grave.

DIMENSIONS OF
FAMILY ADAPTATION

Given the enormity of the challenge, the family facing HIV disease must adapt to continual change and transition over the course of the illness and treatment. The resources of the family will be severely taxed, and these stresses may be particularly overwhelming for low-income, minority families who may already be struggling to meet basic, daily needs. The strength of the particular family therefore depends on its ability to generate alternative transactional patterns when changes in the system demand its reorganization. From this perspective, we consider families to be adapting poorly if they respond to stress by increasing the rigidity of their patterns of behavior and boundaries or by fragmenting and disintegrating. In contrast, families who are able to explore alternatives and generate flexible coping strategies demonstrate a healthier adaptation.

Each family should be approached as a unique cultural system that is influenced by ethnicity, race, religion, and social class. To develop a clinically meaningful picture, three additional dimensions of functioning should be evaluated: (1) the family's developmental level, (2) the family's structure and system of beliefs, and (3) the family's relationship with the treatment setting. Difficulties in functioning emerge when problems in any of these interrelated domains function to keep the family from fulfilling the important task of attending to the sick person without impeding the growth of other family members. The goal of a family systems assessment is to account for the salience of these potential factors and then to generate a dynamic understanding of the sick person in his or her social context.

Family Development

Families, like individuals, move through their own life cycle consisting of different stages marked by specific tasks that must be negotiated. The family life cycle includes the early stage where families come together (for example, marriage, the birth of the first child, family with young children), the middle stage of consolidation and child rearing (entry of children into adolescence, launching children), and the family in later life (becoming grandparents, death and dying). At each point of transition, a realignment of family relationships must occur to support the entry, departure, and development of family members.

Because of the pressing practical demands associated with HIV disease, the normal emotional, practical, and developmental needs of healthy family members can be forced into the background as the family focuses its attention on the patient's care. While many families are able to negotiate new roles and relationships with one another, success cannot always be expected.

LORRAINE

Lorraine, the healthy thirty-four-year-old sister of a young drug-abusing woman with AIDS, devoted herself entirely to taking care of her sister's HIV-infected toddler. A generous and loving woman, Lorraine's commitment was so strong that she left a responsible job in order to provide optimal caretaking to her nephew. In addition, her own teenaged daughter dropped out of school to lend an additional hand, despite having a promising academic future. At the same time that these substantial changes occurred, Lorraine's teenage son also stopped attending school and made a desperate suicide attempt, stating that "there was no one left to look after him." Unfortunately, it was the suicide attempt that brought his family into treatment, not the stress of coping with HIV disease.

Although a family may naturally derail during a period of crisis and ambiguity, clinicians should regularly assess the developmental status of the family as a whole. As an undesired consequence of the illness, otherwise healthy family members may be prematurely forced into self-sufficient positions that they are unable to handle. In the instance of the young adult with HIV disease, his or her parents may be involved in the caretaking of their own parents while being called on to care for their AIDS-stricken adult child. At the same time, a partner, spouse, or sibling may have major responsibilities at home or at work that complicate the task of providing adequate care. Because the timing of the illness is often so out of step with the expected order of things, relatives may discover that they are unable to provide optimal attention without making substantial compromises. Therefore, finding a balance that acknowledges the needs of all family members represents an important aspect of family adaptation.

Family Structure and Beliefs

Another basic premise of the family systems approach is that families function as self-regulating, rule-bound systems. Over the family's life course, stable patterns of behavior evolve between family members that reflect the family's underlying structure. The preferred patterns of interaction in a family (such as who is closer to whom, who leads, who follows, what is disclosed, what is not) provide a clue to those norms that govern the life of the family members.

Researchers have identified four problems often found in families coping with the demands of serious illness:

1. Normative family needs are frequently subordinated to the needs and requirements of the illness.

2. Intra-family coalitions and exclusions often develop in response to or exacerbated by the illness.

3. These patterns of family response are rigidly held, even when there is evidence that these responses are dysfunctional.

4. The rigidity of the family's solutions to the problems posed by the illness is sustained, in part, by the family's relative isolation in managing the stresses of the medical condition.

When news of serious illness is disclosed, a family's equilibrium is challenged. The stress of illness can rigidify the structure of a couple's functioning, leaving them vulnerable to significant distress.

FRANK

Frank, the long-time partner of an HIV-infected gay man, had dedicated himself to the support of his lover throughout his illness. Over time, this previously healthy and protective relationship became dysfunctional, as the exclusive connection between the men made it difficult for other family members to participate in patient care or decision making. When his lover's medical status deteriorated, Frank was overwhelmed with feelings of panic, depression, and isolation. At the same time, he viewed the caretaking efforts made by his partner's parents as a threat to his role in the relationship.

Exclusive caretaker-patient coalitions can create distance from other family members, conflicted relationships within the larger family system. To his credit, the family therapist in this case helped the couple continue to define the boundaries of their relationship while permitting more involvement with the extended family.

When confronting rigid, maladaptive patterns of family functioning, clinicians should also assess the belief systems of relevant family members to determine the extent to which family beliefs may be reinforcing current behaviors. Family members often hold strong beliefs about how to react at a time of crisis and who should take care of the sick. These ideas frequently guide contemporary appraisals of crisis, the means by which resources are called on and managed, and the extent to which positive outcomes can be expected. As a result, family members may relate to a present crisis by relying on strategies that were successful in dealing with previous stressful experiences. Because cultural norms and religious views can be powerful determinants of a family's reaction to HIV disease, the clinician should also assess the family's attitudes toward homosexuality or drug abuse to determine whether or not their beliefs have contributed to their level of involvement.

One way that a family's beliefs can influence their approach to HIV disease may be seen in their failure to grasp crucial aspects that distinguish this illness from others. For example, because of prior experiences with illnesses that were marked by a rapidly deteriorating course, family members may not understand the episodic nature of HIV disease.

DAVID

In the case of David, a recently diagnosed gay man, his parents continued to relate to their asymptomatic son's HIV-positive status with such continuing hopelessness that they failed to identify any opportunities for positive, constructive involvement. A problem-focused exploration of their own histories with illness revealed a number of "sudden" deaths due to malignancies that served as a blueprint for their current responses to David's condition. Because they equated the dreaded HIV-infection with imminent death, they were unable to respond to the longer-term, chronic issues of HIV disease without therapeutic family intervention.

This case demonstrates the importance of assessing intergenerational family patterns and beliefs pertaining to illness and caretaking.

Family's Relationship with the Treatment Setting

It is difficult to overestimate the intensity of the relationships that patients and families develop with the treatment staff where their medical and supportive care is centered. The initial stage of diagnosis and later stages of treatment are largely defined by the unfamiliar environment and customs of the medical setting. Despite whatever welcoming efforts a hospital makes, patients and family members often report feeling like strangers and experiencing helplessness, dislocation, and confusion. At the same time, as the medical staff rapidly assume greater control over the patient's welfare, family members may feel excluded from the focus of care.

Because the person with HIV disease and his or her family are closely linked with many professionals who will influence patient care, it is important that family members form a collaborative partnership with both the hospital and other community-based settings. The current medical culture supports the entry of multiple caregivers by promoting specialization and the identification of a specific kind of helper for every aspect of a problem. The sick person in a modern medical center can expect to be involved with a wide range of professional caregivers, including internists, infectious-disease specialists, oncologists, pulmonologists, fellows, residents, medical students, nurses, dietitians, physical therapists, social workers, clergy, and aides. A similarly wide range of professional caregivers can be expected within social services. Although such a setting can draw out the best in patients and their families, the sheer number of staff can obscure and erode the strengths and resources that family members bring with them.

Life-threatening illness can induce many different reactions in family members, including fearful disengagement, passive acquiescence, rage and hostility, demanding behavior, and flight. The ability of the person with HIV disease and his or her family to understand both the illness and its treatments enables them to shift from an emotional response to effective management of practical problems. Through their interactions with staff, family members indirectly affect the nature of patient care. The sick person, family, and staff can be encouraged to avoid later struggles by making open, respectful collaboration a joint goal.

FAMILY-ORIENTED CONSULTATION AND TREATMENT

Persons with HIV disease and their families may seek consultation for a variety of reasons. These include difficulties in adjusting to the demands of life-threatening illness, dealing with fears of contagion, accepting the sexual orientation of family members, coping with stigma and discrimination, managing conflict among family members and significant others, confronting a time-limited push for reconciliation between family members, preparing for loss and bereavement, dealing with shifting family roles, and providing necessary care and negotiating with external systems. If the family is viewed as the primary unit of care, then consultation regarding these issues should include relevant family members in addition to the sick person.

There are three general goals implicit in a consultation request: to solve the presenting problem, to restore order, and to facilitate family decision making regarding treatment. Families coping with chronic, life-threatening illness can often benefit from different kinds of psychological help, ranging from brief supportive contacts to extended family therapy. Whereas anticipatory guidance and education may be sufficient for many families, others show dysfunction requiring more substantive therapeutic intervention.

Clinical practice from a family systems perspective differs from a standard psychiatric approach in the careful attention paid to the presenting problem and the sick person in the context of a complex social system. In approaching a case, we have aimed to develop interventions that enhance the family's ability to respond to the patient's needs, the staff's ability to meet the patient-family's needs, and the patient-family's ability to meet the staff's needs. The therapist working with HIV disease is best served by drawing on *generic* treatment skills and competencies as well as by drawing on therapeutic strategies that are *stage-specific* or matched to the issues and problems posed by HIV disease at the particular phase of the illness.

Generic Treatment Issues

We have identified a general set of psychosocial issues that emerge when working with families with HIV disease. These themes cut across all types of family constellations and all stages of the illness (acute, chronic, and resolution). We propose that these six generic issues may be addressed through planned therapeutic interventions.

1. *Dealing with loss.* The first component of paramount significance is understanding the impact of loss on each family member from a systemic perspective. We have found that it is important for the therapist to understand that HIV disease is very much about losses of many kinds, including the loss of health, life, longevity, capacities, sexual intimacy, partner, roles in primary and family relationships, career and financial security, recreational and social connections, and physical appearance. Furthermore, it is important to identify the multiple losses experienced by individuals with HIV disease and their family members and to recognize the significance attached to each loss for each person. Cultural variations and age differences can also affect loss reactions and the dynamics of grieving. For example, it is important that clinicians understand that children's and adolescents' grief processes differ from the more mature cognitive processes of adults.

Constructing a multigenerational genogram provides an effective therapeutic intervention that illustrates the pattern of losses and coping strategies within a given family system. In our experience, family members are able to learn from their past experiences about the particular styles of coping with loss that have been characteristic of their family. Including extended family members can also reveal hidden strengths and resources that may not be noticed in times of crisis and distress. We believe that it is important to validate the different adaptive strategies family members have used to manage illness, disability, family transitions, absences, and death. At the same time, we have found that it is essential to differentiate normal symptoms of grief from signs of complicated bereavement (for example, self-destructive behavior and substance abuse).

2. *Creating a safe place for open communication.* Individuals confronting HIV disease are likely to experience extreme feelings that may be distressing or frightening. Because there are multiple participants in couples and family meetings, we have found that the task of conducting the session can be challenging. Couples and family sessions also tend to be noisier and more openly conflictual than the modal individual psychotherapy session, especially when life-and-death issues are at stake.

We have learned that facilitating open communication and creating a safe environment in which to share these feelings must occur so that everyone feels heard and able to "speak the unspeakable." In our work, we support and validate each person, structure and modulate painful affect, and set limits on destructive and unrestrained rage. This aspect of working with families facing death and disintegration requires therapists to tolerate high levels of emotional expression.

3. *Taking a broader view.* It is prudent to remember that referral to treatment may not indicate the presence of HIV disease as the source of conflict or reason for referral. The problem presented to the therapist may be relationship discord, violence, depression, adolescent acting-out, substance abuse, or parenting problems. We have also discovered instances of HIV in families already in ongoing treatment for these types of prob-

lems. At the same time, studies have found that patients with HIV disease may already carry a primary psychiatric diagnosis.

4. *Remaining flexible.* In our work with families facing HIV disease, we have understood the importance of remaining flexible with regard to when and where therapy occurs. Therapists accustomed to fifty-minute hours in comfortable offices may need to adjust to working in other locations, such as HIV clinics, hospital rooms, hospices, or the patient's home. For example, we have experienced the challenge of conducting therapy in a hospital isolation room with everyone but the patient wearing surgical masks that both obscured familiar facial expressions and created an additional interpersonal barrier.

Family meetings may also be intermittent and discontinuous rather than ongoing and consistent. Brief, goal-directed family therapy employed at times of need has been shown to be cost effective and beneficial to the entire family system, especially given the potentially lengthy course of the disease, the growing number of HIV-infected individuals, and possibly limited financial resources.

5. *Integrating an educational approach.* A major role for therapists working with HIV disease is to educate family members and to include education as an essential aspect of treatment. Among the common topics we address are medical aspects of HIV disease, contagion, familial adaptation to acute and chronic stressors, safer sexual behaviors, parenting issues, self-care strategies for caregivers, the dying process, and management of grief and loss. We have found that we must be knowledgeable in these areas and able to present information that is accessible given the patient and family's level of understanding. In particular, using language that is culturally and developmentally appropriate can enhance the effectiveness of educational efforts.

6. *Dealing with our own reactions.* We as therapists are not shielded from the demanding and painful issues that can emerge when confronting HIV disease. Like the patient's family

members, each of us comes to the therapeutic work with our own histories, preferences, and prejudices.

In order to be effective, we must face our own beliefs and attitudes about these provocative issues. By remaining mindful of the myriad ways in which our own biases can affect treatment (both positively and negatively), we may be able to achieve a more balanced and compassionate stance. This constructive approach to strong feelings can also provide a model for family members dealing with similar kinds of emotions. The reader is referred to Chapter One of this book for further discussion of countertransference issues.

Stage-Specific Treatment Issues and Interventions

In addition to considering the general issues just discussed, we have devised clinical interventions that address the particular issues associated with each stage of the illness. In the following section, we highlight those stage-specific issues and interventions.

Acute Stage.   This stage typically begins the initial work-up for and subsequent confirmation of HIV seropositivity, related symptomatology, or AIDS.

1.   *Identifying who is likely to be affected.* We have determined that the most important systemic intervention during the acute stage is to find out who is likely to be affected by the crisis. For example, learning about the patient's family members, support system, and those potentially exposed to the virus enables both patient and clinician to identify sources of conflict and support. After finding out who is going to be affected by the news, we have found it beneficial to then coach the patient about the "if, when, and how" of talking about his or her HIV disease. In working with children diagnosed with HIV disease, helping parents or family members plan how to talk with the child and siblings will be a major initial focus. Role playing these anxiety-laden conversations has also proven to be helpful. In our

experience, it has been valuable to offer a couples or family session in which the therapist can support each partner or family member, facilitate communication, and modulate the intensity of affect.

2. *Modulating emotions.* We have learned that patients and family members experience a range of strong feelings during acute crises that include anger, anxiety, fear, sadness, and helplessness. Rage sometimes explodes from a sense of betrayal if the HIV infection was acquired through sexual activity outside a relationship previously considered to be monogamous. In these situations, disclosure of HIV seropositivity to a partner can amount to a disclosure of infidelity or sexual orientation that often creates an additional crisis for the couple. If the HIV exposure occurred through blood transfusion or a health care accident, anger may be experienced and directed toward the health care system and providers.

Regardless of the source of exposure, we believe that normalizing, pacing, and facilitating the expression of these emotions are critical. The successful clinician must be skillful in validating each person's feelings while limiting destructive styles of expression such as verbal assaults or character assassinations. We have found that with couples, time is required to process their polarized feelings independently before they can join together to support each other. Once the acute crisis has been stabilized, referrals to individual psychotherapy or appropriate community support groups may be necessary. In cases where the disclosure leads to a couple's separation, continued treatment may be important to reduce hostility, facilitate co-parenting, and provide for future support.

3. *Assessing worries and fears.* We have found that a compelling issue emerging in the acute stage involves dealing with fears of contagion and confronting the decision about who in the family needs to be tested for exposure to HIV. For example, if a parent is HIV-positive, the family will need to discuss who

else in the family may need to be tested. In serodiscordant couples, similar fears and concrete decisions should also be anticipated. In addition to addressing these important questions, we often assume an educational role in providing information to family members about risk reduction and modes of HIV transmission.

4.   *Establishing goals.* In the midst of a crisis, family members often feel overwhelmed and confused. Establishing goals and priorities is frequently reassuring and can empower the patient and family to overcome their initial sense of helplessness. These goals can include concrete tasks, such as scheduling meetings with the medical team, learning about the illness, locating additional support, and finding time to rest and refuel. Beginning with small, achievable goals maximizes the chance of success and rebuilds a sense of competence and confidence. Because this initial period is marked by intense stress, we have learned to be prepared for escalations in conflict, potential violence, suicidality, and other serious distress in the family. Providing instruction in cognitive-behavioral strategies focused on stress management can be valuable during this time.

5.   *Anticipating problems.* Although more attention is focused on coping with current issues during the acute stage, we believe it is also essential to help family members identify problems that are likely to emerge in the future. By looking at the family's multigenerational genogram, we highlight the family's previous patterns of illness and caretaking, prior coping strategies, and relevant family beliefs that may predict future difficulties. We have found that this systemic assessment tool helps family members not only to anticipate potential sources of conflict but also to identify valued models of adaptive coping. Because crises and problems can reemerge at any time, we recommend periodic follow-up sessions or let family members know that we are available should additional therapeutic contact be desired.

RANDY AND MARIA

Randy and Maria were teenage sweethearts who married at the age of eighteen. Shortly after their daughter's birth, the couple experienced an escalation in conflict. Randy's family intensified their intrusiveness and controlling behavior after Kathy was born. They implied that Maria was immature and poorly prepared to be a parent. Randy did not support Maria in her parenting efforts; he resented his wife's immersion into caring for the new baby, which he interpreted as withdrawal from him. Randy had abused alcohol as a teenager and again began to drink heavily. In addition, he stayed away from home for extended periods of time. During these absences, Randy had multiple sexual partners, including prostitutes.

Eventually, Randy reconciled his differences with Maria, and they described their reunion as joyful. However, Randy soon became ill with fevers and chronic respiratory infections. He was diagnosed with *Pneumocystis carinii* pneumonia and tested HIV-positive. He was devastated, and Maria was furious upon learning of his relations with numerous sexual partners that placed her and the baby at risk for HIV infection. Randy's illness rapidly progressed. Maria struggled as the primary caregiver, singlehandedly parenting their now three-year-old daughter while continuing to contend with her mother-in-law's intrusive and overprotective behaviors.

Our initial interventions with Randy and Maria, which stabilized the couple's crisis, included (1) normalizing Maria's overwhelming emotions and helping her begin to manage her intense anger and profound sadness; (2) supporting Randy in listening to Maria and expressing his own painful regrets, sadness, and fear; (3) educating the couple about HIV disease and recommending HIV antibody testing for Maria and Kathy; and (4) dealing explicitly with their multiple losses. Through these interventions, the couple was able to calm the feeling of "going crazy," reduce the threat of divorce, and begin to join together to fight the disease. Maria was also referred to her previous individual therapist to sort out her feelings; Randy benefited from joining a support group for newly diagnosed patients.

Additional sessions with the couple and Randy's mother affirmed the couple's identity and Maria's position as primary caregiver, while Randy's mother's learned that her intrusive behavior was indeed problematic for the couple. Acknowledging that the childhood sweethearts had grown to be adults permitted her to step back and reduce her interference. At the same time, this insight provided a new opportunity for Maria and her to negotiate constructive ways of supporting each other. As a result, Randy's mother was given an important role in caregiving for her granddaughter. She also participated in a family support group that encouraged mourning the loss of her son's youth and future. Finally, Randy and Maria learned to reconnect in a safe, physical way that provided comfort and restored intimacy and privacy to their relationship.

Chronic Stage. The chronic stage of HIV disease can be quite lengthy, with many years elapsing between HIV seropositivity and the appearance of AIDS. It has been reported that some HIV-infected individuals are clinically and immunologically healthy ten to fifteen years after seroconversion and that significant numbers of individuals remain asymptomatic more than three years after CD4 cell counts drop below 200—a criteria for the diagnosis of AIDS. Taking these factors into consideration, therapeutic interventions implemented in this stage are meant to facilitate adaptation to the changing demands of the disease.

1. *Dealing with losses.* The continuing issue of paramount significance during this stage involves the numerous, progressive, and cumulative losses. By this point in time, those losses encountered by the patient should be evident to the clinician. However, the partner and family members experience related losses that can include grieving over the relationship that once was, loss of familiar sexual practices, changes in privacy in the couple's and family relationships, and regrets over not being able to have children. Elements of loss thread through virtually every issue faced during this stage.

An important example is the addressing of a couple's grief over the loss of familiar sexual contact. One way that we have supported couples is by instructing them in safer sexual practices and helping them to "eroticize" these new behaviors. This intervention reduces the likelihood of HIV transmission and restores both sexual closeness and emotional intimacy.

2. *Changing roles.* The progression of HIV disease in the chronic phase may prevent some individuals from functioning in their familiar roles in the family system. These role changes require flexibility among all family members in order to accommodate to added responsibilities and the fluctuating course of the disease. However, the dependency of the HIV-infected person on others may also renew dysfunctional aspects of and preexisting conflicts in interpersonal relationships.

In our clinical work, we typically help families to identify role changes, manage conflict, and negotiate new arrangements in caregiving. These interventions normalize psychological distress and provide opportunities to restructure relationships. Therapeutic techniques, such as family sculpting and role-plays, can help rebalance the dynamics exacerbated by the shift in family roles. In addition, because patients and family members may experience a loss of control as roles are rearranged, interventions supporting the discovery of new areas of competency and control are often valuable.

3. *Confronting ambivalence.* Throughout this stage, patients and family members are confronted with the need to make decisions. For example, in serodiscordant couples, there is sometimes ambivalence about continuing the relationship. Dementia may rob the HIV-infected person of the ability to resolve "unfinished business." Patients must decide when to inform and involve members of the extended family.

Serodiscordant couples in particular exhibit a high degree of ambivalence. We have observed that in such cases, an HIV-negative partner may be tempted to leave the relationship, which generates fears of abandonment in the infected partner. The HIV-positive patient may also consider relinquishing the relationship to protect his or her partner, which can also create fear and confusion. Crises may also pull ambivalent partners back into a caregiving mode or cause them to flee.

At times when this ambivalence is heightened, we focus our therapy on carefully delineating the sequence of such events, exploring any secondary gains or manipulative dynamics, sensitively reframing interaction patterns, and facilitating direct negotiation of each person's needs. In general, delayed resolution of ambivalence is risky, particularly given the unpredictable course of HIV disease. The chronic stage offers opportunities for addressing important issues that may not exist during acute crises or the terminal stage of the disease.

4.   *Resolving loyalty conflicts.* As a shift in family roles occurs, the HIV-infected partner may be caught in a loyalty conflict between his or her primary relationship and family of origin. In both gay and unmarried heterosexual couples, the partner may feel marginalized as family members begin to make decisions for and take care of the person with HIV disease. We have found that helping couples define a boundary around their relationship is as important as coaching the parents of adult children in age-appropriate parenting. Because family members must also consider the legal ramifications of various decisions, such as securing certain binding legal documents, wills, power of attorney, and advance directives, therapists can also help the family members face these crucial decisions.

5.   *Reducing stigma.* As the chronic stage of HIV disease progresses and features of the disease become more visible and difficult to disguise (such as noticeable weight loss and wasting, lesions from Kaposi's Sarcoma, and cognitive impairments associated with AIDS dementia), the choice of "who to tell" dramatically changes, and a broader circle of people becomes aware simply through day-to-day contacts. Given the anxieties in soci-

ety regarding contagion, these changes may elicit significant emotional distress for the patient, his or her partner, and their respective families. We have learned that assisting the family in relation to these issues can increase social support and reduce isolation, shame, and discrimination.

6. *Providing support.* We have observed that the ability of couples and families to withstand the continuing demands of the disease is drastically reduced when they lack the support of extended family, friends, and the community. We believe it is important to coach the couple on how to approach other family members by creating and rehearsing the proposed plan of action. At the same time, we do not underestimate the value of our being available to help the couple speak about the unspeakable— death. To discuss what the person with HIV disease desires regarding concrete issues (such as child care, funeral arrangements, and disposition of property) and what must be taken care of by family members are painfully difficult subjects to broach for many families.

COLIN AND TED

Colin and Ted were a gay couple who had maintained a committed relationship for thirteen years while also owning and operating a business together. Colin was forty-two years old and HIV-positive. Ted was fifty-two years old and remained HIV-negative following repeated annual antibody testings. They were well connected in the local gay community and had witnessed the deaths from AIDS of many close friends and social acquaintances.

During the previous four years, Colin had had several opportunistic infections, accompanied by periods of extreme fatigue and depression, that prevented him from participating in many home and work activities. Consequently, Ted assumed a more prominent role at home caring for Colin and running their shared business. Colin missed the sexual intimacy they had shared early in their relationship, which changed with his HIV-positive diagnosis six years ago, and Ted stated that he was no longer interested in sexual activity. This shift left Colin feeling both rejected and relieved that he was not inadvertently exposing Ted to HIV. However, Ted resented his added responsibilities at home and at work when Colin began to engage in unprotected sexual intercourse with other HIV-positive friends. Ted reportedly did not object to Colin's sexual behavior outside the relationship, yet he could not understand Colin's continued risky behavior when he (Ted) was so committed to caring for his partner's health.

Our therapeutic interventions in this case, addressing specific issues that emerged over the prolonged course of Colin's illness, included (1) helping to improve the couple's communication skills (so that Colin and Ted could understand each other's concerns, de-escalate conflict, and elicit caring instead of blame); (2) generating a clearer understanding of the power struggles arising in their relationship from Colin's fluctuating dependency on Ted (which led to improved adaptation to changing roles as well as to enlisting the resources of outside social support services); (3) educating the couple about safer sexual behaviors (which reduced Ted's fear of contagion, allowed Colin to appreciate that Ted's requests were motivated by his desire to preserve Colin's health rather than control his sexual practices and reinstated erotic sexual intimacy in their relationship); and (4) encouraging the couple to address and grieve the numerous and ongoing losses they experienced.

These interventions facilitated communication about the couple's grief—grief that had accumulated over the years and that was anticipated due to Colin's expected death. They reported that their brief course of couples therapy enhanced their emotional closeness, helped them to resolve ongoing losses, and supported their seeking assistance from other family members, such as Colin's mother and sisters, who had been uninvolved in Colin's care.

Resolution Stage. The appearance of serious opportunistic infections or significant decrements in cognitive functioning signal a fatal decline and mark the end of the chronic stage and the beginning of the briefer, more intense terminal phase. As demands mount due to the patient's deteriorating condition, caregivers' sense of themselves as helpful in their patient-care roles often diminishes. Several major stage-specific interventions for the terminal stage are reviewed here.

1. *Enhancing collaboration.* Throughout the course of treatment, we place a high value on close collaboration with the patient's health care providers in order to remain apprised of the individual's changing health status. In the end stage, this partnership becomes even more essential. We have found that by being gently direct and by questioning what the patient and family have been told or believe the outcome will be, we are able to facilitate the open sharing of information about the dying process and impending death.

Because both patient and family may try to protect each other by not acknowledging or openly discussing this process, such questioning can help the family to take advantage of the last opportunity for the completion of unfinished business. In addition, family conflicts left unresolved over "who's in charge" of caregiving and decision making for the dying person are likely to recur. The therapist can help structure these negotiations, reaffirm the boundary around the couple, and support the partner in carrying out the dying person's wishes.

2. *Saying good-byes.* In many instances, we have assisted those who are closely connected to the dying person with saying good-byes. Therapeutically structuring these exchanges, which may include the expression of regrets, appreciations, and departing wishes, can provide a road map for the family through this uncharted territory. For example, both the patient and the caregivers may be exhausted and privately wishing for the death to occur, resulting in feelings of guilt and self-blame. In serocongruent couples, the terminal stage of AIDS may offer a cruel preview for the surviving partner who witnesses his or her partner's

demise. Through open, careful discussion, the clinician can offer validation to the family members as they struggle with the conflicting feelings of wanting to hold onto and be released from their suffering.

3.   *Bereavement counseling.* Bereavement is likely to be complicated given the stigma associated with AIDS, the likelihood that individuals who die from AIDS are often young and their deaths are premature, and the fact that this grief occurs in the context of multiple deaths and losses. Parents of drug users and of those infected by sexual contact often experience excessive guilt because they feel they failed to instill healthy values that might have prevented their child from becoming infected. Bereavement counseling has also been found to reduce psychiatric morbidity in survivors.

We have found it helpful to give specific suggestions aimed at helping family members to interact with the dying person and each other in a comforting way. For couples, the therapist can help the bereaved partner grieve the loss of the couple's identity and begin to form a new individual identity as part of the grief process. In addition, giving "permission" to the bereaved to attend to their own needs and use support from others can reduce isolation and refocus them in pursuing their own life courses.

TINA

Tina was a forty-four-year-old woman with a history of IV drug use and alcohol dependence during her teens and twenties. She was married and divorced three times and had several children. Now clean and sober for six years, Tina had a steady job and enjoyed a satisfying new romance. When she began to suffer from fatigue and an assortment of recurrent infections, she was ultimately hospitalized with a severe case of *Pneumocystis carinii* pneumonia and diagnosed with AIDS. Her health condition was serious and necessitated aggressive and invasive medical procedures.

Although initially numb with shock, Tina displayed calm resignation and surrendered to the potent medications. However, her available family members moved quickly from shock and denial to rage at their rural medical community. They blamed her medical team for everything from the failure to diagnose her condition appropriately in a timely manner to the present insistence on using heroic measures.

In this case, we attempted to intervene at many levels, including the following: (1) stabilizing the crisis between the family and Tina's health care providers by helping the family to express their anger and distress appropriately; (2) mediating between the family and medical personnel to help both systems accurately hear information in order to reduce the powerful emotionality of the moment; (3) highlighting Tina's wishes that no heroic measures be employed and working with the medical staff and Tina's family members to discuss guardianship and guidelines regarding life-threatening medical emergencies; and (4) facilitating an emotionally charged discussion with Tina and her boyfriend about their positive memories and earlier regrets, her anticipated death, and their lost dreams. Frequent meetings with the family were held to discuss Tina's dying, and the family was encouraged to recognize the likelihood that Tina's death might reactivate feelings from previous losses.

Although family members can be burdensome to the sick person, these cases also demonstrate how they can function as caregivers, informants, consultants, and participants in patient care. We have also observed that family members can sometimes be difficult to engage in consultation meetings, despite obvious evidence of the need for such consultation. Among the obstacles we have encountered are the reluctance of family members to change their way of handling the illness; their preference for talking about the pragmatic aspects of the illness rather than emotional issues; the likelihood that some of their distress is related to their experiences with the medical system; the possibility that they may feel criticized by offers of psychological help; problems related to geographic distance; and an inability to find time for an additional illness-related activity.

Effective coping with chronic illness has been described as involving a sense of action on the part of the individual, an ability of the family to simultaneously understand the illness and deny its threat so that the individual's needs can be met, and the family's ability to identify and use sources of support. Although anticipatory guidance and education may be sufficient for some families, these interventions rarely address the family's isolation or their lack of exposure to how other families are coping with similar demands. Multiple-family discussion groups, where four to six families can meet together, provide another format from which families can learn about the course of illness, share their common experiences and problems, and join together in developing more flexible solutions.

Living with a life-threatening illness is fundamentally a solitary experience. Therefore, identifying ways to reduce isolation and enhance supportive connections within the sick person's own family is essential. General family therapy approaches can be modified to suit the task of working with the families of medically ill persons, and several groups have developed more specific guidelines for working with HIV disease. Although there is a range of opinion regarding whether or not to involve all family members in a family consultation, we recommend that treatment teams should include whoever is willing to participate.

Finally, if therapy is indicated, it is advisable to frame the problem as a transitional issue for the whole family that relates to their struggle with the illness. By helping family members view their psychological symptoms as transient signs of distress, the consultant normalizes their experiences. By doing so, the added stigma that accompanies seeing a mental health provider can be mitigated. Seeing themselves as having been destabilized by the stresses associated with HIV disease, the family may be in an opportune position for self-exploration, mobilization, and transformation.

One of the untold stories of the devastating AIDS epidemic has been its catastrophic effect on the families of its victims. We have witnessed how parents, partners, children, siblings, grandparents, and friends are compelled to bear and respond to the extreme practical, existential, economic, and psychosocial consequences of a terrifying life threat. Although there is no typical family of the person with HIV disease, we recognize that such a family is constantly in transition, actively reorganizing itself to master the acute and chronic stresses of the illness. Some families flexibly adapt to these demands, others rigidify or disintegrate under the strain. In our experience, even brief consultations with family members can help them to manage their experience of the illness.

Working with these couples and families, we consider the specific biopsychosocial stage of HIV disease and the family's cultural background, developmental level, structure and beliefs, and relationship with the treatment setting. Our awareness of these factors results in a more comprehensive view of how the family is managing the overpowering impact of the disease. The family-oriented clinician will be immeasurably assisted by a systemic framework that places the sick person in the context of the family, and by drawing both on generic interventions that are common across the stages of illness and on stage-specific strategies.

We also recommend that therapists working with HIV disease recognize two integral aspects of the patient and family's paradoxical circumstances; that what is happening is truly tragic and painful, and that human beings can create competency and are capable of adaptation to even extreme realities. We have been inspired to find in treating these stricken families that although this type of work is demanding and often painful, there are unparalleled opportunities to mitigate effectively the suffering and distress of everyone involved. By respecting the family's style and allying with their sources of strength and resilience, we can assist patients, their families, and those that treat them to master the fundamental challenges associated with HIV disease and its treatment.

NOTES

P. 225, *despite evidence that serious illness can adversely affect family functioning:* Leventhal, H., Leventhal, E. A., & Van Nguyen, T. (1985). Reactions of families to illness: Theoretical models and perspectives. In D. C. Turk & R. D. Kerns (Eds.), *Health, illness, and families: A life-span perspective* (pp. 108–146). New York: Wiley.

P. 225, *there is a growing interest in applying family systems concepts:* Fishman, H. (1979). Family considerations in liaison psychiatry. *Psychiatric Clinics of North America, 2,* 249–263; Sargent, J. (1985, March). *Chronic illness and the family.* Paper presented at New England Deaconess Medical Center, Boston, MA.

P. 226, *With the Centers for Disease Control and Prevention (CDC) reporting that 1 in every 250 persons:* Centers for Disease Control and Prevention (CDC). (1995). *HIV/AIDS Surveillance Report, 7* (2), 13.

P. 226, *Just as the AIDS epidemic . . . human anguish:* Martin, J. L. (1988). Psychological consequences of AIDS-related bereavement among gay men. *Journal of Consulting and Clinical Psychology, 56,* 856–862.

P. 226, *families are being forced to confront difficult practical and interpersonal demands:* Tross, S. (1988). Acquired immunodeficiency syndrome (AIDS). In J. Holland & J. Rowland (Eds.), *Handbook of psychooncology* (pp. 254–270). New York: Oxford Press; Hepworth, J., & Shernoff, M. (1989). Strategies for AIDS education and prevention. In E. D. Macklin (Ed.), *AIDS and families: Report of the AIDS Task Force Groves Conference on marriage and the family* (pp. 39–81). New York: Harrington Park Press.

P. 226, *Studies have shown that the most frequent sources of stress:* Frierson, R. L., Lippman, S. B., & Johnson, J. (1987). AIDS: Psychological stresses on the family. *Psychosomatics, 28,* 65–68.

P. 227, *A study looking at the sequelae of AIDS-related death:* Martin, J. L. (1988). Psychological consequences of AIDS-related bereavement among gay men. *Journal of Consulting and Clinical Psychology, 56,* 856–862.

P. 227, *Several reports on the partners of HIV-infected gay men:* Frierson, R. L., Lippman, S. B., & Johnson, J. (1987). AIDS: Psychological stresses on the family. *Psychosomatics, 28,* 65–68; Martin, J. L. (1988). Psychological consequences of AIDS-related bereavement among gay men. *Journal of Consulting and Clinical Psychology, 56,* 856–862; George, H. (1989). Counselling people with AIDS, their lovers, friends and relations. In J. Green & A. McCreaner (Eds.), *Counselling in HIV infection and AIDS* (pp. 88–108). Worcester, England: Billings.

P. 227, *case studies have described the acute psychological reactions:* Patten, J. (1988). AIDS and the gay couple. *Family Therapy Networker, 12,* 37–39.

P. 227, *Clinical experience suggests . . . common among relatives of heterosexual people with HIV:* Williams, R. J., & Stafford, W. B. (1991). Silent casualties: Partners, families and spouses of persons with AIDS. *Journal of Counseling and Development, 69,* 423–427; Foley, M., Skurnick, J. H., Kennedy, R. V., & Louria, D. B. (1994). Family support for heterosexual partners in HIV-serodiscordant couples. *AIDS, 8,* 1483–1487.

P. 227, *A survey of major pediatric AIDS centers:* Seibert, J. M., Garcia, A., Kaplan, A., & Septimus, A. (1989). Three model pediatric AIDS programs: Meeting the needs of children, families, and communities. In J. M. Seibert & R. A. Olson (Eds.), *Children, adolescents, and AIDS* (pp. 25–61). Lincoln: University of Nebraska Press.

P. 227, *Locating a home and placement for an HIV-infected child:* Beckerman, N. L. (1994). Psychosocial tasks facing parents whose adult child has AIDS. *Family Therapy, 21,* 209.

P. 227, *National Coalition on AIDS and Families issued general principles:* E. D. Macklin (Ed.). (1989). *AIDS and families: Report of the AIDS Task Force Groves Conference on marriage and the family* (pp. 269–270). New York: Harrington Park Press.

P. 227, *the focus of health care policy and patient care:* E. D. Macklin (Ed). (1989). *AIDS and families: Report of the AIDS Task Force Groves Conference on marriage and the family* (pp. 269–270). New York: Harrington Park Press.

P. 229, *individuals who functionally form the system of support:* Curtis, J. H. (1989). Treating AIDS: A family therapy perspective. In C. Kain (Ed.), *No longer immune: A counselor's guide to AIDS* (pp. 169–187). Alexandria, VA: American Association for Counseling and Development.

P. 229, *Family therapists have described this emergent family as the "problem-defined system":* Goolishian, H., & Anderson, H. (1991). Including non–blood-related persons in treatment: Who is the family to be treated? In A. Gurman (Ed.), *Questions and answers in the practice of family therapy.* New York: Brunner/Mazel.

P. 230, *The biopsychosocial paradigm:* Fink, P. J. (1988). Response to the presidential address: Is "biopsychosocial" the psychiatric shibboleth? *American Journal of Psychiatry, 145,* 1061–1067.

P. 231 *A four-step paradigm:* Minuchin, P., & Minuchin, S. (1987). Family as the context for patient care. In L. H. Bernstein, A. J. Grieco, & M. Dete (Eds.), *Primary care in the home setting.* Philadelphia: Lippincott.

P. 232, *The diagnosis also represents a tremendous crisis . . . lovers, family members, and friends:* George, H. (1989). Counselling people with AIDS, their lovers, friends and relations. In J. Green & A. McCreaner (Eds.), *Counselling in HIV infection and AIDS* (pp. 88–108). Worcester, England: Billings and Sons.

P. 232, *Relatives of the recently diagnosed . . . disbelief, powerlessness:* Figley, C., & McCubbin, H. I. (1983). *Stress and the family: Coping with normative transition, coping with catastrophe* (Vol. 2). New York: Brunner/Mazel.

P. 233, *In some families with AIDS, . . . confirmation of illness:* Tiblier, K. B., Walker, G., & Rolland, J. S. (1989). Therapeutic issues when working with families of persons with AIDS. In E. D. Macklin (Ed.), *AIDS and families: Report of the AIDS Task Force Groves Conference on marriage and the family* (pp. 81–129). New York: Harrington Park Press.

P. 233, *Issues of secrecy, ambivalence over homosexuality, and troubles with empathy:* Frierson, R. L., Lippman, S. B., & Johnson, J. (1987). AIDS: Psychological stresses on the family. *Psychosomatics, 28,* 65–68.

P. 233, *there is great potential for feelings of betrayal, shame, and confusion:* Tiblier, K. B., Walker, G., & Rolland, J. S. (1989). Therapeutic issues when working with families of persons with AIDS. In E. D. Macklin (Ed.), *AIDS and families: Report of the AIDS Task Force Groves Conference on marriage and the family* (pp. 81–129). New York: Harrington Park Press.

P. 234, *As with most chronic illnesses:* Patterson, J. M., & McCubbin, H. I. (1983). Chronic illness: Family stress and coping. In C. Figley, & H. I. McCubbin (Eds.), *Stress and the family: Coping with normative transition, coping with catastrophe* (Vol. 2, pp. 21–36). New York: Brunner/Mazel.

P. 234, *The family's social life frequently contracts:* Turk, D. C., & Kerns, R. D. (1985). The family in health and illness. In D. C. Turk & R. D. Kerns (Eds.), *Health, illness, and families: A life-span perspective* (pp. 1–23). New York: Wiley.

P. 234, *capacity to rejoin the family in that role:* Minuchin, S. (1974). *Families and family therapy.* Cambridge, MA: Harvard University Press.

P. 235, *The presence of more visible, . . . (such as wasting . . .):* Tiblier, K. B., Walker, G., & Rolland, J. S. (1989). Therapeutic issues when working with families of persons with AIDS. In E. D. Macklin (Ed.), *AIDS and families: Report of the AIDS Task Force Groves Conference on marriage and the family* (pp. 81–129). New York: Harrington Park Press.

P. 235, *Many family systems, whatever their configuration:* Bor, R., Miller, R., &

Perry, L. (1988). Systemic counseling for patients with AIDS/HIV infections. *Family Systems Medicine, 6,* 21–39.

P. 236, *This chronic period has been described as "neutral time"*: Sourkes, B. (1982). *The deepening shade: Psychological aspects of life-threatening illness.* Pittsburgh, PA: University of Pittsburgh Press.

P. 236, *the capacity of caretakers to feel effective:* Boss, P., Carton, W., Horbal, J., & Mortimer, J. (1990). Predictors of depression in caregivers of dementia patients: Boundary ambiguity and mastery. *Family Proceeding, 29,* 245–254.

P. 237, *sometimes described as a "conspiracy of silence":* Reiss, D., Gonzalez, S., & Kramer, N. (1986). Family process, chronic illness, and death: On the weakness of strong bonds. *Archives in General Psychiatry, 43,* 795–804.

P. 237, *There is no greater problem for the family than death:* Bowen, M. (1976). Family reaction to death. In P. J. Guerin (Ed.), *Family therapy: Theory and practice* (pp. 335–349). New York: Gardner Press.

P. 237, *reinvestment in other relationships and life pursuits:* Walsh, F., & McGoldrick, M. (1988). Loss and the family life cycle. In C. J. Falicov (Ed.), *Family transitions: Continuity and change over the life cycle* (pp. 311–337). New York: Guilford Press.

P. 237, *Clinicians working with the families of AIDS victims:* Walker, G. (1988). An AIDS journal. *Family Therapy Networker, 12,* 20–33.

P. 237, *Researchers have also found greater rates of traumatic stress response:* Martin, J. L. (1988). Psychological consequences of AIDS-related bereavement among gay men. *Journal of Consulting and Clinical Psychology, 56,* 856–862.

P. 238, *changes in the system demand its reorganization:* Gonzalez, S., Steinglass, P., & Reiss, D. (1987). *Family-centered interventions for people with chronic disabilities.* Washington, DC: George Washington University Medical Center.

P. 238, *we consider families to be adapting poorly:* Minuchin, S. (1974). *Families and family therapy.* Cambridge, MA: Harvard University Press.

P. 238, *To develop a clinically meaningful picture:* Rait, D. (1991). The family context of AIDS. *Psychiatric Medicine, 9,* 423–439.

P. 238, *impeding the growth of other family members:* Carter, E. A., & McGoldrick, M. (1980). *The family life cycle: A framework for family therapy.* New York: Gardner Press.

P. 239, *a realignment of family relationships must occur:* Rait, D. S. (1989). A family-systems approach to the patient with cancer. *Cancer Investigations, 7,* 77–81.

P. 239, *the normal emotional, practical . . . patient's care:* Carter, E. A., & McGoldrick, M. (1980) *The family life cycle: A framework for family therapy.* New York: Gardner Press.

P. 240, *Researchers have identified four problems:* Gonzalez, S., Steinglass, P., & Reiss, D. (1987). *Family-centered interventions for people with chronic disabilities.* Washington, DC: George Washington University Medical Center.

P. 241, *The stress of illness can rigidify . . . a couple's functioning:* Minuchin, P., & Minuchin, S. (1987). Family as the context for patient care. In L. H. Bernstein, A. J. Grieco, & M. Dete (Eds.), *Primary care in the home setting* (pp. 83–94). Philadelphia: Lippincott.

P. 241, *the long-time partner of an HIV-infected gay man:* Patten, J. (1988). AIDS and the gay couple. *Family Therapy Networker, 12,* 37–39.

P. 241, *more involvement with the extended family:* Gonzalez, S., Steinglass, P., & Reiss, D. (1987). *Family-centered interventions for people with chronic disabilities.* Washington, DC: George Washington University Medical Center.

P. 242, *who should take care of the sick:* Penn, P. (1983). Coalitions and binding interactions in families with chronic illness. *Family Systems Medicine, 1,* 16–25.

P. 242, *the extent to which positive outcomes can be expected:* Figley, C., & McCubbin, H. I. (1983). *Stress and the family: Coping with normative transition, coping with catastrophe.* (Vol. 2). New York: Brunner/Mazel.

P. 243, *The current medical culture supports the entry of multiple caregivers:* Imber-Black, E. (1985). Families and multiple helpers. In R. Draper & D. Campbell (Eds.), *Applications of systemic family therapy: The Milan method.* Philadelphia: Grune & Stratton.

P. 243, *The ability of the person with HIV disease:* Sargent, J. (1985, March). *Chronic illness and the family.* Paper presented at New England Deaconess Medical Center, Boston, MA.

P. 244, *Persons with HIV disease . . . may seek consultation for a variety of reasons:* Tiblier, K. (1987). Intervening with families with young adults with AIDS. In M. Wright & M. L. Leahey (Eds.), *Families and life-threatening illness.* St. Louis, MO: Springhouse.

P. 244, *There are three general goals implicit in a consultation request:* Wellisch, D., & Cohen, M. (1986). The family therapist as a systems consultant to medical oncology. In L. Wynne, S. McDaniel, & T. Weber (Eds.), *Systems consultation: A new perspective for family therapy.* New York: Guilford Press.

P. 244, *in the context of a complex social system:* Wellisch, D., & Cohen, M. (1986). The family therapist as a systems consultant to medical oncology. In L. Wynne, S. McDaniel, & T. Weber (Eds.), *Systems consultation: A new perspective for family therapy.* New York: Guilford Press.

P. 245, *Constructing a multigenerational genogram:* Walker, G. (1991). *In the midst of winter: Systemic therapy with families, couples, and individuals with AIDS infections.* New York: Norton.

P. 246, *high levels of emotional expression:* Rait, D. S. (1995). The therapeutic alliance in couples and family therapy: Theory in practice. *Psychotherapy in Practice, 1,* 59–72.

P. 247, *studies have found that patients . . . a primary psychiatric diagnosis:* Perry, S., Jacobson, L., Fishman, B., Frances, A., Bobo, J., & Jacobsberg, B. K. (1990). Psychiatric diagnosis before serological testing for the human immunodeficiency virus. *American Journal of Psychiatry, 147,* 89–93.

P. 247, *Brief, goal-directed family therapy:* Bor, R., Miller, R., Salt, H., & Scher, I. (1991). The relevance of a family counseling approach in HIV/AIDS: Discussion paper. *Patient Education and Counseling, 17,* 235–242.

P. 248, *coach the patient about the "if, when, and how":* Mansergh, G., Marks, G., & Simoni, J. M. (1995). Self-disclosure of HIV infection among men who vary in time since seropositive diagnosis and symptomatic status. *AIDS, 9,* 639–644.

P. 249, *disclosure of HIV seropositivity to a partner:* Earl, W. L. (1990). Married men and same sex activity: A field study on HIV risk among men who do not identify as gay or bisexual. *Journal of Sex and Marital Therapy, 16,* 251.

P. 252, *It has been reported that some HIV-infected individuals:* Buchbinder, S. P., Katz, M. H., Hessol, N. A., O'Malley, P. M., & Holmberg, S. D. (1994). Long term HIV-1 infection without immunologic progression. *AIDS, 8,* 1123–1128.

P. 252, *significant numbers of individuals remain asymptomatic:* Hoover, D. R., Rinaldo, C., He, Y., Phair, J., Fahey, J., & Graham, N. M. H. (1995). Long-term survival without clinical AIDS after CD4+ cell counts fall below 200 × 106/l. *AIDS, 9,* 145–152.

P. 253, *restores both sexual closeness and emotional intimacy:* Myers, M. F. (1991). Marital therapy with HIV-infected men and their wives. *Psychiatric Annals, 21,* 466–470.

P. 253, *we typically help families to identify role changes:* Leigh, J. P., Lubeck, D. P., Farnham, P. G., & Fries, J. F. (1995). Hours at work and employment status among HIV-infected patients. *AIDS, 9,* 81–88.

P. 254, *cognitive impairments associated with AIDS dementia:* Zeifert, P., Leary, M., & Boccellari, A. A. (1995). *AIDS and the impact of cognitive impairment: A treatment guide for mental health providers.* San Francisco: University of California, San Francisco, AIDS Health Project; Ackerman, F. (1989). Case report: Family-systems therapy with a man with AIDS-Related Complex. *Family Systems Medicine, 7,* 292.

P. 255, *the ability of couples and families to withstand the continuing demands of the disease:* Maloney, B. D. (1988). The legacy of AIDS: Challenge for the next century. *Journal of Marital and Family Therapy, 14,* 143–150.

P. 258, *Bereavement counseling has also been found:* Bor, R., Miller, R., Salt, H., & Scher, I. (1991). The relevance of a family counseling approach in HIV/AIDS: Discussion paper. *Patient Education and Counseling, 17,* 235–242.

P. 258, *specific suggestions aimed at helping family members:* Tiblier, K. B., Walker, G., & Rolland, J. S. (1989). Therapeutic issues when working with families of persons with AIDS. In E. D. Macklin (Ed.), *AIDS and families: Report of the AIDS Task Force Groves Conference on marriage and the family* (pp. 81–129). New York: Harrington Park Press.

P. 259, *they can function as caregivers:* McDaniel, S., Campbell, T. L., & Seaburn, D. B. (1990). *Family-oriented primary care: A manual for medical providers.* New York: Springer-Verlag.

P. 259, *family members can sometimes be difficult:* Gonzalez, S., Steinglass, P., & Reiss, D. (1987). *Family-centered interventions for people with chronic disabilities.* Washington, DC: George Washington University Medical Center.

P. 260, *Effective coping with chronic illness:* Sargent, J. (1985, March). *Chronic illness and the family.* Paper presented at the New England Deaconess Medical Center, Boston, MA.

P. 260, *Multiple-family discussion groups . . . flexible solutions:* Gonzalez, S., Steinglass, P., & Reiss, D. (1987). *Family-centered interventions for people with chronic disabilities.* Washington, DC: George Washington University Medical Center.

P. 260, *Therefore, identifying ways to reduce isolation . . . is essential:* McDaniel, S., Campbell, T. L. & Seaburn, D. B. (1990). *Family-oriented primary care: A manual for medical providers.* New York: Springer-Verlag.

P. 260, *Although there is a range of opinion . . . in a family consultation:* Tiblier, K. B., Walker, G., & Rolland, J. S. (1989). Therapeutic issues when working with families of persons with AIDS. In E. D. Macklin (Ed.), *AIDS and families: Report of the AIDS Task Force Groves Conference on marriage and the family* (pp. 81–129). New York: Harrington Park Press.

P. 260, *it is advisable to frame the problem as a transitional issue:* Minuchin, P., & Minuchin, S. (1987). Family as the context for patient care. In L. H. Bernstein, A. J. Grieco, & M. Dete (Eds.), *Primary care in the home setting.* Philadelphia: Lippincott.

P. 261, *actively reorganizing itself to master the acute and chronic stresses of the illness:* Minuchin, P., & Minuchin, S. (1987). Family as the context for patient care. In L. H. Bernstein, A. J. Grieco, & M. Dete (Eds.), *Primary care in the home setting.* Philadelphia: Lippincott.

P. 261, *capable of adaptation to even extreme realities:* Sargent, J. (1985, March). *Chronic illness and the family.* Paper presented at the New England Deaconess Medical Center, Boston, MA.

8

TREATING HIV IN DUAL DIAGNOSIS PATIENTS

Philip A. Bialer, Steven Bluestine, and Jeffrey J. Richards

The term *dual diagnosis* is usually used when describing patients presenting with symptoms and history indicative of a substance use disorder (SUD) plus a psychiatric disorder. One example would be that of a person who chronically abuses alcohol and has also developed a phobic disorder unrelated to the alcohol abuse. On the other hand, some chronic mentally ill patients may abuse drugs or alcohol either to self-medicate or in response to the underlying symptoms of their illness.

Dual diagnosis for the purpose of this chapter, however, will refer to patients with a diagnosis of HIV/AIDS disease plus an additional diagnosis of either SUD or chronic mental illness (CMI). This chapter will provide further diagnostic clarification in the context of HIV and discuss assessment and general treatment approaches for these populations, including pharmacologic management. We will also give attention to the special HIV-related risk behaviors associated with SUD and CMI.

In addition to a brief review of the literature, much of this chapter will be based on our experience at the Krueger Clinic for the Treatment of Immunological Disorders of the Beth Israel Medical Center, which was founded in 1988. Located in the Lower East Side of Manhattan, this clinic serves more than two thousand active patients with HIV/AIDS. More than 70 percent of these patients have a significant history of SUD; 25

percent of the clinic population are women. The Krueger Psychiatric Outpatient Clinic was begun in 1988 by Dr. Bialer to provide on-site psychiatric consultation, long-term individual and group treatment, and staff support. In addition to our work at this clinic, we also see many people with HIV/AIDS in the inpatient setting and in our private practices. Our collective total of over fifteen years of work treating thousands of patients in an epicenter of the AIDS epidemic has, ironically, provided us with vast clinical experience in the midst of this tragedy. The dedication of our co-workers and, more important, the courage of our patients has made this experience enormously gratifying.

Although the chapter will address SUD and CMI as separate subjects, patients rarely fit into neat categories. Many patients we see actually have a triple diagnosis of HIV, substance abuse, and psychiatric disorder, as in the following case.

ROBERT

Robert is a thirty-three-year-old Jewish white gay male, HIV-positive, who has a known history of Bipolar Disorder. While in his twenties he dropped out of psychiatric treatment and would often abuse drugs such as Ecstasy or cocaine, especially when his mood was low and when "partying" with friends. He also found that alcohol was helpful for "taking off the edge" or for getting to sleep. He admitted to numerous unsafe sexual encounters during this time period.

After learning of his HIV-positive status at the age of thirty, his drug and alcohol abuse as well as his cycling mood symptoms escalated during the next two years. When a close friend died from complications of AIDS, Robert finally felt that his own death was imminent if he didn't get help, so he "crawled" into a treatment facility.

Robert successfully completed a detox and rehabilitation program that included Twelve-Step groups and individual therapy. In addition, the Bipolar Disorder was treated with a combination of medications, and he was also started on antiretroviral therapy. He has remained in treatment, has stayed sober for one year, and currently has no obvious HIV symptoms, although he complains of mild memory problems.

HIV AND SUBSTANCE USE DISORDERS (SUD)

We have found that the psychotherapeutic treatment of SUD among people with HIV/AIDS is one of the most problematic areas of mental health care. Patients with SUD may frustrate us as therapists because they frequently seem to be resistant to our interventions. However, we have also seen patients for whom HIV served as an impetus to change their habits and thus become more amenable to help. In the following discussion, we will attempt to address the complex dynamics involved in order to assist you in the treatment of this population.

Epidemiology

First, we can look at the rates of drug abuse in persons with HIV, and the rates of HIV in persons with drug abuse. The rate of HIV infection in a particular group is also known as the *seroprevalence rate*. In 1994, 27 percent of all AIDS cases reported to the Centers for Disease Control and Prevention (CDC) identified IV drug use as the primary risk factor, and an additional 4.8 percent reported both male homosexual or bisexual contact and IV drug use. One study in a Bronx, New York, methadone maintenance treatment program found that 39.4 percent of the patients were HIV-positive; another study in San Francisco found seroprevalence rates of 12 percent. In both of these studies, the overwhelming majority of subjects were Black or Hispanic. This was found to be due to the higher frequency with which Blacks and Hispanics shared needles with strangers, higher numbers of injections in "shooting galleries," higher numbers of sex partners who used IV drugs, and lower socio-economic status. In addition, the San Francisco group found that those who used cocaine daily had a significantly higher rate of seropositivity.

Epidemiologic research has also demonstrated a high prevalence of co-morbid mental illness among substance abusers. A study in Toronto found that 78 percent of patients at one treatment facility had some psychiatric disorder during their lifetime, and 65 percent had a current mental disorder. The most common disorders in the sample were Antisocial Personality Disorder (36.2 percent), phobias (28.8 percent), Generalized Anxiety Disorder (26.1 percent), and Major Depression (20.0 percent). Of course, the presence of multiple coexisting problems further complicates treatment.

The significance of SUD in the HIV population is multifold. First, patients who use substances have impaired judgment and poor impulse control, due to both their craving for substances and the direct mind-altering effects of intoxication. This may impede the practice of safe behaviors and lead to more dangerous ones, such as exchanging unsafe sex for drugs or money. Second, such impaired judgment and erratic behavior often present an obstacle to entering into and complying with medical treatment. Finally, for patients with the stress of chronic and life-threatening illness, the mental and physical changes produced by substance use can further decrease their quality of life.

Defining SUD

Defining SUD is more difficult than it first appears. Not all use of illicit substances creates a problem with functioning, and many legal drugs that have legitimate medical uses, such as benzodiazepines, can also be abused. Furthermore, there is a continuum among such phenomena as use, misuse, abuse, dependence, and addiction. Unfortunately, many clinicians automatically label most substance use as abuse or dependence without first doing the necessary evaluation.

The most recent *DSM-IV* criteria for Substance Dependence have been useful clinically to distinguish truly problematic use. A patient must meet at least three of the following seven criteria during a twelve-month period:

1. Tolerance: the substance needs to be taken in progressively larger amounts to achieve the same effect, or taking the same amount results in diminished effect.

2. Withdrawal: stopping the substance results in the characteristic withdrawal syndrome for the substance.

3. The substance is taken in larger amounts or over a longer period than was intended.

4. There is a persistent desire or unsuccessful efforts to cut down or control substance use.

5. A great deal of time is spent in activities necessary to obtain the substance, use the substance, or recover from its effects.

6. Important social, occupational, or recreational activities are given up or reduced because of substance use.

7. Substance use is continued despite knowledge of having a persistent or recurrent physical or psychological problem that is likely to have been caused or exacerbated by the substance.

The behavior common to each of these criteria is an inability to cut down on intake of a substance despite adverse consequences. Note also that the presence of tolerance or withdrawal alone is no longer sufficient to diagnose Substance Dependence. These phenomena can occur with the use of medications that are not abused as well as with drugs that have potential for both legitimate use and abuse. For instance, patients given opiates for chronic pain may develop both tolerance and dependence with prolonged use. However, many of these patients never develop the dysfunction and impairment in daily functioning that differentiate pathological from appropriate use.

The *DSM-IV* criteria for Substance Abuse differ from Substance Dependence in that they do not include tolerance, withdrawal, or a pattern of compulsive use. Instead, they focus on the harmful consequences of repeated use.

Assessment of SUD

As noted above, there is a high prevalence of co-morbid mental disorders among substance users. For this reason, a comprehensive evaluation is necessary and should include assessment of the following: substance use; chronic personality traits that may or may not constitute a personality disorder; and such symptoms as depression or anxiety, which may be due to mental illness, coping problems, or the effects of substance use.

The traditional approach to assessing substance use has been to quantify the amounts of substances used, the routes of administration, the frequency and duration of use, and the time since last use. This information is important, but it does not necessarily address the definition of SUD, which relies on change in functioning. For this reason, we have always found it important to ask about such issues as changes in work, mood, activities, and sleep. One method for doing this is the so-called CAGE questionnaire:

1. Have you ever felt the need to *C*ut down on drinking?
2. Have you ever felt *A*nnoyed by criticisms of drinking?
3. Have you ever had *G*uilty feelings about drinking?
4. Have you ever taken a morning *E*ye opener?

Because many patients are in denial about how drugs are affecting their life, it is usually necessary to obtain collateral information (with the patient's permission) from family, friends, or co-workers. They are usually able to give a clearer picture of changes in functioning, relationships, and personality.

Diagnosing active substance abusers is difficult because of the varied effects of the substances used. In general, acute intoxication with stimulating substances such as cocaine or amphetamine causes anxiety, agitation, insomnia, and, occasionally, full manic symptoms. Withdrawal from these substances causes depression, irritability, and lethargy. Conversely, acute intoxication with sedating substances such as alcohol, benzodiazepines, barbiturates, heroin, and marijuana causes depression, mental slowing, and sedation; withdrawal causes agitation, irritability, and insomnia. However, in actual clinical practice, because patients with chronic use go through varying cycles of intoxication and withdrawal during the course of a day or week, they can present with almost any of the previously mentioned psychiatric symptoms. It can be very difficult, especially on an initial visit, to determine what role substances play in the patient's clinical picture. Most substance-induced syndromes usually remit after a week or two of abstinence, but abstinence cannot be ensured if a patient is in a nonrestrictive environment.

Sometimes a patient's picture changes during the course of treatment because of new information. It is important to be flexible enough to alter the treatment and to set limits as needed. The following case exemplifies this approach.

JULIO

Julio, a thirty-eight-year-old gay Latino male with a known past history of crack and heroin abuse, presented to our clinic with a month of poor sleep, which he attributed to the worsened health status of his partner. On initial evaluation, he denied any use of illicit drugs or alcohol for the past five years. He then developed a depression with prominent insomnia that only partially responded to medication. After missing several appointments, the patient admitted that he had been using crack every two to three days since one month before our first appointment.

Initially, the therapist explained that Julio's symptoms would not respond to medications unless he was drug free. Considering that the therapist had now seen Julio for five months, the therapist decided to see him one more time rather than terminate treatment.

When the patient returned and admitted that his crack use had worsened, the therapist refused to medicate him or see him for psychotherapy, while emphasizing the need for drug treatment. Despite Julio's protests, the therapist held firm that the insomnia, depression, and anxiety would never properly respond to treatment unless the patient was drug free.

When Julio returned two months later, he reported that he had been abstinent from crack since the last psychiatric appointment. He had no further symptoms of anxiety, insomnia, or depression, and he no longer needed medication.

In this case, all of the patient's symptoms were drug induced, but this was not apparent initially. His treatment had to be modified once this became clear.

We should also mention that evaluation can be particularly difficult in cases of multiple effect, wherein a patient is using a substance for more than one reason. For instance, one patient was using marijuana for both nausea relief and to escape from the reality of his situation. When other treatments for nausea were proposed, he did not want to consider them, because this would mean giving up his "high."

Treatment Approaches

Treatment approaches for HIV-positive patients with SUD are far from straightforward. Some therapists feel that patients should always be challenged on the issue of their substance abuse, maintaining that they cannot otherwise be treated effectively. Others feel that it is important to keep patients in treatment at any cost; they fear that refusing to work with patients who have not given up drug or alcohol use will alienate them. Unfortunately, there are no easy guidelines. Many patients will not accept that they have a substance abuse problem, especially initially, and the clinician's suggesting that they get help for this may drive them out of needed care. However, as in the previous case example, a health professional's insistence that a person enter drug or alcohol treatment can also be a powerful tool.

Countertransference issues are very important to acknowledge and resolve when dealing with HIV-positive substance abusers. For instance, many people have negative feelings, which can be quite intense, about substance abusers with HIV, feeling that "they brought this on themselves." Others feel that because these patients have a fatal illness, it is cruel to confront them or try to force them to get off drugs. The clinician should remember that HIV is not imminently fatal, that most people with HIV live for many years after diagnosis, and that life span after diagnosis continues to increase thanks to medical advances. We believe such statements as "He's dying anyway, so why bother fighting over drug use?" to be dismissive.

Clinicians can also inhibit proper treatment with the belief that because so many of the people with dual diagnosis have had very hard lives, with histories of physical abuse, sexual molestation, poverty, and so on, they are "entitled" to use drugs now that they have HIV as well. Although well meaning, conceptualizing patients as "victims" is the sort of enabling that helps to prolong SUD. Patients with SUD can usually find a stressor to rationalize their continued drug or alcohol use. This does not change the fact that substance abuse or dependence causes significant impairment in a person's life. Regardless of HIV serostatus, such persons deserve to have that impairment addressed. Patients are entitled to live their lives, no matter how long or how short, with as much quality and as little impairment as possible, and the therapist has an obligation to aid in this endeavor.

In our experience, the most helpful approach is to determine whether SUD is the primary diagnosis. This can be difficult, either because of a patient's poor reliability or because of a mixed picture, such as a sleep disorder and alcohol abuse presenting simultaneously. If SUD is the primary diagnosis, then abstinence is required before treatment can continue. Whether or not the therapist can work with the patient in the face of continued use of drugs or alcohol depends on the therapeutic relationship, the nature of the substance use, and the patient's symptoms and clinical picture.

A full discussion of treatment of SUD as a primary problem is beyond the scope of this chapter, but we can say that options include the following: brief inpatient detoxification for patients with physiologic dependence on substances such as heroin or alcohol; outpatient rehabilitation or therapeutic communities, for longer-term intensive treatment; methadone maintenance for heroin users; and Twelve-Step programs such as Alcoholics Anonymous (AA) or Narcotics Anonymous (NA), which stress that participants must admit they have lost control over their lives because of substance abuse, and then give them the tools to change this situation.

All of these modalities offer group settings, which address the difficulties in interpersonal relationships so common among these patients. They also offer the support and advice of others who are further along in their recovery, so that patients have role models who can offer concrete advice. Twelve-Step programs are available everywhere and do not have a waiting list or exclusion criteria, so they offer readily accessible treatment for patients who do not qualify for or cannot immediately access other substance treatment modalities.

It is important to have lists of these referrals readily available, because patients tend to have brief "windows of opportunity" when they are willing to accept these services. For some patients, the diagnosis of HIV can be an impetus to changing various maladaptive aspects of their lives, and the clinician should take advantage of this opportunity if possible. A case example follows.

MICHAEL

Michael, a forty-year-old gay white male with a twenty-year history of alcohol and cocaine abuse, was diagnosed with HIV. Several months later, he decided to become abstinent and to begin attending regular Alcoholics Anonymous meetings, going to several different ones in the course of a week. He began to speak of changing other aspects of his life and of the need to stop lying to himself as well as to others, and to realize that much of the histrionic and disorganized features that had characterized his behavior were largely due to substance use. He was referred to psychiatry for treatment of depression, which responded well to medication.

The therapist continued seeing him weekly, working on issues of coping with his illness and integrating the changes in his life necessitated by giving up substance use. Although Michael died approximately eighteen months after beginning therapy, he frequently spoke of how much happier he was living without drugs and without the associated maladaptive behavior patterns.

This example shows how patients can have dramatic changes in long-standing coping styles if they are willing to address substance abuse and remain abstinent. They can then begin to make other positive changes in their lives, including changes in areas that seemed to be related to chronic "personality traits" but were in fact largely caused or maintained by the substance use.

The treatment of SUD in individual therapy takes several forms, with multiple approaches often required. Supportive therapies bolster healthy defenses and help patients cope with stressors directly related to HIV and illness progression as well as other social stressors. Cognitive therapies teach patients new ways to cope with negative thoughts and difficult emotions so that they no longer turn to drugs to avoid uncomfortable feelings. Interpersonal therapies teach them different ways of relating to others. And exploratory therapies examine early life experiences such as physical or emotional abuse and sexual molestation, which are very common in this population. The therapist must be prepared to be flexible and to incorporate whichever form of treatment (or combination of treatments) is most useful for a particular patient at a particular time.

If substance use is not the primary diagnosis, frequently the patient can be medicated and worked with in therapy. However, it is important to make a proper diagnosis, and not blindly accept such complaints as "depression" or "anxiety." In the following case, a patient with a past history of substance abuse also had a panic disorder, a form of anxiety that required specific treatment.

ELLEN

Ellen, a forty-year-old white female with a past history of intravenous heroin use, presented at our clinic with a clear-cut new onset of panic attacks. She had not used heroin or other drugs for several years, but in consideration of her past drug use, the therapist initiated treatment with nortriptyline because it has no abuse potential. However, this did not help her panic symptoms, and the patient pleaded for something that would help immediately, as she had by this point had several weeks of ineffective treatment.

Reluctantly, the therapist began Klonopin and Prozac. Within a few weeks the patient reported a significant positive response, with complete resolution of her panic attacks and great improvement in her mood. She subsequently decreased the dose of both medications on her own, and at no time was there any evidence of misuse.

Ellen continued weekly treatment for problems coping both with her HIV and her mother's chronic mental illness.

This case also illustrates how flexibility is needed when using medications for these patients, and how medications are often only a partial treatment for patients with complicated problems.

Difficult Cases

One of the most difficult aspects of working with patients with SUD and HIV/AIDS is that they are not all treatable. Some patients, such as the person in the following example, do not accept that substances are responsible for their complaints and symptoms, and therefore psychiatric treatment cannot be successful.

DWAYNE

Dwayne, a forty-five-year-old Black male, demanded Prozac for his "depression." Evaluation revealed that Dwayne had a long history of heroin, cocaine, and crack use, and that this use continued during previous treatment with Prozac. Dwayne was found to be very angry, but his continuous substance abuse prevented making any diagnosis other than Substance-Induced Mood Disorder.

The therapist explained that he could not give Dwayne further medication, as it was clearly of no benefit in reducing drug use and it would not help his depression in this context. The patient became enraged, insisting again that he needed the Prozac to treat his "depression," and stormed out of the office. Discussion with the patient's primary physician revealed that Dwayne had never shown any motivation or interest in stopping his drug use, but had always maintained that he had a "depression." Dwayne was very frustrating for everyone in the clinic to treat, because he kept insisting he needed our help yet would not accept our recommendations.

This example shows that some patients with active substance use cannot be properly treated with medication (because it is not indicated) or psychotherapy (because they do not want anything but medications). However, other patients who struggle with active substance use will be able to work profitably with a therapist, as the following case illustrates.

JORDAN

Jordan, a forty-year-old white male, was referred to our clinic for treatment of depression, which responded partially to medication. However, in assessing the patient it became clear that there were

long-standing issues of dependency, passivity, and difficulty inter-
acting with others. He described heroin as making him more social
and outgoing. The patient had a twenty-five-year history of intravenous heroin use, although he had continued to work during this
time. Over the course of two years of psychotherapy, there would be
an episode of heroin use approximately every three months. After
each episode the patient was remorseful; he was able to engage in a
discussion about what had led him to use and how to try to prevent
it in the future. This patient remained clearly motivated to engage
with the therapist, kept all appointments on time, and never accepted
the "victim" role. For these reasons, he was able to benefit from
therapy, despite his periods of active drug use.

This case shows how each patient must be evaluated individually, rather than being lumped in a group such as "active user"
or "untreatable." It also illustrates that sometimes, even patients
who initially seem very problematic can ultimately be rewarding
to work with.

As we stated previously, patients with a dual diagnosis of HIV
and SUD are among the most difficult to treat. They need to be
approached with a delicate mixture of limit setting and flexibility.
Some patients will be unwilling to give up drug or alcohol use,
and these patients may not be accessible for psychological intervention. We must be ever vigilant for evidence of substance
abuse or dependence and at the same time be willing to allow
patients to make "mistakes" and still get the necessary treatment.
Approached in this manner, many patients will be able to use
various therapeutic interventions.

CHRONIC MENTAL ILLNESS (CMI), HOMELESSNESS, AND HIV

There are many neuropsychiatric and psychological complications related to HIV that can arise in the course of an infected
individual's illness. Depression, mania, delirium, psychosis, and

dementia can present alone or in combination even in a patient who may have no prior psychiatric history. The situation becomes more complex when the patient has a pre-existing CMI or is homeless. In this section, we review what is known about the co-morbidity of CMI, homelessness, and HIV. We will discuss assessment methods and treatment strategies for reducing risk, increasing compliance with medical treatment, and minimizing the impact of psychopathology on HIV/AIDS in this unique and often underserved population.

HIV Seroprevalence Among the Homeless and the Mentally Ill

How many homeless people are mentally ill? How many of those who are homeless and mentally ill are infected with HIV? These are two extremely difficult questions to answer, largely because this transient population lacks adequate access to resources for medical and mental health care, making it difficult to obtain an accurate census.

Data from communities throughout the United States indicate that about one-third to one-half of the total homeless population suffers from a co-morbid CMI. Conversely, homelessness rates among the mentally ill in one study of patients in San Francisco ranged from 22 percent to 57 percent, depending on the definition of *homeless.*

The answer to our second question is equally variable. One report indicates that between 6 and 19 percent of homeless adults with psychiatric disorders in New York City are infected with HIV. Other studies, conducted in psychiatric hospitals in New York City, have revealed an HIV seroprevalence among the chronic mentally ill of 5 to 7 percent.

HIV infection rates among the chronic mentally ill and homeless are of great concern, and the need to address the mental health care needs of this population is imperative. We can begin this process by examining risk factors that may predispose mentally ill patients to HIV or increase the spread of HIV by those already infected.

Risk Behaviors Associated with CMI and Homelessness

When a person with CMI develops a serious medical illness such as AIDS, management is often complicated by the nature of the psychiatric symptoms. For example, psychosis or mania may render a patient unable to understand the nature and severity of his or her medical problem and the treatment that may be necessary. Cognitive impairment and compromised judgment may result from the direct effect of HIV, from the patient's pre-existing psychiatric disorder, or both. As a result, it may be difficult to convey information about HIV and associated risk factors to this patient population.

One recent study revealed that women in a psychiatric outpatient setting for CMI patients scored significantly lower on an "AIDS knowledge" questionnaire than did a matched control group of medical outpatients. Similarly, in another study, 43 percent of mentally ill patients (with and without HIV) believed that heterosexual women cannot get AIDS. Furthermore, 45 percent of patients surveyed believed that a person's appearance signals whether he or she has HIV. Some patients believe that birth control pills can prevent infection. Others may integrate issues about HIV into their delusional systems, as did one patient who believed that AIDS does not exist because "the disease is part of a conspiracy by the surgeon general and condom manufacturers to make a profit."

In addition to their lack of knowledge about HIV transmission, mentally ill persons have been shown to be less likely to use condoms, to have more IV drug–using sexual partners, and to use drugs or alcohol more frequently in conjunction with sex. Schizophrenics, for example, tend to have more frequent sexual encounters (when compared to matched controls), and bipolar manic patients tend to display more hypersexual behaviors and higher rates of sex with prostitutes and homosexual activity. It has also been shown that patients with a CMI are often victims of childhood sexual abuse, which has been linked to repeated engagement in sexually promiscuous, impulsive, and dangerous behaviors in adulthood.

Substance abuse can further increase this population's risk for HIV. Schizophrenic patients may "self-medicate" their symptoms with drugs or alcohol, and depressed patients tend to use more IV drugs than do matched controls. Even non-IV drug users are at risk, as substance intoxication can impair judgment and lead to unsafe sexual behavior.

Another risk factor for patients with CMI may be the increased incidence of sexually transmitted diseases (STDs) among this population. Data from an urban study in the Midwest showed that 33 percent of twenty subjects reported being diagnosed and treated for another, non-HIV STD at some point during the course of their mental illness. These results are not surprising given the greater number of sexual contacts among these patients, particularly in the context of unstable and often transient relationships.

In addition to adults, an estimated one to two million runaway youths are homeless. HIV seroprevalence studies of this population have shown rates that are higher than among adolescents and young adults in other settings. In one study, 11 percent of youth surveyed had known HIV-risk exposures that included IV drug use, homosexual or bisexual activity, having a partner with known HIV-risk exposures, and unprotected intercourse. The seroprevalence rate for this sample was 2.3 percent.

Another important issue among homeless youth is the exchange of sex for drugs or money. Because adolescents who prostitute themselves most often do so out of necessity, they are more likely to engage in risky sexual behaviors. This, coupled with the sense of invulnerability perceived by this age group, increases the chance for HIV infection among youth, particularly in larger urban centers.

Assessing the Patient with CMI and HIV

Patients with CMI often present at our facilities with an exacerbation of their psychiatric disorder in the face of having HIV/AIDS. Because infection with HIV can itself cause neuropsychiatric problems, it may be difficult to determine the precise etiology of the presenting symptoms. Is this a relapse of the patient's Schizophrenia or Bipolar Disorder, or is this psychosis or mania related to the effects of HIV?

In order to answer these questions as accurately as possible, we always obtain a comprehensive psychiatric history. This includes collateral history from the patient's family and friends whenever possible, as well as from the patient's medical caregivers. In our AIDS clinic, for example, psychiatrists, social workers, and primary caregivers take a multidisciplinary approach and communicate with each other regularly about patient treatment. The temporal relationship between the patient's psychiatric symptoms and HIV seroconversion can help determine if the patient had symptoms at some point prior to infection or if the current symptoms are a new manifestation of AIDS.

In patients with CMI, we continually assess for psychiatric symptoms that can place the patient at risk for HIV infection or foster spread of HIV if the patient is already infected. During active psychotic states, patients may exhibit poor judgment and diminished insight, which can lead to risky behaviors such as drug use and promiscuity. Acute manic states may result in hypersexuality, self-destructive behavior, and poor impulse control. Persons with CMI often have impaired cognition, which interferes with information processing and may limit the patient's appreciation of associated risks. Negative symptoms such as poor social problem-solving, lack of assertiveness, and difficulty establishing stable relationships can further contribute to HIV risk. For instance, patients may enter into risky situations because they are unable to resist coercion or feel they cannot be loved in more fulfilling ways other than through repeated, anonymous sexual liaisons.

Homelessness among the chronic mentally ill often leads to further isolation and poor social supports. This subgroup may be even more difficult to reach in the way of prevention programs and risk management. As with other mentally ill persons, the homeless often exhibit low self-esteem and live in poverty. A recent study showed that of 106 homeless persons surveyed (60 percent of whom had a diagnosis of Schizophrenia or Schizoaffective Disorder), the average monthly spending allowance was $92.30 per person. Only 68 percent were receiving some sort of local or federal aid. Thus, the necessity for food or money increases the chance that patients will trade sexual favors for these basic needs. Similarly, homeless substance abusers often exchange sex for drugs and money, and, in the context of already compromised judgment, increase their risk for HIV.

Chronic mentally ill and homeless patients often do not comply with their treatment, which can lead to decompensation and multiple hospital admissions. As a result, patients may be lost to follow-up, or may drop out of various community outreach programs that provide the social support and problem-solving skills necessary to limit risky behaviors. Self-neglect may also result because of psychosis or frank denial of their illnesses, both mental and physical. Psychiatric symptoms that occur as a result of the patient's chronic illness may also interfere with medical treatment for HIV-related illness. The following case study illustrates how an exacerbation of CMI can present an obstacle to the medical treatment of AIDS patients.

TAYLOR

Taylor, a fifty-three-year-old homeless African-American male with AIDS and a history of chronic paranoid schizophrenia, was emergently admitted to the intensive care unit for treatment of a large pericardial effusion. Cultures of the fluid grew *Mycobacterium* tuberculosis, requiring that the patient receive a minimum of nine months of anti-TB medication. Prior to admission, treatment with various antipsychotics had resulted in partial remission of the schizophrenia, although he remained paranoid.

During the mental status exam at admission, Taylor was found to be alert and oriented. He was irritable and minimally cooperative. His thoughts were disorganized and often illogical, with paranoid delusions that "someone [was] trying to starve" him. When discussing his cardiac condition, Taylor stated that he "no longer had a heart" and that it had been removed and "replaced with a box." He denied any auditory or visual hallucinations. He was not suicidal or homi-cidal. The dose of his antipsychotic medication was increased, but he often refused to take it.

Approximately four weeks into his admission, Taylor requested to leave against medical advice. Because of his history of noncom-pliance and risk for worsening of his illness if left untreated, it was determined that Taylor was dangerous to himself and that he should be involuntarily admitted to the psychiatry service. Further adjust-ments in his medication helped to reorganize his thought process enough to allow him to understand the need for compliance with the prescribed regimen. Eventually, Taylor was stabilized and trans-ferred to a long-term care facility for continuation of his medical and psychiatric treatment.

Given the cognitive and social barriers faced by persons with CMI, we find that it is imperative to assess the basic coping and social skills of patients who are at risk for or who have HIV. We also ask patients about their frequency of sexual contact; the number, gender, and potential risk behaviors of their partners; their use or lack of use of condoms and other contraceptive methods; and their awareness of safer sex guidelines. We discuss patients' use of intravenous and other drugs and needle sharing practices. In addition, we inquire about patients' knowledge regarding AIDS and, if not already known, their HIV status. Finally, patients are asked about a history of sexual or physical abuse (either as a child or an adult) and whether they have ever acquired any other STDs. These basic inquiries reveal a great deal about patients and how their mental illness may relate to HIV-risk behaviors. Such knowledge enables us to make inter-ventions to prevent the spread of HIV.

Clinical Interventions for Prevention and Treatment

Despite the large numbers of chronic mentally ill and homeless with HIV/AIDS, few programs exist, to our knowledge, that are specifically designed to teach this population about HIV risk factors, treatment, and prevention. This process can and should begin during the initial assessment of the patient. When inquiring about sexual practices and use of drugs and alcohol, we provide simple, straightforward answers about HIV and AIDS as well as prevention techniques. Our clinic distributes condoms to patients as part of their ongoing treatment plan. Inpatient units in one major metropolitan center use staff members and audiovisual materials to educate patients about HIV.

A specific area that is often neglected among the chronic mentally ill is sex education. Historically, these patients, particularly schizophrenics, have been viewed as "asexual." Sexuality is often not discussed or even considered when treating such patients. Studies throughout the years, however, have refuted this notion. Indeed, schizophrenic patients are often actively interested in or engage in sexual activity, even when acutely psychotic. Nevertheless, mental health staff often feel that chronically ill patients are unable to tolerate any form of sex education, fearing that they may regress or be unable to understand the material being presented.

Several studies have shown, however, that sex education among this population has been successful. Such material must be tailored to the individuals' level of functioning. When conducting education meetings, for example, we have found it helpful to divide patients into small groups of no more than six to eight people (including facilitators) to minimize overstimulation. Severely psychotic patients who may be too disorganized to process the information should first be treated with appropriate medication until their symptoms have diminished enough to allow participation.

Those who can participate and understand should be taught in short (no more than one-hour) sessions in a succinct and repetitive manner. Audiovisual aides are invaluable to sustain interest and attention. Safer sex practices, including demonstration of how to apply a condom, should be clearly described. In addition, the effects of drug and alcohol use on patients' judgment and ability to make decisions in the "heat of the moment" should be discussed.

Patients may engage in unsafe sexual activity for other reasons as well. In addition to poor insight or judgment, patients may act out of impulsivity as a component of their psychosis or severe personality disorder. Because being HIV-positive may not produce symptoms, at least early on, patients often deny that they have the illness or that they can infect others. A sense of invulnerability may accompany mental illness, especially if a patient is delusional. All of these issues must be addressed when educating and treating CMI, with or without HIV.

CMI patients often suffer low self-esteem in addition to other debilitating symptoms. They may feel out of control with respect to their own behavior, either due to active psychosis or because of negative symptoms of isolation, withdrawal, and disconnectedness. This can leave patients feeling demoralized and helpless. For patients who have AIDS or are at risk for infection, being faced with potentially lethal consequences because of sex can exacerbate these feelings and be overwhelming. Programs should incorporate modified cognitive-behavioral skills to help alleviate as much anxiety around issues of sex and HIV as possible. This may include eliciting thoughts and feelings about HIV and sex in order to help patients understand the myths versus the facts. Patients can also have many misconceptions about what is safe or unsafe sexual behavior; repetitive informational sessions can decrease unnecessary anxiety. Assertiveness training classes can also help patients to resist coercion into risky behaviors and to say no when faced with a potentially dangerous situation.

Allowing patients to ask questions in a nonthreatening atmosphere and receive appropriate information from sensitive staff fosters self-esteem. Regular, brief follow-up meetings that allow patients to talk about personal experiences and behaviors can empower patients, giving them a sense of control over their own bodies. These strategies not only foster a sense of autonomy among patients but also increase compliance with medical and psychiatric treatment.

Programs that incorporate these principles may not be suitable for severely psychotic or manic patients who also have HIV, however. In such cases, one must treat the psychiatric illness before any meaningful education and risk prevention can be initiated.

The most difficult subpopulation to reach may be the homeless mentally ill with concomitant HIV. Such patients are unlikely to take advantage of the traditional health care system. Street-based programs that distribute condoms and information on risk reduction have been shown to be effective for such disaffiliated groups.

MEDICATIONS

Treatment with psychotropic medications for patients with a double or triple diagnosis of HIV infection plus SUD, CMI, or both is an important and often necessary modality. As physicians, we receive most patient referrals because of this need for medication. However, for several reasons, we believe that *all* clinicians must be aware of the basic principles of medication management:

1. To have a better understanding of the symptoms and syndromes that medication can successfully treat, and thus to know when to refer patients for medication
2. To be aware of the side effects and interactions of the medications and, if necessary, alert the physician to developing complications
3. To coordinate, along with the physician and patient, the most comprehensive treatment plan

In general, when medicating patients with HIV/AIDS, we adhere to the rule of thumb "start low and go slow." This means using low doses of medication initially and being cautious about raising the doses. Even if a patient has been taking a medication for many years, we are very careful to monitor for side effects. As HIV illness progresses, the basic pharmacodynamics and metabolism of psychotropic medications may be affected by changes in body mass from wasting or by problems with absorption due to opportunistic infections in the gastrointestinal system.

In addition, infection of the central nervous system (CNS) by HIV early in the course of illness has now been well demonstrated. Although HIV's exact effects on normal CNS anatomy and physiology can only be hypothesized, it appears that the subcortical structures are most involved. Clinically, this results in patients being more sensitive to both the beneficial effects and the side effects of psychotropic medications. Chronic drug or alcohol use may also result in CNS damage, with subsequent effects on the efficacy of psychotropics. Current, active drug use is likely to interfere with or obscure the results of psychotropic treatment.

The interactions of psychotropics with the numerous medications used for HIV-related conditions require special attention and may produce unexpected results. Patients' current social circumstances and environment must also be taken into account when adding psychotropic medications to their treatment regimen.

Schizophrenia

It is clear that HIV-associated cognitive/motor complex (also known as AIDS Dementia Complex or HIV encephalopathy) can produce symptoms that mimic schizophrenia. Certain patients with a previously known history of schizophrenia may also be at risk for HIV infection. During the asymptomatic phase of HIV disease, one can most often maintain the schizophrenic patient on his or her usual medication without changing the dosage. As the patient develops symptoms related to HIV, however, the clinician may wish to consider adjusting the dosage or even changing the medication depending on the presentation.

High-potency neuroleptics such as haloperidol (Haldol) or fluphenazine (Prolixin) are more likely to cause extrapyramidal side effects (EPS) in the general population. Examples of EPS include tremors, muscular rigidity, and dystonic reactions (severe and painful contractions of muscles in the eyes, tongue, neck, or limbs). AIDS patients have been shown to be extremely sensitive to EPS, and dosages of neuroleptics often have to be reduced. Low doses of amantadine (Symmetrel) may be added to treat the side effects. Although benztropine (Cogentin) is also effective in treating EPS, the anticholinergic profile of this medication can contribute to cognitive impairment and other neuropsychiatric complications in AIDS patients.

Alternatively, low-potency neuroleptics such as chlorpromazine (Thorazine) or thioridazine (Mellaril) may be used, as they tend to produce much less EPS. The sedating side effects of low-potency neuroleptics may also be useful for patients experiencing high levels of anxiety or mild agitation. Disadvantages of the low-potency neuroleptics include a higher anticholinergic profile and lowering of the seizure threshold, which is a particular problem for patients with brain lesions. Once again, the use of much lower dosing than one would use in the non–HIV-infected population may overcome some of the potential problems.

Some authors strongly advocate for the use of "mid-potency" antipsychotics such as perphenazine (Trilafon) or molindone (Moban) because they tend to produce less extreme side effects. However, based on our experience, one should not expect these medications to be free from complications, especially if patients develop HIV-related medical problems. The following case provides an example.

WILLIAM

William was a forty-year-old man with a history of chronic, undifferentiated schizophrenia diagnosed in his early twenties. His psychiatric course had been very stable for the past five years while he was living in an adult home run by the Salvation Army and taking Haldol 20 mg per day. He was known to be sexually active with other men and had tested positive for HIV three years before he was admitted to our hospital for the treatment of *Pneumocystis carinii* pneumonia. His Haldol was discontinued at the time of admission because he had developed Parkinsonian tremors and rigidity.

William responded well to medical treatment, but three weeks into his hospital course, his thought process was found to be much more disorganized, and he was becoming withdrawn. We decided to treat him with Moban 10 mg twice daily, which was roughly half the equivalent dose of the Haldol he had been taking. His mental status returned to baseline over the next two weeks with no noticeable side effects from the Moban. William returned to our hospital two weeks later because of a severe dystonic reaction in his right arm and shoulder; he was also noted to be somewhat confused. The Moban was discontinued, and William was treated with amantadine for the next week before the dystonia completely cleared. An MRI of his head revealed a new finding of progressive multifocal encephalopathy (PML).

Over the next few weeks with no antipsychotic medication, William again became disorganized and mildly agitated. A very low dose (12.5 mg) of Thorazine was started at bedtime with fair results. He was discharged back to his adult home one week later on 25 mg Thorazine. William died three months later as a result of the PML; however, his mental status remained relatively stable on the low dose of Thorazine, which was well tolerated.

This example illustrates how HIV-related illnesses can dramatically alter the clinical course of patients with CMI. At times it may not be possible to determine if changes in mental status are a result of exacerbation of the underlying psychiatric illness, HIV-related brain disease, or a combination of both. The case also illustrates that doses of medications much lower than those usually used in the non–HIV-infected chronic mentally ill can have serious side effects. These medications can be used beneficially as long as the patient is carefully monitored.

Recent reports have indicated that the new antipsychotic risperidone (Risperdal) may be effective for HIV-infected patients with few side effects even among patients who have experienced side effects with other medications. Risperdal has been recommended for the treatment of the negative symptomatology of schizophrenia, and it remains to be seen if this medication can affect the withdrawn, apathetic behavior of AIDS dementia. As with the other neuroleptics, we have found that AIDS patients respond to lower doses of Risperdal (1–3 mg per day) than non-HIV patients.

Two final caveats: (1) because of the increased risk of serious side effects from neuroleptics among AIDS patients, we avoid the use of depot preparations such as Haldol Decanoate; and (2) clozapine (Clozaril), which has been found to be effective for some treatment-resistant schizophrenic patients, is contraindicated for HIV-infected patients due to the increased risk of bone marrow suppression.

Depression

Some studies have demonstrated a higher lifetime prevalence of depressive disorders among the HIV population compared to the general population, and estimates of current depression have ranged from 2 percent to 21 percent of patients evaluated. Several antidepressants, including imipramine (Tofranil) and fluoxetine (Prozac), have proven to be effective treatment in both clinical research and practice. We usually choose an antidepressant based on the patient's clinical presentation and how a particular medication's side-effect profile will affect the patient. Selective serotonin reuptake inhibitors (SSRI) such as Prozac, sertraline (Zoloft), and paroxetine (Paxil) are often prescribed for HIV patients because of fewer overall side effects. These medications are not free of side effects, however, and once again, lower doses are often required for patients with AIDS. We have also had good, albeit limited, experience using venlafaxine (Effexor) for some of our patients. At the time of this writing, we are unaware of the efficacy of nefazodone (Serzone) for the HIV population, but its low side-effect profile makes it a promising treatment choice.

Some have also advocated the use of psychostimulants such as methylphenidate (Ritalin) for depressed HIV patients, although we recommend reserving these medications primarily for patients whose mood changes are secondary to AIDS dementia. Recently, we have also seen some male patients' mood improve after treatment with testosterone, a finding corroborated by others.

Bipolar Disorder

Although manic symptoms can be a manifestation of AIDS dementia, some reports indicate that a previous history of Bipolar Disorder may also be associated with increased risk for HIV infection. Presumably this could result from the increased drug use, hypersexuality, and poor impulse control of manic episodes. One report on a small series of patients implied that patients whose manic syndrome appeared to be due to HIV responded more effectively to treatment with valproic acid (Depakote) than with lithium, but either agent appears to be effective for patients with a known history of Bipolar Disorder. This corresponds with our experience in treating chronic bipolar patients.

If lithium is given, serum levels must be monitored very carefully, especially during acute medical illness. Although Depakote has a broader therapeutic index of safety than lithium, its use can cause liver damage, which can be problematic in combination with some HIV-related medications, such as Zidovudine (AZT), or among patients with a history of chronic alcohol abuse. Similarly, we avoid using Depakote in patients with chronic active hepatitis. We have often found that lower than previously used doses of lithium or Depakote may be effective once the patient has developed AIDS. In some cases, combinations of clonazepam

(Klonopin) and a low-dose neuroleptic may be the safest, most effective treatment choice for bipolar, manic patients with AIDS.

Substance Use Disorder

Abstinence should be the primary goal of pharmacotherapy of SUD. Although methadone maintenance of heroin-dependent patients does not result in absolute abstinence from opiates, it has been shown to be effective in reducing IV drug use and the associated antisocial behavior of maintaining a "habit." In addition, many methadone clinics in New York City have developed programs to provide primary medical care for patients with HIV as well as directly observed therapy (DOT) programs for HIV patients needing treatment of tuberculosis. We feel these secondary benefits of methadone maintenance outweigh the drawbacks of continued opioid dependence.

Recently, naltrexone (REVIA), an opioid antagonist, was approved for the treatment of alcohol dependence. Because it blocks the euphoric effects of opiates, it may also be useful for the treatment of narcotic addiction, although this has not yet been proven in clinical trials. Liver toxicity is a potential adverse effect of REVIA, which may pose a problem for patients taking other hepatotoxic HIV-related medication.

Research involving the use of antidepressants such as desipramine (Norpramin) for the treatment of cocaine addiction has produced mixed results. In our experience, cocaine (especially crack cocaine) dependence and its associated psychiatric complications are the most resistant to pharmacologic management. Any treatment plan for this or other substance use disorders must include a comprehensive, structured drug treatment program.

Anxiety and insomnia are the most common chief complaints among patients referred for psychiatric consultation at our AIDS clinic. The majority of these patients have a co-morbid SUD. The evaluation of these complaints is complex because anxiety and insomnia may be related to HIV-related medications, medical illness, HIV encephalopathy, or active substance abuse itself. For the treatment of insomnia we have had good results with the sedating antidepressant trazodone (Desyrel) used in doses that are subtherapeutic for the treatment of depression.

Anxiety may be more difficult to treat in this population. Although buspirone (Buspar) has been shown to be effective in treating a small sample of anxious HIV-positive SUD patients, our experience indicates that many patients cannot tolerate the delayed effect of this medication and do not comply with treatment. Frank Fernandez has recommended low-dose neuroleptics for chronic anxiety, but as we have already discussed, there are potential problems with these medications in the HIV population.

Antidepressants are effective in the treatment of Panic Disorder and, in some cases, chronic anxiety, and we often offer these as treatment for SUD patients complaining of anxiety. We, and others, have reported on the substantial prescribing of benzodiazepines for anxious HIV patients. However, because of the potential for abuse of these medications, strict ground rules for compliance and follow-up must be instituted. Following is an example of a patient with SUD for whom a benzodiazepine was indicated, with a good outcome.

CLAIRE

Claire was a forty-two-year-old female with a history of heroin dependence dating back to her teenage years. Upon entering into a methadone maintenance program, she was tested for HIV and found to be seropositive. At the time of psychiatric consultation she had been maintained successfully on methadone for five years with no relapses of IV drug use. Although her CD4 count was below 500, she had no HIV-related symptoms. Her primary physician prescribed diazepam (Valium) for complaints of anxiety, and evaluation revealed that she did in fact meet diagnostic criteria for Generalized Anxiety Disorder. The Valium was continued, and biweekly supportive psychotherapy sessions were initiated. The patient developed a strong therapeutic alliance, and treatment has continued for five years. Although there was one episode of antisocial acting out, involving shoplifting, this was interpreted in treatment. She has remained remarkably compliant, and her anxiety has been controlled.

Although the patient in this case illustrates that safe and adequate treatment of anxiety may be accomplished with long-term benzodiazepine use, we generally try to avoid this. The side effects of benzodiazepines, which include behavioral disinhibition and cognitive impairment, are often more problematic than the anxiolytic benefits. Character pathology may further complicate the picture of patients with SUD, making it difficult for them to comply with the ground rules of treatment and thus leading to abuse of the benzodiazepines. Following is an example of such a patient.

JENNIFER

Jennifer was a thirty-year-old female graduate student who had a previous history of IV drug use and was known to have been HIV-positive for four years at the time of referral. Her primary physician had also prescribed Valium because of complaints of extreme anxiety and insomnia. Psychiatric evaluation revealed features consistent with Borderline Personality Disorder.

Treatment with Valium was continued; however, she was rarely compliant with dosage recommendations and would run out of medication before her appointments. She would blame the "pressures of school" and perceived rejections from friends due to her HIV status as reasons for needing increasing doses of Valium.

When limit setting and psychoeducation failed to bring the Valium use under control, it was suggested that she be admitted to the hospital for detox and subsequent drug rehab. The patient responded by leaving treatment after devaluing the therapist as incompetent.

Unfortunately, the poor outcome exemplified by this patient is probably more typical of our experience treating patients with anxiety and SUD than is the favorable outcome of the patient in the previous case. Although we do prescribe benzodiazepines in selected cases, we cannot recommend this as standard clinical practice.

Side Effects of HIV Medications and Interactions with Psychotropics

When evaluating the chronic mentally ill or substance-abusing patient, the clinician must take into account the HIV-related medications being taken. Almost all of the medications taken by HIV patients can have neuropsychiatric side effects in toxic doses, but a few are worth mentioning because of more frequent problems. Both Zidovudine (AZT) and didanosine (ddI) can cause anxiety, agitation, and insomnia, and AZT has been reported to cause frank mania in a few cases. On the other hand, these antiretrovirals can also produce lethargy and malaise.

Medications used to treat tuberculosis such as INH, ethambutol, and rifampin can cause mild agitation and confusion. Cycloserine, which is sometimes used to treat drug-resistant TB, can commonly produce frank psychosis. Also, rifampin has been shown to induce hepatic metabolism of methadone, and patients on maintenance may need their doses of methadone increased.

Alpha interferon, used in the treatment of Kaposi's Sarcoma, can produce symptoms indistinguishable from clinical depression. Medications such as gancylcovir (DHPG), foscarnet, acyclovir, pentamadine (intravenous), and even Bactrim have all been known to cause delirium in HIV patients. Also, pentamadine and ddI can cause acute pancreatitis and must be used cautiously in patients who are actively abusing alcohol.

Some psychotropic medications, such as Paxil, inhibit hepatic metabolism of other medications; others, such as Depakote, induce hepatic metabolism, and this must be taken into account in the overall treatment of HIV patients. Conversely, ketoconazole, which is used in the treatment of fungal infections, may cause increased serum levels of some antidepressants and benzodiazepines.

Although extremely challenging, working with patients with SUD, CMI, and HIV/AIDS can also be gratifying to the same extent. The multidisciplinary and comprehensive assessment and treatment approaches that we have outlined here offer the best opportunity for improved quality of life for these afflicted populations.

NOTES

P. 270, *Many patients we see actually have a triple diagnosis:* Batki, S. L. (1990). Drug abuse, psychiatric disorders, and AIDS: Dual and triple diagnosis. *Western Journal of Medicine, 152,* 547–552.

P. 271, *In 1994, 27 percent of all AIDS cases:* Centers for Disease Control and Prevention. (1994). *HIV/AIDS Surveillance Report, 6*(2), 10.

P. 271, *One study in a Bronx, . . . treatment program:* Schoenbaum, E., Hartel, D., Selwyn, P., Klein, R. S., Davenny, K., Rogers, M., Feiner, C., & Friedland, G. (1989). Risk factors for human immunodeficiency virus infection in intravenous drug users. *New England Journal of Medicine, 321,* 874–879.

P. 271, *another study in San Francisco:* Chaisson, R., Bacchetti, P., Osmond, D., Brodie, B., Sande, M. A., & Moss, A. R. (1989). Cocaine use and HIV infection in intravenous drug users in San Francisco. *Journal of the American Medical Association, 261,* 561–565.

P. 272, *A study in Toronto found:* Ross, E., Glaser, F., & Germanson, T. (1988). The prevalence of psychiatric disorders in patients with alcohol and other drug problems. *Archives of General Psychiatry, 45,* 1023–1031.

P. 273, *The most recent* DSM-IV *criteria:* American Psychiatric Association. (1994). *Diagnostic and statistical manual of mental disorders* (4th ed.). Washington, DC: Author.

P. 273, *The* DSM-IV *criteria for Substance Abuse:* American Psychiatric Association. (1994). *Diagnostic and statistical manual of mental disorders* (4th ed.). Washington, DC: Author.

P. 274, *One method for doing this . . . CAGE questionnaire:* Ewing, J. (1984). Detecting alcoholism: The CAGE questionnaire. *Journal of the American Medical Association, 252,* 1905–1907.

P. 279, *Cognitive therapies teach patients:* Toneatto, T. (1995). The regulation of cognitive states: A cognitive model of psychoactive substance abuse. *Journal of Cognitive Psychotherapy, 9,* 93–104.

P. 283, *Data from communities throughout the United States:* Bachrach, L. L. (1992). What we know about homelessness among mentally ill persons: An analytical review and commentary. *Hospital and Community Psychiatry, 43,* 453–464.

P. 283, *homelessness rates among the mentally ill:* Bachrach, L. L. (1992). What we know about homelessness among mentally ill persons: An analytical review and commentary. *Hospital and Community Psychiatry, 43,* 453–464.

P. 283, *One report indicates that between 6 and 19 percent:* Torres, R. A. (1990). Human immunodeficiency virus infection among homeless men in a New York City shelter. *Archives of Internal Medicine, 150,* 2030–2036.

P. 283, *Other studies, conducted in psychiatric hospitals:* Kalichman, S. C., Kelly, J. A., Johnson, J. R., & Buto, M. (1994). Factors associated with risk for HIV infection among chronic mentally ill adults. *American Journal of Psychiatry, 151,* 221–227; Empfield, M., Cournos, F., Meyer, I., McKinnon, K., Horuath, E., Sicver, M., Schrage, H., Herman, R. (1993). HIV seroprevalence among homeless patients admitted to a psychiatric inpatient unit. *American Journal of Psychiatry, 150,* 47–52.

P. 284, *One recent study revealed that women in a psychiatric outpatient setting:* Aruffo, J. F., Coverdale, J. H., Chacko, R. C., & Dworkin, R. J. (1990). Knowledge about AIDS among women psychiatric outpatients. *Hospital and Community Psychiatry, 41,* 326–328.

P. 284, *43 percent of mentally ill patients:* Kelly, J. A., Murphy, D. A., Bahr, G. R., Brasfield, R. L., Davis, D. R., Hauth, A. C., Morgan, M. G., Stevenson, L. X., & Filers, M. K. (1992). AIDS/HIV risk behavior among the chronic mentally ill. *American Journal of Psychiatry, 149,* 886–889.

P. 284, *Others may integrate issues about HIV into their delusional systems:* Carmen, E., & Brady, S. M. (1990). AIDS risk and prevention for the chronic mentally ill. *Hospital and Community Psychiatry, 41,* 652–657.

P. 284, *mentally ill persons have been shown to be less likely:* Kalichman, S. C., Kelly, J. A., Johnson, J. R., & Buto, M. (1994). Factors associated with risk for HIV infection among chronic mentally ill adults. *American Journal of Psychiatry, 151*, 221–227.

P. 284, *Schizophrenics, for example, tend to have:* Seeman, M. V., Lang, M., & Rector, N. (1990). Chronic schizophrenia: A risk factor for HIV? *Canadian Journal of Psychiatry, 35*, 765–768; Kelly J. A., Murphy, D. A., Bahr, G. R., Brasfield, R. L., Davis, D. R., Hauth, A. C., Morgan, M. G., Stevenson, L. X., & Filers, M. K. (1992). AIDS/HIV risk behavior among the chronic mentally ill. *American Journal of Psychiatry, 149*, 886–889.

P. 284, *bipolar manic patients tend to display more:* McDermott, B. E., Sautter, F. J., Winstead, D. K., & Quirk, T. (1994). Diagnosis, health beliefs, and risk of HIV infection in psychiatric patients. *Hospital and Community Psychiatry, 45*, 580–585.

P. 284, *patients with a CMI are often victims of childhood sexual abuse:* Carmen, E., & Brady, S. M. (1990). AIDS risk and prevention for the chronic mentally ill. *Hospital and Community Psychiatry, 41*, 652–657.

P. 284, *sexually promiscuous, impulsive, and dangerous behaviors:* Ricker P. P., & Carmen E. (1986). The victim-to-patient process: The disconfirmation and transformation of abuse. *American Journal of Orthopsychiatry, 56*, 360–370.

P. 285, *depressed patients tend to use more IV drugs:* McDermott, B. E., Sautter, F. J., Winstead, D. K., & Quirk, T. (1994). Diagnosis, health beliefs, and risk of HIV infection in psychiatric patients. *Hospital and Community Psychiatry, 45*, 580–585.

P. 285, *Data from an urban study in the Midwest:* Kelly J. A., Murphy, D. A., Bahr, G. R., Brasfield, R. L., Davis, D. R., Hauth, A. C., Morgan, M. G., Stevenson, L. X., & Filers, M. K. (1992). AIDS/HIV risk behavior among the chronic mentally ill. *American Journal of Psychiatry, 149*, 886–889.

P. 285, *an estimated one to two million runaway youths:* Rotheram-Borus, M., Koopman, C., & Ehrhardt A. (1991). Homeless youth and HIV infection in the United States. *American Psychologist, 46*, 1188–1197.

P. 285, *HIV seroprevalence studies of this population:* Rotheram-Borus M., & Koopman C. (1991). Sexual risk behaviors, AIDS knowledge, and beliefs about AIDS among runaways. *American Journal of Public Health, 81*, 208–210.

P. 285, *In one study, 11 percent of youth surveyed:* Allen, D. M., Lehman, S., Green, T. A., Lindegren, M. L., Onerato, I. M., Forestor, W., & the Field Services Branch. (1994). HIV infection among homeless adults and runaway youth, United States 1989–1992. *AIDS, 8*, 1593–1598.

P. 286, *Acute manic states may result in hypersexuality:* Gewirtz, G., Horwath,

E., Cournos, F., & Empfield, M. (1988). Patients at risk for HIV. *Hospital and Community Psychiatry, 39,* 1311–1312.

P. 286, *impaired cognition, which interferes with information processing:* Baer, J. W., Dwyer, P. C., & Lewitter-Koehler, S. (1988). Knowledge about AIDS among psychiatric inpatients. *Hospital and Community Psychiatry, 39,* 986–988.

P. 286, *Negative symptoms such as poor social problem-solving:* Kelly, J. A., Murphy, D. A., Sikkema, K. J., Somcai, A. M., Mulry, G. W., Fernandez, M. I., Miller, J. G., & Stevenson, L. Y. (1995). Predictors of high and low levels of HIV risk behavior among adults with chronic mental illness. *Psychiatric Services, 46,* 813–818.

P. 286, *A recent study showed that of 106 homeless:* Lehman, A. F., Kernan, E., DeForge, B. R., & Dixon, L. (1995). Effects of homelessness on the quality of life of persons with severe mental illness. *Psychiatric Services, 46,* 922–926.

P. 287, *homeless substance abusers often exchange sex for drugs:* Carmen, E., & Brady, S. M. (1990). AIDS risk and prevention for the chronic mentally ill. *Hospital and Community Psychiatry, 41,* 652–657.

P. 287, *Chronic mentally ill and homeless patients often do not comply:* Dickson, L. R., & Neill, J. R. (1987). When schizophrenia complicates medical care. *American Family Physician, 35,* 153–159.

P. 289, *Our clinic distributes condoms:* Goisman, R. M., Kent, A. B., Montgomery, E. C., Cheevers, M. M., & Goldfinger, S. M. (1991). AIDS education for patients with chronic mental illness. *Community Mental Health Journal, 27,* 189–197.

P. 289, *Inpatient units in one major metropolitan center:* Baer, J. W., Dwyer, P. C., & Lewitter-Koehler, S. (1988). Knowledge about AIDS among psychiatric inpatients. *Hospital and Community Psychiatry, 39,* 986–988.

P. 289, *schizophrenic patients are often actively interested:* Seeman, M. V., Lang, M., & Rector, N. (1990). Chronic schizophrenia: A risk factor for HIV? *Canadian Journal of Psychiatry, 35,* 765–768.

P. 289, *sex education among this population:* Pepper, E. (1988). Sexual awareness groups in a psychiatric day treatment program. *Psychosocial Rehabilitation Journal, 11,* 45–52; Wasow, M. (1980). Sexuality and the institutionalized mentally ill. *Sexuality and Disability, 3,* 3–16.

P. 290, *CMI patients often suffer low self-esteem:* Cohen, C. I., & Thompson, K. S. (1992). Homeless mentally ill or mentally ill homeless? *American Journal of Psychiatry, 149,* 816–823.

P. 290, *They may feel out of control:* Bachrach, L. L. (1992). What we know about homelessness among mentally ill persons: An analytical review and commentary. *Hospital and Community Psychiatry, 43,* 453–464.

P. 291, *Street-based programs that distribute condoms:* Empfield, M., Cournos, F., Meyer, I., McKinnon, K., Horuath, E., Sicver, M., Schrage, H., & Herman, R. (1993). HIV seroprevalence among homeless patients admitted to a psychiatric inpatient unit. *American Journal of Psychiatry, 150,* 47–52.

P. 292, *infection of the central nervous system:* Perry, S. (1990). Organic mental disorders caused by HIV: update on early diagnosis and treatment. *American Journal of Psychiatry, 147,* 696–710; Brew, B. J. (1993). HIV-1–related neurological disease. *Journal of Acquired Immune Deficiency Syndromes,* 6(Suppl. 1), S10–S15.

P. 293, *AIDS patients have been shown to be extremely sensitive:* Swenson, J. R., Erman, M., Labelle, J., & Dimsdale, J. E. (1989). Extrapyramidal reactions: Neuropsychiatric mimics in patients with AIDS. *General Hospital Psychiatry, 11,* 248–253.

P. 293, *Some authors strongly advocate:* Fernandez, F., & Levy, J. K. (1993). The use of molindone in the treatment of psychotic and delirious patients infected with the human immunodeficiency virus: Case reports. *General Hospital Psychiatry, 15,* 31–35; Janicak, P. G. (1995). Psychopharmacotherapy in the HIV-infected patient. *Psychiatric Annals, 25,* 609–613.

P. 295, *the new antipsychotic risperidone (Risperdal) may be effective:* Gilmer, W., Ferando, S., Jong, M., & Goldman, J. (1995). Risperidone in the treatment of psychiatric symptoms in patients with AIDS (Poster NR 407). *Proceedings and Abstracts of the 148th Annual Meeting of the American Psychiatric Association,* Miami, FL; Singh, A. N., & Catalan, J. (1994). Risperidone in HIV-related manic psychosis. *Lancet, 344,* 1029–1030.

P. 295, *a higher lifetime prevalence of depressive disorders:* Atkinson, J. H., Grant, I., Kennedy, C. J., Richman, D. D., Spector, S. A., & McCutchan, A. (1988). Prevalence of psychiatric disorders among men infected with human immunodeficiency virus. *Archives of General Psychiatry, 45,* 859–864; Williams, J. B. W., Rabkin, J. G., Remien, R. H., Gorman, J. M., & Ehrhardt, A. A. (1991). Multidisciplinary baseline assessment of homosexual men with and without human immunodeficiency virus infection: Standardized clinical assessment of current and lifetime psychopathology. *Archives of General Psychiatry, 48,* 124–130; Maj, M., Janssen, R., Starace, F., Jaudig, M., Satz, P., Sughowhabirom, B. Luabeya, M. K., Rieder, R., Ndetei, D., Calil, H. M., Bing, E., St. Louis, M., & Sartorius, N. (1994). WHO neuropsychiatric AIDS study, cross-sectional phase I: Study design and psychiatric findings. *Archives of General Psychiatry, 51,* 39–49.

P. 295, *estimates of current depression:* Lyketsos, C. G., Hoover, D. R., Guccione,

M., Senterfitt, W., Dew, M. A., Wesch, J., VanRaden, M. J., Treisman, G. J., & Morgenstern, H. (1993). Depressive symptoms as predictors of medical outcomes in HIV infection. *Journal of the American Medical Association, 270,* 2563–2567; Bialer, P. A., Wallack, J. J., Prenzlauer, S. L., Bogdonoff, L., & Willets, I. (in press). Psychiatric comorbidity among hospitalized AIDS patients vs. non-AIDS patients referred for psychiatric consultation. *Psychosomatics;* Maj, M., Janssen, R., Starace, F., Jaudig, M., Satz, P., Sughowhabirom, B. Luabeya, M. K., Rieder, R., Ndetei, D., Calil, H. M., Bing, E., St. Louis, M., & Sartorius, N. (1994). WHO neuropsychiatric AIDS study, cross-sectional phase I: Study design and psychiatric findings. *Archives of General Psychiatry, 51,* 39–49.

P. 295, *Several antidepressants:* Rabkin, J. G., Rabkin, R., Harrison, W., & Wagner, G. (1994). Effect of imipramine on mood and enumerative measures of immune status in depressed patients with HIV illness. *American Journal of Psychiatry, 151,* 516–523; Levine, S. H., Anderson, D., Bystritsky, A., & Baron, D. (1990). A report of eight HIV-seropositive patients with major depression responding to fluoxetine. *Journal of Acquired Immune Deficiency Syndromes, 3,* 1074–1077; Hintz, S., Kuck, J., & Peterkin, J. J. (1990). Depression in the context of human immunodeficiency virus infection: Implications for treatment. *Journal of Clinical Psychiatry, 51,* 497–501; Markowitz, J., Rabkin J. G., & Perry, S. (1994). Treating depression in HIV-positive patients. *AIDS, 8,* 403–412.

P. 296, *Some have also advocated the use of psychostimulants:* Fernandez, F., Levy, J. K., & Galizzi, H. (1988). Response of HIV-related depression to psychostimulants: Case reports. *Hospital and Community Psychiatry, 39,* 628–631; Fernandez, F., & Levy, J. K. (1994). Psychopharmacology in HIV spectrum disorders. *Psychiatric Clinics of North America, 17,* 135–148; White, J. C., Christensen, J. F., & Singer, C. M. (1992). Methylphenidate as a treatment for depression in acquired immune deficiency syndrome: An n-of-1 trial. *Journal of Clinical Psychiatry, 53,* 153–156.

P. 296, *a finding corroborated by others:* Rabkin, J. G., Rabkin, R., & Wagner, G. (1995). Testosterone replacement therapy in HIV illness. *General Hospital Psychiatry, 17,* 37–42.

P. 296, *manifestation of AIDS dementia:* Boccelari, A., Dilley, J. W., & Shore, M. D. (1988). Neuropsychiatric aspects of AIDS Dementia Complex: A report on a clinical series. *Neurotoxicology, 9,* 381–390; El-Mallakh, R. S. (1991). Mania in AIDS: Clinical significance and theoretical considerations. *International Journal of Psychiatric Medicine, 21,* 383–391; Kieburtz, K., Zettelmaier, A. E., Ketonen, L., Tuite, M., & Caine, E. A. (1991). Manic syndromes in AIDS. *American Journal of Psychiatry, 148,* 1068–1070; Lyketsos, C. G., Hanson, A. L., Fishman, M., Rosenblat, A., McHugh, P. R., &

Taeisman, G. J. (1993). Mania early and late in the course of HIV infection. *American Journal of Psychiatry, 150,* 326–327.

P. 296, *some reports indicate that a previous history of Bipolar Disorder:* Cournos, F., Empfield, M., Horuath, E., & Shrage, H. (1990). HIV infection in state hospitals: Case reports and long-term management strategies. *Hospital and Community Psychiatry, 41,* 163–166

P. 296, *One report on a small series:* Halman, M. H., Worth, J. L., Sanders, K. M., Aenshaw, P. F., & Murray, G. B. (1993). Anticonvulsant use in treatment of manic syndromes in patients with HIV-1 infection. *Journal of Neuropsychiatry and Clinical Neurosciences, 5,* 430–434.

P. 297, *Although methadone maintenance:* Cooper, J. R. (1989). Methadone treatment and acquired immunodeficiency syndrome. *Journal of the American Medical Association, 262,* 1664–1668; Batki, S. L. (1988). Treatment of intravenous drug users with AIDS: The role of methadone maintenance. *Journal of Psychoactive Drugs, 20,* 213–216.

P. 297, *Research involving the use of antidepressants:* Levin, F. R., & Lehman, A. F. (1991). Meta-analysis of desipramine as an adjunct in the treatment of cocaine addiction. *Journal of Clinical Psychopharmacology, 11,* 374–378.

P. 298, *Although buspirone (Buspar) has been shown:* Batki, S. L. (1990). Buspirone in drug users with AIDS or AIDS-Related Complex. *Journal of Clinical Psychopharmacology 10*(suppl.), 111S–115S.

P. 298, *Frank Fernandez has recommended low-dose neuroleptics,* Fernandez F. (1989). Anxiety and the neuropsychiatry of AIDS. *Journal of Clinical Psychiatry, 50*(suppl.), 9–14; Fernandez, F., & Levy, J. K. (1990). Psychiatric diagnosis an pharmacotherapy of patients with HIV infection. In A. Tasman, S. M. Goldfinger, & C. A. Kaufman (Eds.). *Review of Psychiatry* (Vol. 9). Washington, DC: American Psychiatric Press.

P. 298, *substantial prescribing of benzodiazepines:* Bialer, P. A., Wallack, J. J., & Snyder, S. L. (1991). Psychiatric diagnosis in HIV-spectrum disorders. *Psychiatric Medicine, 9,* 361–375; O'Dowd, M. A., Natali, C., & McKegney, F. (1991). Characteristics of patients attending an HIV-related clinic. *Hospital and Community Psychiatry, 42,* 615–619; Freedman, J. B., O'Dowd, M. A., McKegney, F., Kaplan, I. J., Bernstein, G., Biderman, D. J., Gomez, M. F. (in press). Managing benzodiazepine abuse in an AIDS-related clinic with a high percentage of substance abuse. *Psychosomatics;* Hintz, S., Kuck, J., & Peterkin, J. J. (1990). Depression in the context of human immunodeficiency virus infection: Implications for treatment. *Journal of Clinical Psychiatry, 51,* 497–501.

P. 300, *Almost all of the medications:* Katz, M. H. (1994). Effect of HIV treatment on cognition, behavior, and emotion. *Psychiatric Clinics of North America,*

17, 227–230; Wallack, J. J., Bialer, P. A., & Prenzlauer, S. L. (1995). Psychiatric aspects of HIV infection and AIDS: An overview and update. In A. Stoudemire & B. S. Fogel (Eds.). *Medical Psychiatric Practice* (Vol. 3). Washington, DC: American Psychiatric Press.

P. 300, *AZT has been reported to cause frank mania:* Maxwell, S., Scheftner, W. A., Kessler, H. A., & Busch, K. (1988). Manic syndrome associated with Zidovudine treatment [letter]. *Journal of the American Medical Association*, *259*, 3406–3407; O'Dowd, M. A., & McKegney, F. (1988). Manic syndrome associated with Zidovudine. *Journal of the American Medical Association, 260*, 3587.

9

LEGAL AND ETHICAL ISSUES IN THE TREATMENT OF HIV

Jeff Stryker

This chapter on the ethical and legal ramifications of treating people with HIV is the caboose here, but do not be misled. Attention to ethical and legal concerns cannot be an afterthought for mental health professionals who care for people living with or at risk for HIV disease. The dire nature of the illness, the stigma that shrouds it, the infectiousness that renders it a societal as well as individual concern—all of these factors combine to pose daily dilemmas.

ETHICAL AND LEGAL PERSPECTIVES

The same ethical principles that guide all health care practice apply in the care of individuals with HIV disease: autonomy, confidentiality, truth telling, beneficence, nonmaleficence, and justice.

Ethical Principles

The principle of *autonomy*, or respect for persons, states that competent adults, once properly informed, have a right to make decisions about their bodies and health care—even if these decisions have negative consequences for health, functioning, or even continued life.

An outgrowth of autonomy is the concept of *informed consent*, an ethical precept well recognized by the law, which requires that health care providers obtain the express consent of the patient, once the patient has been fully informed of the risks and benefits of treatment.

The principle of *confidentiality* recognizes the sensitive, private nature of the relationship between a patient and health care provider; it is the oxygen that permits this relationship to thrive, fostering the sharing of personal information critical to treatment. A related principle, *truth telling*, requires the health care provider to share with the patient all relevant information about his or her care.

Beneficence requires professionals to act in the best interests of their patients, and *nonmaleficence* is the injunction commonly rendered as "First, do no harm."

As stated here, these principles may seem a little arid, or perhaps formulaic or boilerplate. They come roaring to life, however, when they clash in their application to the dilemmas facing health care providers charged with caring for those living with HIV disease.

Legal Rules

Ethical beacons are not the only lights guiding caregivers. The law has much to say about the dilemmas practitioners face.

During the late 1980s, there were more than a thousand bills each year considered in state legislatures related to AIDS; hundreds achieved passage, resulting in a large body of law on HIV-related issues such as insurance, liability for transmission, and needle availability and condom distribution, to name just a few issues. The courts have also weighed in, making AIDS the most litigated disease in American history.

There are many laws directly impinging on mental health care professionals' practice with people at risk for or infected by HIV.

The variations in the law from state to state are considerable; mental health care professionals who encounter HIV-related legal dilemmas are advised to seek advice and counsel on the law in the state where they practice.

DUTY TO TREAT

The discomfort felt by the American public about AIDS and those at heightened risk for it (especially gay men and drug users) is shared to some extent by health and mental health professionals.

Fear

Several studies have revealed reluctance among many health care providers surveyed to be willing to care for people with HIV disease, in part rooted in fears of contracting the disease from patients (exacerbated by worries that should they become infected through their work, they may then pose a risk to their own families and intimate associates).

Reluctance to care for people with HIV disease has a number of sources. Some health care workers harbor negative attitudes about homosexuality or may be frustrated in treating drug users who find it difficult or impossible to forgo drug use. Health care workers who have contact with blood and bodily fluids risk occupational HIV transmission. However, health care workers tend to overestimate the risk of contracting HIV, while underestimating the threat of less stigmatized but more infectious diseases, such as hepatitis B.

Health care givers may be intimidated by the complexity of AIDS care, believing it is only for specialists with greater training or experience. These tensions are often compounded by anxieties involved in treating relatively young individuals who may be terminally ill.

Prejudice

Prejudice associated with homosexuality and drug use may be expressed in subtle devaluations of stigmatized patients in ways that providers may not even realize. When patients sense that their caregivers are uncomfortable discussing sensitive topics, they may be unwilling to share information about their lifestyle that is relevant to their health care.

Unwillingness to care for people with HIV disease may result in a broad range of harm. Health care professionals' refusal to treat HIV disease can lead to systematic denial of access and to substandard care. People who are refused care may ultimately never find it, or they may be harmed by delays if their condition worsens as a result. Being refused care further stigmatizes patients and adds to the considerable psychological burdens of living with HIV disease. In the medical care setting, such refusals exacerbate the risk of nosocomial infection for the remaining health care professionals who are steadfast in their willingness to treat and, hence, assume a disproportionate burden of caring for people with HIV disease.

Mental health professionals who work in nonmedical settings do not have to contend with issues of occupational risk for HIV infection, as they are unlikely to come in contact with any blood or bodily fluids of HIV-infected patients. Nevertheless, they too are subject to the same feelings and prejudices.

Much of the research on professional attitudes in treating HIV disease relies on questions posed about hypothetical cases, rather than on what providers actually do when confronted with HIV disease. The other part of the story involves those who have dedicated themselves to AIDS care, often at great personal and emotional risk. Many gay men, themselves infected or at risk, have struggled with their own responses to AIDS while trying to help others. These stalwart professionals include many mental health care providers. In fact, it is the particular expertise of mental health care professionals that can help clinicians and patients alike cope with difficulties related to the social aspects of HIV.

BARRIERS TO TESTING

The stigma associated with AIDS that has played a part in care-givers' attitudes has also kept people from seeking health care, including testing for antibodies to HIV.

The HIV antibody test was first licensed in the spring of 1985. The test quickly proved to be a double-edged sword. The test was of great benefit in protecting the blood supply; it also permitted public health officials to track the spread of disease. Yet unwanted disclosure of results in a variety of contexts wrought much social harm. In the early years of the test's availability, many gay activists counseled against taking it, arguing that finding out one's infection status was not worth the risk of discrimination. After all, the advice—to practice safer sex and avoid sharing needles—would be the same whatever the results.

The backdrop of the debate about HIV antibody testing and screening has changed considerably in the second decade of AIDS. Every year there is more to offer those who test HIV-positive. Considerable gains have been made with preventive treatments to ward off the development of some of the opportunistic infections that characterize AIDS, such as *Pneumocystis carinii* pneumonia (PCP) and *Mycobacterium avium complex* (MAC). A new class of drugs known as protease inhibitors is the source of renewed hope for people with HIV disease, offering even more reason for people to find out as early as possible in the course of the disease if they are HIV infected. Still, many at high risk remain unaware of their HIV status.

These clinical advances have fueled calls for more widespread routine and, in some cases, mandatory testing. The issue of how far to cast the HIV screening and testing net is perhaps the most enduring of the AIDS epidemic. Just consider the range of population groups that at one time or another have been the subject of mandatory testing programs or proposals: health care workers, hospital patients, marriage license applicants, military recruits, "source patients" in needlestick accidents, and accused or convicted perpetrators of sexual offenses. The list could go on and on, and so far, those at highest risk haven't even been mentioned—men who have sex with men and IV drug users. Aside from screening blood, organs, and tissues, mandatory screening approaches are by and large quixotic efforts, likely to result in a backlash that further deters people from seeking care and support.

Mandatory programs are difficult to justify; on the other hand, efforts to encourage people to be tested voluntarily have not yet fulfilled their promise. The National AIDS Behavioral Survey of more than thirteen thousand adults examined whether those at highest risk were using public programs for counseling and testing. As of the early 1990s, an "alarmingly high" proportion (more than 60 percent of those at highest risk) had not yet been tested for HIV antibody. Furthermore, as many as a third of those who are tested through the alternative test system—a federally funded network of anonymous testing sites—fail to return for their test results. These figures have contributed to support for making other testing options available, such as home test kits to be sold over the counter and through the mail.

Mental health professionals have a key role to play in helping people overcome fear, denial, or other psychological or emotional factors that may keep those at high risk from seeking testing. In order to do so, mental health professionals need to be aware of a wide range of information related to HIV testing: the clinical meaning of a positive (or negative) result, including the nature of the "window" period between infection and the development of measurable antibodies; test sensitivity and specificity, and any other limitations on interpretation of results; and how and where test results are recorded.

MANAGING TEST RESULTS AND DISEASE PROGRESSION

Mental health care professionals may have ongoing opportunities to help clients deal with the many ramifications of learning they are HIV-positive. Establishing early links with medical caregivers is essential for HIV-positive clients. So too is the task of attending to the potential social and emotional fallout from an HIV diagnosis.

Psychological Health

Part of the role of the mental health counselor is to assess the psychological health of the HIV-positive client. There is no consistent pattern of psychiatric disorders experienced by those with HIV disease, nor any "typical" diagnosis. In fact, patients with AIDS suffering from multiple physical problems, personal losses, and social stresses exhibit a surprisingly low rate of psychological problems. Depression, although not the norm in this population, can be treated in patients with HIV. Because many of the symptoms of depression and HIV disease are the same, assessment by an experienced diagnostician is crucial.

In many ways the psychological concerns of HIV-positive individuals, including depression, anxiety, and fear, are inextricable from ethical and legal questions that flow from a diagnosis of HIV disease. HIV-positive clients live in a wider society; much of their ability to cope with their illness and maintain optimal mental health will depend on their relationships with immediate family and loved ones, as well as with a wide range of other individuals who are significant in their lives, such as friends, coworkers, and neighbors.

Social Ramifications

HIV disease often threatens these family, work, and social relationships. Individuals may choose different courses of action regarding which family and friends to disclose their status to, in what order, and by what means. Such disclosures can be explosive. Although there are no studies to document its extent with any certainty, a number of researchers have suggested that HIV-positive women are at increased risk of domestic violence, underscoring the need for sensitivity and understanding in discussing with patients how and when to disclose their status.

The social ramifications of HIV disease are heightened when AIDS is diagnosed and, later, when individuals with AIDS approach death. HIV-positive individuals typically live for years without displaying any outward symptoms of the disease. Once symptoms develop, bouts of illness may be interspersed with long periods of relative good health.

The rocky course of the disease may pose difficult challenges in the employment context. One's job and income are important, not only to pay the bills and survive, but also to fulfill various psychological needs. The stresses of trying to hold on to a job or deciding when to leave it once the illness becomes too debilitating are likely to be part of discussions between mental health care workers and HIV-positive clients.

A significant step toward the protection of the rights of people living with HIV disease is the federal Americans with Disabilities Act (ADA). This law, phased into effect between 1992 and 1994, extends prohibitions against discrimination based on HIV infection or AIDS—formerly available only to government employees and contractors—to private sector employees. Mental health care workers should be aware of the existence of such laws forbidding employment discrimination, as well as where to refer clients who encounter such problems. Many local bar associations provide low-cost or pro bono legal services and provide a good starting point for inquiry.

CONFIDENTIALITY

Because of the stigma associated with AIDS, significant efforts have been made to provide for the confidentiality of information about risk-group identification, HIV testing, and the results of such tests in medical records. Most states have specific laws to detail the circumstances in which HIV test results may be recorded and with whom they may be shared. Early in the epidemic, a few jurisdictions even made it illegal to enter a patient's HIV status into a medical record without the express written consent of the patient.

There is a range of third parties who may have an interest in an individual's HIV status, some legitimate, some not. In all states, health care providers must report cases of AIDS (with named identifiers) to local public health authorities, who pass the information along to the Centers for Disease Control and Prevention as part of its surveillance efforts. In approximately half the states, the names of HIV-positive individuals known to health care providers are reportable to health authorities. (Most of these states also provide for anonymous testing, which precludes such reporting, however.)

Mental health care workers must be careful in how they maintain records of treatment of HIV-positive individuals. As with other sensitive information, regarding topics such as other sexually transmitted diseases, drug abuse, or homosexuality, part of securing informed consent for treatment will necessarily involve a discussion with the patient concerning how such information is to be recorded and stored and whether it is ever subject to release.

Computerized medical records, when not protected properly, can also abet unauthorized disclosures. Nor is unauthorized access to medical records the only source of untoward disclosures. Idle gossip and careless chatter by caregivers, office staff, and others with varying levels of patient contact frequently result in confidentiality breaches. Mental health care workers have a responsibility to ensure that office staff are sensitive to HIV confidentiality concerns.

Patients should be made aware of specific circumstances in which HIV-related information may be required or requested by third parties, such as insurers, employers, or police officials. Insurers may have legitimate needs for diagnostic information. In the era of managed care, however, the distinction between insurer and employer is not always a clear one, raising concerns about the uses of HIV-related information.

Mental health care providers also face particular dilemmas when HIV becomes a factor in group therapy or residential treatment settings. This is of particular concern in drug treatment facilities, where group encounters are often part of the therapeutic regimen.

DUTY TO WARN

One of the most common ethical dilemmas facing psychologists and other health care professionals who treat people with HIV disease is how to behave when the patient or client's behavior poses a threat to others. There are many variations on this theme. Consider these not-so-hypothetical hypotheticals: A married man discloses in the course of mental health counseling that he has had (unsafe) sexual relationships with men during the course of the marriage. He refuses to be tested for HIV or to tell his wife of his extramarital sexual activity. He also refuses to wear a condom when having sex with his wife. The counselor believes the patient may be putting his wife at great danger, yet worries that if the wife is informed it may spell an end to the therapeutic relationship.

Other concerns may involve less specific harms. For example, a letter to a professional journal inquired about the ethics of treatment of an HIV-positive individual for sexual dysfunction. The patient, a fifty-five-year-old man, had been promised a vacuum-type device known as an "Erectaid" to treat erectile dysfunction resulting from diabetes. When the clinic staff learned of his HIV-positive status, they balked at giving him the device, aware that he had frequented bathhouses in the past and concerned that "he made no commitment to the sexual dysfunction clinic staff to use his newly functioning penis inside a condom."

Medical ethics and the law may leave health care providers with considerable doubt about whether their duty is to protect a patient's privacy or to protect a third party from becoming infected with a dread disease. One legal commentator described health care professionals as being "between a rock and a hard place"—an especially apt description in a few particular jurisdictions where judge-made common law directs disclosing of HIV status to third parties at risk, and a statute says to keep a secret.

Some ethicists take a hard line on patient confidentiality. Philosopher Michael Kottow maintains that any limitations or exceptions put on confidentiality would destroy it, calling confidentiality an "intransigent and absolute obligation." Under this view, any occasional benefits to third parties or the broader society would not be worth jeopardizing the integrity of confidential relationships.

Although such an absolutist view has the appeal of recognizing a time-honored professional value and removing any ambiguity, it fails to account adequately for the interests of specific individuals who may be put at risk for becoming infected with a potentially lethal virus because of a patient's irresponsible behavior. Moreover, certain specific exceptions to confidentiality—such as the reporting of gunshot wounds, elder abuse or child abuse—are already mandated. Such mandated reporting does not seem to have destroyed our basic values of respect for privacy and the confidentiality of sensitive health information.

At the other extreme, some have argued that health care providers should be legally *required* to warn third parties of risk, urging that notifying spouses and other sexual partners of a patient's antibody status should be the rule and not the exception. Although this polar view also has the virtue of simplicity, the drawbacks are numerous. The knowledge that confidences are routinely violated is likely to deter many from seeking professional care or from sharing personal information.

The weight of law and ethics would seem to support a position somewhere between the polar extremes described above. About half of the states have specifically addressed this issue in HIV privacy or public health statutes. In almost all such instances, physicians are given the discretion to disclose, without fear of incurring a legal penalty for choosing either course. Some state statutes are narrowly drawn, permitting notification only of specific individuals with whom the patient is likely to have unprotected sex or share needles in the future, and then only after the patient has been counseled and warned that the notification is to take place. These laws often require that the patient's identity not be revealed.

For mental health care providers faced with deciding where the tradeoff lies between obligations to respect the confidentiality of the clinician-patient relationship versus the duty to the wider society, there are a number of key factors to consider.

To warrant breaching confidentiality, there should be an identifiable individual at risk, for whom disclosure can make a difference in how he or she behaves. There should be good reason to believe that such a person is in danger and that the risk is of serious bodily harm. The obligation to disclose is also more compelling if the individual being put at risk is unwitting and has no particular reason to otherwise be on guard or take measures to protect himself or herself. (The converse is also true—there is less reason to disclose if the third party has reason to know he or she is potentially at risk.)

The two cases cited above represent the different ends of the spectrum. The first case involves an unwitting, identifiable individual at risk, offering a more compelling case for disclosure than the second, in which the future threat is much more abstract.

Counselors should start by encouraging their patients or clients themselves to disclose their HIV status to the third parties they may be putting at risk. The client should be offered not just encouragement but practical support in doing so, perhaps in a session with the counselor. Mental health care providers in some jurisdictions may be able to rely on public health officials to disclose to third parties that they have been put at risk, without revealing the identity of the patient.

If a mental health care worker decides disclosure is the proper course and that he or she is the appropriate person to make the disclosure, it should be done in such a way as not to worsen the situation. A private channel of communication should be relied on to avoid inadvertent disclosure to other parties. The mental health care worker should not send letters nor leave phone messages unless there is a way to know that they cannot be intercepted.

END-OF-LIFE DECISIONS

AIDS takes its toll on families as well as individuals. In particular, mental health care professionals should be aware of the ethical and legal issues parents encounter when they face a terminal illness. In some ways the issues are those faced by *all* parents. Who knows when an accident or illness may claim a parent? Parents should be prepared for any eventuality with documented plans for their children's future.

Parental Concerns

The fear that they may not live long enough to see their children into adulthood, that someone will have to stand in and fulfill the parenting role, is a profound implication of AIDS for HIV-positive parents. Parents with HIV may delay making such arrangements because doing so reminds them of their own mortality. Parents may want to disclose their status to their children, but fear that it would unduly upset them or risk further disruptive disclosures.

Mental health professionals can help clients with such issues, which are difficult to discuss but critical to resolve. Broaching these topics directly and forthrightly is likely to be appreciated by parents, especially when the discussion is respectful and informed. Mental health professionals should be aware of the legal issues involved in custody and guardianship, as well as the resources and agencies available to help.

Parents may also balk at making guardianship arrangements because they fear that involvement with lawyers and courts will force them to share information about their HIV status more widely. Parents may be wary of their treatment at the hands of the judicial system.

Many parents opt for a middle course of disclosing a terminal illness, but not AIDS itself. Prospective guardians deserve to be apprised of the possibility that a medical condition may call for their assuming guardianship duties soon rather than later, although they may not need to know the exact nature of the diagnosis.

Parents can designate a legal guardian for their children through a will, an option that avoids immediate contact with the court system and does not transfer guardianship rights until after death. Of course, such a document will not necessarily defeat another biological parent's right to custody, and if there is a conflict, the courts will conduct an inquiry as to the best interests of the child.

In most states, parents also have the option of appointing a guardian for their children in order to plan for their children's future care and to make sure that their wishes will be honored. However, such a plan involves the immediate transfer of parental rights, including day-to-day decision making regarding child rearing. In some instances parents have been able to avoid this by informal agreements that guardianship would not actually be transferred until the parent is physically unable to care for the child.

Such informal agreements to delay transfer of parental rights and responsibilities are not binding, however. This scenario prompted New York, California, and a number of other states to adopt so-called standby guardianship laws. These statutes allow terminally ill parents and legal guardians to designate provisional guardians for their children without initiating a court proceeding. The parent simply designates a standby guardian whose authority commences upon some specified triggering event— when the parent becomes physically or mentally disabled, consents in writing, or dies. Once the triggering event occurs, the designated standby guardian has a specified amount of time to file a regular guardianship proceeding.

In all such decision making, parents should involve children who are old enough in discussions about their future. In most states, children fourteen years or older have the right to consent or object in writing to the appointment of a legal guardian. It is in the best interest of everyone involved to discover how a child feels about any particular future care arrangement; mental health professionals can be critical in helping children express their desires.

Decisions About Life-Sustaining Treatment

Only a competent adult patient can accept or reject treatment. *Competence* is a legal concept implying the ability to understand one's situation, the benefits of treatment, and the risks of refusal. HIV-related neurologic manifestations may affect competence. However, psychiatric disorders and organic brain syndromes do not necessarily preclude competence. Disturbances of affect may complicate assessment of patient preference, but they do not necessarily vitiate competence. In other words, schizophrenic, demented, or depressed patients may be competent to refuse treatment, even life-sustaining treatment.

The law presumes competence unless the courts have determined otherwise. Non-emergency therapies cannot be administered to patients whose competence is in question. State laws vary in the breadth of authorization for emergency treatment when the patient refuses and competence is uncertain.

The courts have recognized the expressed preferences of incompetent patients if the preferences were expressed before the patient became incompetent, particularly preferences about limiting aggressive, technologically oriented care.

Surrogate Decision Making

HIV disease may involve as long as a decade or more between infection and the development of symptoms. AIDS itself typically involves waxing and waning of symptoms over a lengthy time period. This type of disease progression affords much opportunity for individuals to reflect on the desired course of treatment should they become incompetent and hence unable to express their contemporaneous desires about treatment options such as ventilators, resuscitation orders, chemotherapy, and narcotic drugs.

Studies of the preferences of gay men with AIDS for life-sustaining therapies have shown that people with AIDS are eager to discuss end-of-life care with their providers, and indeed, when such discussions take place, they are often at the behest of the patient.

Patients can execute advance directives to ensure that their wishes regarding life-sustaining treatment are honored. They may, through living will–style documents, specify the range of treatments they are willing to undergo under what circumstances. Another alternative is to designate a surrogate decision maker with sufficient knowledge of the individual's values and desires to be able to speak on his or her behalf.

Executing the appropriate legal documents and otherwise making wishes known regarding terminal care is of particular concern for people with AIDS. There is little recognition in law and society for even long-standing gay relationships, and courts may not recognize same-sex partners as proxy decision makers without specific supporting documentation. Mental health professionals can help people with AIDS in preparing for their death by encouraging them to make their wishes known both to loved ones and health care providers.

Assisted Death

HIV disease has played a significant part in a growing societal debate over the ethics of end-of-life care, including the legality of physician-assisted suicide for the terminally ill. Over the years, Michigan physician Jack Kevorkian has propelled this debate by providing assistance in dying to a number of terminally ill patients.

Opponents of physician-assisted suicide have objected to the use of active measures to end life, actions that might pervert or mock the physician's role as a healer. Objections also arise from very pragmatic concerns regarding the potentially deleterious social consequences should the practice of medically assisted death be societally recognized and institutionalized.

Suicide rates greater than among age-matched controls in the general population have been found among people with chronic and terminal illnesses, including AIDS. As with all patients, mental health professionals must assess suicidality in HIV-positive clients and be able to respond to it. In so doing, it is critical to distinguish acute suicidality from an expression of intent to take one's life should the pain become unbearable, the indignities too great, or the disease reach a certain stage or have particular manifestations, such as blindness or disfigurement. Many patients appreciate the opportunity to discuss the possibility of suicide under such circumstances, even if caregivers are sometimes reluctant.

Often patients are seeking a degree of control, and merely being able to have a frank discussion of suicide may reduce stress and allay fears. When patients actually reach the milestones they once thought would be triggers for suicide, they may still find reason to live on, discovering new ways to cope with their illness and striking a new bargain about the manner of their death.

HIV presents the clinician with many potential ethical and legal dilemmas. The stigma and controversy surrounding HIV disease has made these concerns greater still. Practitioners should be aware of those instances in which ethical or legal questions are raised, even if they are not always able to determine their own clear solutions. In such cases, consultation is often necessary, and as with many ethical considerations, consensus may be the best assurance we have that we are operating in support of treatment and public health. In the course of resolving each of these decisions is the opportunity to further the best interests of the client and the public.

NOTES

P. 309, *ethical principles that guide all health care practice:* Beauchamp, T. L., & Childress, J. F. (1994). *Principles of biomedical ethics* (4th ed.). New York: Oxford University Press.

P. 310, *the most litigated disease in American history:* Gostin, L. O. (1990). The AIDS litigation project: A national review of courts and human rights decisions. Part I: The social impact of AIDS. *Journal of the American Medical Association, 264,* 1261–1266.

P. 311, *discomfort felt . . . about AIDS:* Herek, G., & Glunt, E. (1988). An epidemic of stigma: Public reactions to AIDS. *American Psychologist, 43,* 886–891; Herek, G. & Cogan, J. (1995). *AIDS and stigma: A review of the scientific literature.* San Francisco: Public Media Center.

P. 311, *Several studies have revealed reluctance among many health care providers:* Crawford, I., Humfleet, G., Ribordy, S. C., Ho, F. C., & Vickers, V. L. (1991). Stigmatization of AIDS patients by mental health professionals. *Professional Psychology: Research and Practice, 5*, 357–361; Fliszar, G. M., & Clopton, J. R. (1995). Attitudes of psychologists in training toward persons with AIDS. *Professional Psychology: Research and Practice, 26*, 274–277.

P. 312, *they too are subject to the same feelings and prejudices:* Dhooper, S. S., Royse, D. D., & Tran, T. V. (1987–1988, Fall/Winter). Social work practitioners' attitudes toward AIDS victims. *Journal of Applied Social Sciences, 12*(1), 109–123; Kegeles, S. M., Coates, T., Christopher, T. A., & Lazarus, J. L. (1989). Perceptions of AIDS: The continuing saga of AIDS-related stigma. *AIDS 3*(suppl.), S253–S258; Crawford, I., Humfleet, G., Ribordy, S. C., Ho, F. C., & Vickers, V. L. (1991). Stigmatization of AIDS patients by mental health professionals. *Professional Psychology: Research and Practice, 5*, 357–361; Fliszar, G. M., & Clopton, J. R. (1995). Attitudes of psychologists in training toward persons with AIDS. *Professional Psychology: Research and Practice, 26*, 274–277.

P. 313, *many at high risk remain unaware of their HIV status:* Higgins, D. L., Galavotti, C., O'Reilly, K. R., Schnell, D. J., Moore, M., Rugg, D. L., & Johnson, R. (1991). Evidence for the effects of HIV antibody counseling and testing on risk behaviors. *Journal of the American Medical Association, 266*, 2419–2429; Berrios, D. C., Hearst, N., Coates, T., Stall, R., Hudes, E. S., Turner, H., Eversley, R., & Catania, J. (1993). HIV antibody testing among those at risk for infection: The National AIDS Behavioral Surveys. *Journal of the American Medical Association, 270*, 1576–1580.

P. 314, *The National AIDS Behavioral Survey of more than thirteen thousand adults:* Berrios, D. C., Hearst, N., Coates, T., Stall, R., Hudes, E. S., Turner, *New England Journal of Medicine, 314*, 457–460.H., Eversley, R., & Catania, J. (1993). HIV antibody testing among those at risk for infection: The National AIDS Behavioral Surveys. *Journal of the American Medical Association, 270*, 1576–1580.

P. 314, *as many as a third of those who are tested:* Valdiserri, R. O., Moore, M., Gerber, A. R., Campbell, C. H., Jr., Dillon, B. A., & West, G. R. (1993). A study of clients returning for counseling after HIV testing: Implications for improving rates of return. *Public Health Reports, 108*, 12–18.

P. 314, *support for making other testing options available:* Bayer, R., Stryker, J., & Smith, M. D. (1995). Testing for HIV infection at home. *New England Journal of Medicine, 332*, 1296–1299.

P. 315, *researchers have suggested that HIV-positive women:* Rothenberg, K. H., & Paskey, S. J. (1995). The risk of domestic violence and women with HIV infection: Implications for partner notification, public policy, and the law. *American Journal of Public Health, 85,* 1569–1576.

P. 317, *Mental health care workers must be careful in how they maintain records:* Siegler, M. (1982). Confidentiality in medicine: A decrepit concept. *New England Journal of Medicine, 307,* 1518–1521; Cohen, J. D. (1990). HIV/AIDS confidentiality: Are computerized medical records making confidentiality impossible? *Software Law Journal, 4,* 93–107; Pfaff, D. (1991, March 18). AIDS leaks viewed as symptoms of systemic sickness. *Daily Journal* (San Francisco), pp. 8–9; Doughty, R. (1994). The confidentiality of HIV-related information: Responding to the resurgence of aggressive public health interventions in the AIDS epidemic. *California Law Review, 82,* 111–184.

P. 318, *how to behave when the patient or client's behavior poses a threat to others:* Stanard, R., & Hazler, R. (1995). Legal and ethical implications of HIV and duty to warn for counselors: When does Tarasoff apply? *Journal of Counseling and Development, 73,* 397–400; Friedman, A. L., & Hughes, R. B. (1994). AIDS: Legal tools helpful for mental health counseling interventions. *Journal of Mental Health Counseling, 3,* 291–303.

P. 318, *letter to a professional journal:* Lightfoote-Young, B. (1989). Ethical issues in the treatment of sexual dysfunction in HIV-seropositive patients [letter]. *Western Journal of Medicine, 150,* 93–94.

P. 318, *Philosopher Michael Kottow maintains:* Kottow, M. (1986). Medical confidentiality: An intransigent and absolute obligation. *Journal of Medical Ethics, 12,* 117–122.

P. 321, *a profound implication of AIDS for HIV-positive parents:* Pinoty, M. (1995). Future care and custody planning: The legal issues. In W. Odets & M. Shernoff (Eds.), *The second decade of AIDS: A mental health practice handbook.* New York: Hatherleigh Press.

P. 322, *Only a competent adult patient can accept or reject treatment:* Buchanan, A. E., & Brock, D. W. (1989). *Deciding for others.* New York: Cambridge University Press; Appelbaum, P. S., & Grisso, T. (1988). Assessing patient's capacities to consent to treatment. *New England Journal of Medicine, 319,* 1635–1638.

P. 323, *HIV-related neurologic manifestations may affect competence:* Zeifert, P., Leary, M., & Boccellari, A. A. (1995). *AIDS and the impact of cognitive impairment: A treatment guide for mental health providers.* San Francisco: University of California, San Francisco, AIDS Health Project.

P. 323, *Studies of the preferences of gay men with AIDS:* Steinbrook, R., Lo, J., & Moulton, J. (1986). Preferences of homosexual men with AIDS for life-sustaining treatment. *New England Journal of Medicine, 314,* 457–460.

P. 323, *Patients can execute advance directives:* Teno, J., Fleishman, J., Brock, D. W., & Mor, V. (1990). The use of formal prior directives among patients with HIV-related diseases. *Journal of General Internal Medicine, 5,* 490–494.

P. 324, *HIV disease has played a significant part in a growing societal debate:* Werth, J. L. (1995). Rational suicide reconsidered: AIDS as an impetus for change. *Death Studies, 19,* 65–80; Gold, J. A., Jablonski, D. F., Christensen, P. J., Shapiro, R. S., & Schiedermayer, D. L. (1990). Is there a right to futile treatment? The case of a dying patient with AIDS. *Journal of Clinical Ethics, 1,* 1923.

P. 324, *Suicide rates greater than among age-matched controls:* Cote, T. R., Biggar, R. J., Dannenberg, A. L. (1992). Risk of suicide among persons with AIDS. *Journal of the American Medical Association, 268*(15), 2068; Marzuk, P. M., Tierney, H., Tardiff, K., Gross, E. M., Morgan, E. B., Hsu, M. A., & Mann, J. (1988). Increased risk of suicide in persons with AIDS. *Journal of the American Medical Association, 259,* 1333–1337; Rabkin, J. G., Remien, R. H., Katoff, L., & Williams, J. B. W. (1993). Suicidality in AIDS long-term survivors: What is the evidence? *AIDS Care, 5,* 401–411.

Selected List of Medications Used in HIV and Their Mental Health Consequences

The following list contains only the most commonly used medications in HIV infection and their most common neuropsychological effects. The medications are organized into three groups: antiretrovirals, drugs for opportunistic diseases, and drugs used to treat wasting. They are listed alphabetically by their generic name or description; trade names are shown in parentheses.

None of the information provided here is intended to recommend specific drugs for any particular HIV-related condition. For more complete information about approved and experimental treatments for HIV infection, please consult your physician and refer to *AIDS Treatment News*, published by John S. James, P.O. Box 411256, San Francisco, CA 94141; *BETA*, published by the San Francisco AIDS Foundation and available through Infocom Group, 1250 45th Street, Suite 200, Emeryville, CA 94608–2924; and *Treatment Issues*, published by Gay Men's Health Crisis (GMHC), 129 W. 20th Street, New York, NY 10011. In addition, Project Inform has recently published *The HIV Drug Book*, a compendium of information about all drugs used in the treatment of HIV and its related illnesses. It is highly recommended and can be ordered through Simon & Schuster, 200 Old Tappan Road, Old Tappan, NJ 07675.

ANTIRETROVIRALS

Acyclovir (Zovirax).   Antiviral medication used most commonly to treat herpes simplex and other viruses. Sometimes used in conjunction with AZT to boost antiretroviral activity.

Neuropsychological consequences: reported to cause depression, agitation, auditory and visual hallucinations, depersonalization, confusion, hyperaesthesia, hyperacusis, insomnia, headache.

AZT (Retrovir, Zidovudine).   The first antiretroviral drug approved for treatment of AIDS and HIV infection; inhibits reverse transcriptase (RT), an enzyme required in the replication cycle of retroviruses, by substituting for the naturally occurring nucleoside building blocks of DNA, thereby blocking further activity of RT. Effectiveness of all the nucleoside RT inhibitors is limited by the virus's ability to mutate into resistant forms, as well as by significant side effects such as anemia and myopathy.

Neuropsychological consequences: reported agitation, mania, headache, insomnia, muscle pain and weakness, peripheral neuropathy. Has been used to treat HIV-related encephalopathy, AIDS-Related Dementia. Crosses blood-brain barrier.

d4T (Zerit, Stavudine).   Another nucleoside RT inhibitor of HIV replication; usually given in combination with AZT or to persons who have developed resistance to AZT treatment.

Neuropsychological consequences: neuropathy, headache, nausea.

ddC (Hivid).   Another RT inhibitor of HIV replication used to treat HIV, usually in combination with AZT.

Neuropsychological consequences: the most significant side effect of ddC is peripheral neuropathy, which is nerve damage that typically includes numbness, tingling, or sharp burning pain in the feet, legs, or hands. In addition, ddC can cause pancreatitis, a painful and serious inflammation of the pancreas, which can be accompanied by nausea, vomiting, and depression.

ddI (Videx). Another nucleoside RT inhibitor. Usually given in combination with AZT or another RT inhibitor, as resistance is less likely to occur when the combination is given.

Neuropsychological consequences: neuropathy, headache, pancreatitis.

3TC (Lamivudine). Another nucleoside RT inhibitor, usually used in combination with AZT and increasingly with a protease inhibitor as well. Well tolerated, with fewer side effects than the earlier RT inhibitor drugs.

Neuropsychological consequences: neuropathy, headache.

Non-nucleoside reverse transcriptase inhibitors (Delavirdine, Nevirapine, Atevirdine, Loviride). A new class of RT inhibitors that work at the same site as AZT and other nucleoside RT inhibitors but have a different structure and, one hopes, different patterns of resistance and side effects. These drugs are being tested in combination with AZT or other nucleoside RT inhibitors due to the rapid development of resistance when given alone. It is too early to report on any specific neuropsychological toxicities of these drugs.

Protease inhibitors (Saquinavir or Invirase, Crixivan or Indinavir, Ritonavir). A very new class of antiretroviral drugs that work at a completely different molecular site in the HIV life cycle than the RT inhibitors, and thus have different patterns of resistance and toxicity. The protease inhibitors all work by binding to the active site of the HIV viral protease, thus blocking the processing of viral-coded proteins within the cell and preventing the production of viable virus. The most effective way to give these drugs is in combination with one or more RT inhibitors (such as AZT, 3TC, or both) in order to reduce the development of resistance and produce the most rapid and sustained reductions in viral load. Although these drugs look very promising in early clinical trials, there is as yet little if any clinical data to indicate that they are effective in terms of slowing the progression to AIDS or the development of opportunistic infections in persons with AIDS. There is also very limited information at this time on their side-effect profiles, but all seem to interact with other drugs in this list to cause potential increased toxicities.

DRUGS FOR OPPORTUNISTIC DISEASES

Ciprofloxacin (Cipro). A broad-spectrum antibiotic used for various infections, including those of the lung, urinary, and digestive tracts, and *Mycobacterium avium* complex (MAC) infections. Commonly used to prevent or treat "traveler's diarrhea."

Neuropsychological consequences: nausea, diarrhea, headache, restlessness. Less commonly can cause convulsions, psychosis, tremor, light-headedness, confusion, hallucinations.

Clarithromycin (Biaxin). A derivative of erythromycin used to treat mild-to-moderate bacterial infections of the respiratory tract, skin and soft tissue, or as part of combination therapy to treat or prevent MAC infection.

Neuropsychological consequences: nausea, vomiting, and, more rarely, hearing loss.

Diaminodiphenysulfone (Dapsone). An alternative preventive treatment for PCP and occasionally for mycobacterial and other protozoal infections in persons with HIV/AIDS.

Neuropsychological consequences: anemia, peripheral neuropathy, muscle weakness, nausea, vomiting, inflammation of the pancreas, vertigo, blurred vision.

Erythropoietin (Epogen, Procrit). A protein that stimulates the production of red blood cells and is used to treat the anemia caused by HIV or by the drugs used to treat HIV infection that can cause anemia (AZT, dapsone, and so on).

Neuropsychological consequences: fever, fatigue, headache, nausea, muscle weakness, dizziness.

Fluconazole (Diflucan). A potent antifungal drug that is used to treat cryptococcal meningitis, histoplasmosis, candidal infections of the esophagus, mouth, and throat (thrush), and vaginal candidiasis.

Neuropsychological consequences: nausea, headache, abdominal pain, diarrhea.

Ganciclovir (Cytovene). The first drug approved for the treatment of CMV retinitis, a particularly serious infection that can rapidly cause blindness in immunosuppressed persons. This drug is usually given intravenously, but it was recently approved for both oral administration and eye implants that can deliver the drug directly to the retina.

Neuropsychological consequences: headache, confusion, anemia, malaise.

Interferons (Interferon alfa-2, Intron A, Roferon-A). A class of naturally occurring immune-modulating substances that have been used to treat Kaposi's Sarcoma and other conditions in AIDS patients.

Neuropsychological consequences: depression, confusion, delirium, memory and psychomotor impairment, fatigue, acute encephalitis, muscle and joint pain, headache, dizziness and balance problems, mania, psychosis.

Isoniazid (INH) (Nydrazid, Rifamate, Rifater). A commonly used anti-TB drug. Usually used in combination with other anti-TB drugs, such as rifampin, pyrazinamide, and ethambutol.

Neuropsychological consequences: depression, agitation, visual and auditory hallucinations, paranoia, peripheral neuropathy, and memory impairment. Vitamin B$_6$ deficiency can develop in persons on high doses of INH, which is preventable by taking oral vitamin supplements.

Itraconazole (Sporanox). A broad-spectrum antifungal drug used for the treatment of histoplasmosis, blastomycosis, cryptococcal meningitis, and fluconazole-resistant candidiasis.

Neuropsychological consequences: nausea, vomiting, headache, diarrhea, high blood pressure, fatigue, malaise, dizziness, sleepiness, impotence.

Nystatin (Mycostatin, Pedi-Dri). An alternative to fluconazole for the treatment of thrush and other fungal infections.
Neuropsychological consequences: nausea, diarrhea, stomach upset, vomiting. Allergic reactions common.

Pentamidine (NubuPent, Pentam, Pentacarinat). An antiprotozoal drug used for the treatment and prevention of PCP, administered either by injection or as an aerosol treatment.
Neuropsychological consequences: fatigue, shortness of breath, dizziness, nausea, chest pain, night sweats, chills, vomiting. Rarely associated with hallucinations, pancreatitis, irregular heart rhythms.

Prednisone (Deltasone, Meticorten, Orasone). A potent corticosteroid used to treat a large variety of inflammatory conditions; most commonly used to counteract allergic drug reactions and as part of combination treatment of AIDS-related lymphoma and PCP.
Neuropsychological consequences: over long periods, may cause mood swings, bone or muscle weakness, fluid retention, diabetes, facial rounding, abnormal hair growth, and high blood pressure. Use for long periods can also be associated with immune suppression, which can exacerbate the effects of HIV on the immune system.

Pyrazinamide. Another anti-TB drug, usually administered as part of a combination treatment with INH and rifampin.
Neuropsychological consequences: nausea, vomiting, joint and muscle pain, loss of appetite, fever, sensitivity to light, difficulty urinating, rashes, itching, reduced blood cell and platelet counts.

Pyrimethamine (Fansidar). Another antiprotozoal drug used as part of combination therapy for toxoplasmosis and to prevent malaria.

Neuropsychological consequences: allergic reaction, loss of appetite, vomiting, anemia, abnormal heart rhythms, and more rarely insomnia, diarrhea, headache, light-headedness, dry mouth, fever, malaise, depression, seizures, breathing disorders.

Rifampin (Rifadin, Rimactane). Used in combination with other antibiotics primarily for the treatment of pulmonary TB.

Neuropsychological consequences: headache, fatigue, loss of appetite, drowsiness, blurred vision, numbness, and visual disturbances.

Trimethoprim and sulfamethoxazole (TMP and SMX) (Bactrim, Septra). A combination of two antibiotics (TMP and SMX), used as a preventive treatment against *Pneumocystis carinii* pneumonia (PCP) and other bacterial infections.

Neuropsychological consequences: psychosis, mutism, bizarre behaviors, depression, insomnia, apathy, headache, nerve pain.

DRUGS USED TO TREAT WASTING IN HIV ILLNESS

Anabolic steroids (Durabolin, oral methyltestosterone, intravenous testosterone, testosterone patches). Anabolic steroids help to treat wasting by increasing the levels of testosterone or its metabolites, which results in weight gain, increased appetite, increased sex drive, and increased energy and concentration. Approximately half of the men with CD4 counts below 200 have testosterone deficiencies, which are often associated with weakness and loss of muscle mass in HIV-related wasting.

Neuropsychological consequences: headache, anxiety, depression, masculinization.

Dronabinol (Marinol, Delta-9-THC). A synthetic version of the active ingredient in marijuana, dronabinol is used to treat weight loss caused by vomiting and loss of appetite in HIV-related illness.

Neuropsychological consequences: elation, easy laughing, dizziness, confusion, drowsiness.

Megestrol (Megace). A synthetic derivative of the hormone progesterone, it has been used for weight gain and improved well-being in persons with wasting.

Neuropsychological consequences: impotence, insomnia, nausea.

About the Authors

Philip A. Bialer, M.D., formerly served as the director of the AIDS psychiatry program at Beth Israel Medical Center in New York City and is currently the chief of the division of consultation-liaison psychiatry at the same hospital. He is an assistant professor of psychiatry at the Albert Einstein College of Medicine.

Steven Bluestine, M.D., received training in AIDS care at Memorial Sloan Kettering Cancer Center in New York City and then served as the director of a Ryan White–funded AIDS psychiatry clinic at Elmhurst Hospital in Queens, New York. He is currently the director of the AIDS psychiatry program at Beth Israel Medical Center and is an assistant professor of psychiatry at the Albert Einstein College of Medicine.

Steven A. Cadwell, Ph.D., has a practice in individual and group therapy and consultation in Boston, Massachusetts. He is the co-editor of *Therapists on the Front Line: Psychotherapy With Gay Men in the Age of AIDS* (American Psychiatric Press, 1994).

Kathleen J. Goggin, Ph.D., is an Aaron Diamond Foundation Postdoctoral Research Fellow at the New York State Psychiatric Institute. She has been engaged in HIV/AIDS research and clinical work since 1988.

Fernando J. Gutierrez, Ed.D., J.D., is a psychologist and attorney in San Jose, California. His psychology practice emphasizes HIV/AIDS, chemical dependency, and gay, lesbian, bisexual, and couples therapy. His legal practice emphasizes family, immigration, conservatorship, guardianship, juvenile, and mental health law.

Heather Huszti, Ph.D., is currently an associate professor in the Department of Pediatrics and a clinical associate professor in the Department of Psychiatry and Behavioral Sciences at the University of Oklahoma Health Sciences Center. She is a licensed clinical psychologist. She has worked extensively with children and adolescents with chronic illnesses, including HIV/AIDS. She has developed, implemented, and evaluated HIV risk-reduction programs for adolescents with HIV.

Michael F. O'Connor, Ph.D., is clinical assistant professor of psychiatry and behavioral sciences at the Stanford University School of Medicine and maintains a private practice in Palo Alto, California. He is the former co-director of the HIV program at Pacific Graduate School of Psychology, Palo Alto, and former director of the California AIDS Education Project for Sheltered and Incarcerated Youth.

Roberta Ann Olson, Ph.D., is currently an assistant professor in the Department of Psychology Counseling at the Oklahoma City University. She is a licensed clinical psychologist. She has worked extensively with children and adolescents with chronic illnesses, including HIV/AIDS. She was a member of the American Psychological Association's Task Force on Pediatric AIDS. She is currently the president of the Oklahoma Psychological Association.

David G. Ostrow, Ph.D., M.D., is professor of psychiatry and mental health sciences and is mental health core director, Center for AIDS Intervention Research (CAIR) at the Medical College of Wisconsin in Milwaukee. He is the author or editor of nine books and over 135 articles, most related to HIV and AIDS, and is the recipient of numerous awards for his extensive efforts in this area. He is currently the editor of the journals *AIDS* and *AIDS Care*, and series co-editor for *AIDS Mental Health and Prevention*.

Jeffrey T. Parsons, Ph.D., is currently an assistant professor in the Department of Psychology at Jersey City State College. He is a developmental psychologist. He has worked extensively with adolescents with HIV infection and with adolescents with diverse sexuality. He has developed, implemented, and evaluated HIV risk-reduction programs for adolescents with HIV.

Judith G. Rabkin, Ph.D., M.P.H., is professor of clinical psychology in psychiatry, College of Physicians and Surgeons, Columbia University. She has been engaged in HIV-related epidemiological and clinical research since 1987.

Douglas S. Rait, Ph.D., is director of the family therapy program at the Palo Alto Veterans Administration Health Care System in California and the chief of the couples and family therapy clinic in Stanford University's Department of Psychiatry and Behavioral Sciences. He is also a clinical assistant professor of psychiatry and behavioral sciences at Stanford University School of Medicine.

Stephen M. Rao, Ph.D., obtained his doctoral degree from Binghamton University–The State University of New York, Binghamton. His predoctoral internship was completed at the Palo Alto Veterans Administration Health Care System in California. He is currently a Postdoctoral Fellow at the Stanford University School of Medicine in the Department of Psychiatry and Behavioral Sciences. He has trained extensively in the psychological and neuropsychological issues of HIV/AIDS; the evaluation and formulation of the interaction between medical conditions and the family; and with an emphasis on engaging in systemic interventions.

Jeffrey J. Richards, M.D., is currently completing a consultation-liaison AIDS psychiatry fellowship at Beth Israel Medical Center and is an instructor of psychiatry at the Albert Einstein College of Medicine.

Joan M. Ross, R.N., M.S.N., MFCC, is senior supervisor in the family therapy program at the Palo Alto Veterans Administration Health Care System and has served as a member of the infectious disease clinic team. She is also a lecturer in psychiatry and behavioral sciences at Stanford University School of Medicine and a consultant in the department's couples and family therapy clinic.

Jeff Stryker, B.A., is a researcher at the Center for AIDS Prevention Studies (CAPS) at the University of California, San Francisco. He has served on the staffs of the National Commission on AIDS, the Congressional Office of Technology Assessment, and the Institute of Medicine. He is co-editor (with Albert R. Jansen) of *The Social Impact of AIDS in the United States* (National Academy Press, 1993). His writings have appeared in the *Journal of the American Medical Association,* the *New England Journal of Medicine,* and the *New York Times.*

INDEX